ABDOMINAL SURGERY

Of

INFANCY and CHILDHOOD

By

WILLIAM E. LADD, M.D., F.A.C.S.

William E. Ladd Professor of Child Surgery at Harvard Medical School; Chief of
Surgical Service, The Children's Hospital, Boston

and

ROBERT E. GROSS, M.D.

Associate in Surgery, the Harvard Medical School; Associate Visiting Surgeon,
The Children's Hospital; Associate in Surgery, The Peter
Bent Brigham Hospital, Boston

ILLUSTRATED

PHILADELPHIA AND LONDON

W. B. SAUNDERS COMPANY

1941

PREFACE

At the turn of the century the practice of medicine was so conducted that little distinction was made between the treatment of surgical diseases of the child and those occurring in the adult. It was soon discovered, however, that the mortality rates in the younger group were extraordinarily high and that, if improved results were to be expected, the infant or small child could not be treated as though he were a diminutive man or woman. It became evident that children were not only heirs to most of the pathologic states found in older individuals, but in addition were subject to types of infection and congenital abnormalities which were seldom encountered in later life.

With the intention of developing better methods of examination, more detailed preoperative and postoperative care, and a more specialized and delicate operative technic, the surgical staff members of the Boston Children's Hospital began to devote the major part of their time to Pediatric Surgery. This trend, which was first fostered twenty-five years ago by the late Dr. James S. Stone, has been amply justified by a striking betterment in mortality statistics. This does not imply that Pediatric Surgery should always be set apart as a separate specialty, but it does indicate that infants and children can obtain improved surgical care if an appropriate number of men in each community will take a particular interest in this field and give it the attention which it rightfully deserves.

The present book is devoted to that part of children's surgery which involves the abdomen. In addition to giving the details of pre- and postoperative care and of the operative technic, the book is intended to be a statistical portrayal of experiences which have been accumulated by our surgical staff during the past twenty-five years. Reference to the literature has been made only when necessary to supplement our own material. In presenting a treatise in such a form we do not wish to minimize the importance of the writings of others who have contributed to the field; our aim is rather to set forth personal observations and practices so that they will be available to the obstetrician, pediatrician, general practitioner, and general surgeon who must diagnose and treat abdominal conditions in infancy and childhood.

The visiting and resident members of our surgical group, by their constant interest and efforts, have helped to make possible the results which are recorded here. Dr. Kenneth D. Blackfan and his associates have been most helpful whenever special pediatric advice and treatment have been required. Advances in surgery must usually be founded upon pathologic studies, and we have been particularly dependent upon Dr. S. Burt Wolbach and Dr. Sidney Farber for their unexcelled preparation, description, and preservation of surgical material in a way which will be of permanent value to all departments of the hospital. Dr. Edward C. Vogt and Dr. George M. Wyatt often aided in roentgenologic investigations, and the latter has provided the films which have been included in the various chapters. Miss Etta Piotti has executed the drawings with precision and gracefulness. Mr. Ferdinand Harding photographed the clinical subjects and pathologic specimens. Finally, the work would not have been completed without the secretarial assistance of Miss Joanne Carpenter, who has diligently collected data, prepared the manuscript, and assembled the index.

For several years we had intended to gather the subject matter which is here assembled in book form. The project was always frustrated because of inadequate financial backing and it was not until a generous grant was received from the Godfrey M. Hyams Trust Fund that serious work could be undertaken and pushed to completion. It would have been impossible to make this contribution to medical literature without such support, and we gratefully express our indebtedness and appreciation.

Some of the illustrations have previously appeared in publications by members of the staff. They are reproduced here by generous permission of the various journals as follows. Journal of the American Medical Association: Fig. 21, from "Congenital Obstruction of the Small Intestine," *101*: 1453, 1933. Pennsylvania Medical Journal: Figs. 37 and 38, from "The Acute Surgical Abdomen in Children," *34*: 153, 1930. Surgery, Gynecology & Obstetrics: Figs. 52 to 65, inclusive, from "Surgical Treatment of Duplications of the Alimentary Tract," *70*: 295, 1940; and Figs. 181 to 190, inclusive, from "Omphalocele in the Newly Born," *71*: 520, 1940; and Fig. 234 from "Granulosa Cell and Brenner Tumor of the Ovary," *61*: 250, 1935, by Bland and Goldstein. The New England Journal of Medicine: Figs. 11 and 30 from "Congenital Obstruction of the Duodenum in Children," *206*: 277, 1932; Figs. 42, 46, and 51 from "Meckel's Diverticulum in Children," *208*: 525, 1933, by Hudson; Figs. 197 to 202, inclusive, from "Congenital Diaphragmatic Hernia," *223*: 917, 1940; Figs. 168, 169, and 170 from "Congenital Patent Urachus," *215*: 193, 1936, by Mahoney and Ennis; and Fig. 242 from "Exstrophy of the Bladder and Epispadias," *222*: 130, 1940, by Ladd and Lanman. The Archives of Surgery: Figs. 70 and 71 from "Intussusception in Infancy and Childhood," *29*: 365, 1934; and Fig. 162 from "Congenital Anomalies of the Gallbladder," *32*: 131, 1936. The American Journal of Surgery: Fig. 116 from "Congenital Malformations of Anus and Rectum," *23*: 167, 1934; and Fig. 138 from "Indications for

Splenectomy in Childhood," *39:* 400, 1938, by Diamond. The Journal of Pediatrics: Fig. 157 from "Idiopathic Dilatation of the Common Bile Duct," *3:* 730, 1933; and Fig. 230 from "Hydrometrocolpos in Infancy," *17:* 772, 1940, by Mahoney and Chamberlain. The Annals of Surgery: Figs. 150, 152, and 154 from "Congenital Obliteration of the Bile Ducts," *102:* 742, 1935. The American Journal of Diseases of Children: Figs. 233, 267, and 268 from "Neoplasms Producing Endocrine Disturbances in Childhood," *59:* 579, 1940.

It is a pleasure to thank the W. B. Saunders Company for their warm cooperation in this undertaking and for their sincere efforts in producing a book of attractive appearance which is in keeping with the highest standards of the publisher's art.

WILLIAM E. LADD, M. D.
ROBERT E. GROSS, M. D.

Boston, Massachusetts,
   June, 1941.

CONTENTS

Chapter XXV

Abdominal Surgery of Infancy and Childhood

CHAPTER I

CONGENITAL HYPERTROPHIC PYLORIC STENOSIS

Congenital hypertrophic stenosis of the pylorus is the most common condition which requires surgical treatment in the first few months of life. The baby with this lesion has a marked increase in size of the pyloric musculature, so that the lumen of the gut at this level is compressed and partially obstructed. The clinical findings include all of the cardinal symptoms and signs of mechanical obstruction at the outlet of the stomach.

The operative attack on pyloric stenosis marks one of the greatest advances in abdominal surgery in the last twenty-five years. Prior to 1912, when the operation of pyloromyotomy was adopted, following the work of Fredet in 1908 and Rammstedt in 1912, the mortality in this condition varied from 50 to 75 per cent or more; whereas today proper surgical technic combined with adequate preoperative and postoperative care has reduced the mortality in competent hands to 1 or 2 per cent. The experiences gained from the operative treatment by pyloromyotomy in 765 cases form the basis of the following presentation.

PATHOLOGY

Gross Pathology.—The important pathologic finding is hypertrophy of the circular pyloric muscle and an actual increase in the number of smooth muscle fibers. This hyperplasia and hypertrophy produces an olive-sized, bulbous or fusiform mass which has a smooth external surface. The *dimensions* of this swelling vary somewhat with the age of the baby and with the degree of hypertrophy which is present. In an average case, the swollen pylorus is about ¾ inch in length and about ⅝ inch in diameter.

The pylorus is quite firm. Its external surface is smoothly covered by serosa. A longitudinal hemisection shows the *musculature* to be of such thickness that it pushes the mucosa inward and thereby greatly diminishes the lumen of the stomach at this point. The great bulk of muscular tissue, which is unyielding, impedes the passage of curds from the stomach into the duodenum. When the thickened musculature is examined in cross section, it is found to be gray, quite firm, and to have a gristly consistency.

A longitudinal section of the hypertrophied pylorus shows one important anatomic difference in the configuration of the mucosa at the gastric and duodenal ends. As shown in Fig. 1, the lumen of the stomach is grad-ually reduced in size toward the pylorus, but *the lumen of the duodenum assumes its full size at once,* due to the abrupt termination of the pyloric sphincter at its distal end. It is important to remember this during opera-tion, for there is great danger of sweeping a scalpel into the duodenal lumen at the point where it balloons out just beyond the pylorus.

Microscopic Pathology.—Microscopic sections of specimens which have come to autopsy without surgical intervention do not show any increase in nerves, nor is there any other neurologic abnormality to suggest that mus-cular hypertrophy is brought about by a neurologic disturbance. In the specimens which are obtained from infants under a week or ten days of age, the mucosa and submucosa are essentially normal. After this time, the

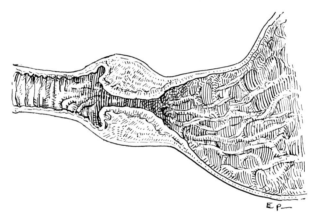

Fig. 1.—Longitudinal section from a case of pyloric stenosis, showing the hypertrophy of musculature at outlet of the stomach. The thickened muscle tapers off gradually on its gastric end, but ends abruptly on the duodenal end.

forcing of curds through the small opening brings about *edema of the mucosa* and a slight increase in the *leukocytic infiltration* of this layer. This mechanical irritation therefore produces a thickening of the mucosa, which further reduces the size of the pyloric lumen. It is for this reason that infants do not exhibit signs of obstruction until they are about two weeks of age, in spite of the fact that the hypertrophied muscle has been present since birth.

Dependent upon the obstruction of the pylorus, there are also changes of less importance in the wall of the gastric antrum and fundus. These are characterized by mild hypertrophy of the muscular coats of the stomach and an increase in size of the mucosal rugae. These changes are similar to those which are found in any portion of the gastro-intestinal tract above the level of a longstanding mechanical obstruction.

ETIOLOGY

There is no satisfactory theory to explain the etiology of congenital hypertrophic stenosis of the pylorus. Some individuals have propounded the theory that injury to the central nervous system *during birth* might be an etiologic factor, but the absence of other signs of cerebral damage in the great majority of cases tends to refute this view. It has been suggested that this disease might be analogous to conditions such as megalo-ureter or Hirschsprung's disease of the colon. We have no reason to condemn this theory, nor do we have any evidence to support it.

Some pediatricians regard pyloric stenosis as the end result of a *pre-existing pyloric spasm*. In other words, the muscle, which has been active for long periods of time, now becomes hypertrophied. Such muscular spasm could have been originally brought about by abnormal reflex disturbances which are occasionally seen in other parts of the gastro-intestinal tract, for example, at the gastric cardia. While this theory might be attractive, it does not appear to be entirely plausible, because the pyloric hypertrophy can be found so early in life that there could hardly be time for a pre-existing spasm. There is no racial predisposition to this condition.

In short, we are at a loss to explain the hypertrophy of the pylorus, and regard this problem as one of only academic interest which is far over-shadowed by practical considerations of the surgical treatment.

SYMPTOMS

The symptoms are all indicative of a high obstruction and of a severe loss of body fluids and electrolytes.

Vomiting seldom occurs before the ninth or tenth day after birth, and usually not before the child is two weeks of age. At first vomiting may be little more than a regurgitation after feeding, but soon it becomes more forceful and projectile in type; at the start it may be infrequent, but later it appears after most of the feedings, and is the outstanding complaint. Since the obstruction is at the distal end of the stomach, the vomitus does not contain bile. The child is continually hungry, because little food passes into the intestine to be absorbed. He will therefore eagerly nurse or take the bottle, even after vomiting.

The amount of *fecal residue* decreases as the pyloric obstruction increases; the stools become less frequent and more scanty. In occasional cases, however, the baby may have a so-called "starvation diarrhea" which is accounted for by the passage of accumulated intestinal juices, or by the previous administration of cathartics.

With continued *starvation*, failure to gain weight or the loss of weight is always seen. There is a loss of subcutaneous fat. Marked *dehydration* is evidenced by wrinkles appearing on the face, neck, and extremities. If vomiting has been long continued and severe, *alkalosis* may result in hyperpnea or other respiratory disturbance.

PHYSICAL FINDINGS

Inasmuch as four fifths of the patients with pyloric stenosis are males, the *sex* of the patient is of some importance. The majority of patients are from four to six weeks of *age* when first seen (Fig. 2).

The *general physical appearance* of patients who are brought to the physician early may show little variation from the normal. However, signs of weight loss, wrinkling of the skin, sunken appearance to the eyes, and a

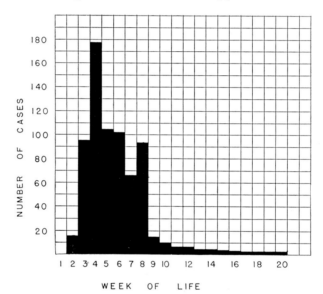

Fig. 2.—Chart showing age of patients at time of admission to hospital for treatment of pyloric stenosis.

decrease of subcutaneous fat (Fig. 3) are more characteristic of advanced stages. Practically all patients have evidence of dehydration, which is best determined by the pliability of the skin. In the normal infant, the skin of the chest, abdomen, or extremity can be rolled up with the fingers and when released it will immediately sink back into its normal position. In contrast to this, the dehydrated baby has a skin of thinner texture which falls back into its normal contour very slowly.

Examination of the abdomen is of greatest importance. If there is any distention it is confined to the epigastrium overlying the stomach area. Inspection shows gastric waves passing from left to right if the baby has been recently fed. Palpation may show a distended stomach if the child has recently nursed.

Most important is the *palpation of the right upper quadrant* with the tip of one finger in the attempt to feel the hypertrophied pylorus. In well over 95 per cent of the cases, the pyloric "tumor" can be felt through the abdominal wall; in occasional cases it can be felt only after repeated examinations. If the tumor cannot be detected, feedings of a milk formula,

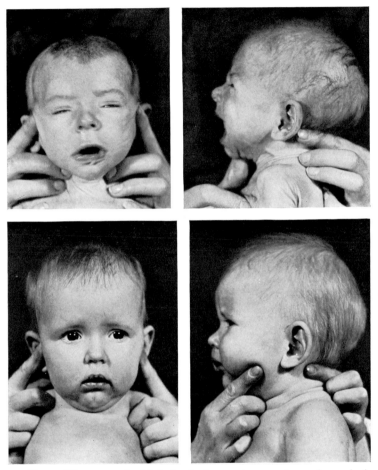

Fig. 3.—*Above,* Three-month-old baby before pyloromyotomy for pyloric stenosis. There is obvious weight loss, atrophy of the subcutaneous tissues, and wrinkling of the skin. *Below,* Same patient, after operation, at eleven months of age. The nutrition is improved and the wrinkling of the skin has disappeared.

sterile water, or dilute orange juice will relax the abdominal wall and give the best conditions for satisfactory examination. The feeding should be continued until the baby vomits, because this is followed by a momentary period of great relaxation during which the abdominal viscera can be best palpated. The vomitus, of course, does not contain bile, a fact which clearly indicates that the obstruction is above the ampulla of Vater.

If the child has been untreated for a long time, the recurring loss of hydrochloric acid brings about *alkalosis,* so that hypertonicity or respiratory disturbances may be found.

It is surprising to find that such starvation over long periods does not produce nutritional *edema.* In only one case have we observed marked edema—serum protein level of 4.9 mg. per cent—which could be explained only on the basis of starvation. This explanation was further supported by the fact that there was no reappearance of edema subsequent to operative relief of pyloric obstruction.

DIFFERENTIAL DIAGNOSIS

Pylorospasm must be differentiated from pyloric stenosis. Babies with pylorospasm are apt to have generalized muscular hypertonicity of the trunk and extremities. The vomiting tends to appear in spells; that is, the child will vomit for two or three days and then be spontaneously relieved for several days before vomiting reappears. No pyloric tumor can be felt by abdominal palpation. The symptoms vary from day to day, whereas they are continually progressive with pyloric stenosis. Furthermore, pylorospasm symptoms can be relieved by using atropine compounds, particularly when they are employed in conjunction with sedatives such as phenobarbital.

Intracranial injury or hemorrhage which results from birth trauma is a frequent cause of vomiting and may have to be considered in the differential diagnosis. In children so afflicted, the vomiting is not apt to be as forceful as that seen with mechanical obstruction. Furthermore, the vomiting is more likely to be in small amounts and to appear at irregular intervals, unrelated to the ingestion of food. Vomiting may be the only symptom or sign of intracranial pathology, but one is more likely to find other evidence of neurologic disease, such as convulsions, spasticity, hypotonicity, bulging fontanel, or possibly bloody cerebrospinal fluid.

Other types of intrinsic intestinal obstruction must be considered in the differential diagnosis. It is important to remember that intrinsic obstruction (*atresia* or *stenosis*) of the esophagus, duodenum, or intestine produces vomiting within the first day or two of life. This is in sharp contrast to the vomiting which occurs in pyloric stenosis, which seldom begins before the ninth or tenth day. Furthermore, these other forms of congenital obstruction are apt to have findings which are not encountered in obstruction at the pylorus. If atresia exists in the esophagus, there may be a communication between the esophagus and the trachea, or else there is a spilling over of saliva into the larynx, so that respiratory difficulties are common. If an atresia exists in the duodenum or lower portion of the intestinal tract, the vomitus will contain bile or fecal material, which clearly indicates that the obstruction is below the pylorus.

Extrinsic forms of congenital obstruction, induced by *incomplete rotation* of the intestinal tract, almost invariably give signs within the first day or two of life. An incompletely rotated intestine commonly lies across and compresses the duodenum below the level of the papilla of Vater, so that the vomitus contains bile. In these cases, the onset of vomiting is within the first twenty-four or forty-eight hours of life, which is in contrast to the later vomiting of pyloric stenosis. In questionable cases, roentgenologic studies are of value.

Poor feeding regimens may bring about vomiting in the second or third week of life, with clinical findings much like those of pyloric stenosis. Unduly long feedings at the breast or the administration of too concentrated or too bulky formulas are apt to produce vomiting which occurs shortly after feeding. Therefore, it is necessary to review the feeding history, to eliminate the possibility of incompatible amount or type of food. Not infrequently patients are admitted to the hospital with a presumptive diagnosis of pyloric stenosis, only to find that institution of a rational feeding regimen completely abolishes the vomiting.

ROENTGENOLOGIC EXAMINATION

Since the symptoms and signs in most cases of pyloric stenosis are sufficient to establish definitely the proper diagnosis, roentgenologic examination is not necessary. There are, however, some cases in which the history is atypical, or the physical examination is unsatisfactory. Under such circumstances the diagnosis is in doubt and it is best to obtain additional information by x-ray examination. In our last 342 cases, x-ray examination has been performed only twenty times.

Methods and Findings.—Two methods of examination are available. A *film* of the abdomen without contrast medium will often show a large, dilated, gas-filled stomach, with relatively little gas in the intestine beyond the pylorus (Fig. 4). If the stomach is not thus outlined with entrapped air, a routine gastro-intestinal examination may be done with the use of contrasting barium, which is incorporated in the formula. The *fluoroscopic* findings thus observed may be listed as: (1) an enlarged stomach with rounded pyloric end (due to a ballooning of the antrum forward and to the right); (2) greatly increased peristaltic activity; (3) passage of the barium to the pylorus but little or no escape of it into the duodenum.

Films taken some hours after the ingestion of barium indicate how much gastric retention is present. Normally, a baby's stomach is completely empty in three hours, and the retention of a large part of the barium after this time is indicative of pyloric obstruction (Fig. 5).

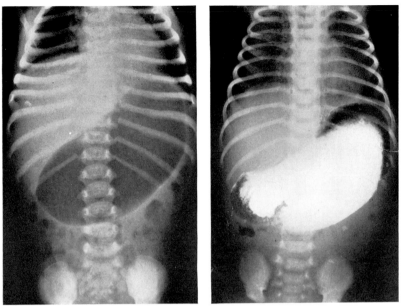

Fig. 4.   Fig. 5.

Fig. 4.—Roentgenogram from a patient with pyloric stenosis, showing the marked gaseous distention of the stomach.

Fig. 5.—Roentgenogram, following barium meal, in a patient with pyloric stenosis, showing complete retention of barium in the stomach. In the great majority of cases the diagnosis of pyloric stenosis can be made from clinical findings, and x-ray examination is not necessary.

PREOPERATIVE CARE

Since the adoption of pyloromyotomy as the treatment of choice for pyloric stenosis, further reduction in mortality has been accomplished by a better preoperative care. Attention is directed toward abolition of ketosis and at replacement of lost body fluids, electrolytes, and carbohydrate stores. The management of this regimen may be in the hands of the surgeon alone or may be under the combined direction of a pediatrician and surgeon.

In our clinic the entire preoperative care has now been handed over to the *surgical staff,* and with the exclusive management by one service there has been a marked increase in efficiency. This plan is practical only when members of the surgical staff devote a large proportion of their time to the treatment of childhood conditions, and are well equipped to cope with the feeding problems and fluid administrations in babies.

Administration of Parenteral Fluids.—The giving of parenteral fluids is the greatest factor in improving the general condition of these dehydrated patients, and two or three days are well spent in thus strengthening the child; indeed, in extreme cases four or five days may be required to get the baby into optimum condition.

Appropriate fluids should be administered morning and night of each preoperative day. At each of these times an intravenous injection is given, and this is immediately followed by a hypodermoclysis. For *intravenous* injection 10 per cent glucose in sterile water is given, in the proportions of 10 cc. of this solution per pound of the baby's body weight. For the *hypodermoclysis,* physiologic saline—and on rare occasions Hartmann's solution—is used, in amounts equaling 15 cc. per pound of body weight.

This combination of intravenous and subcutaneous fluids appears to be unquestionably superior to the administration of fluids solely by the subcutaneous route. However, in general practice or in general hospitals, where comparatively little infant work is done, difficulties with intravenous infusion may arise. Under such circumstances, all of the parenteral administrations may be given by *subcutaneous routes* if the sites of injection are frequently changed from the pectoral region to the back and to the thighs. When the subcutaneous route is the only one employed, 5 per cent glucose in sterile water or 3 per cent glucose in physiologic saline can be given. The guiding rule should be to maintain the infant's fluid intake at 2½ or 3 ounces per pound of body weight per twenty-four hours.

Transfusion.—Transfusion is occasionally of considerable help in preparing the undernourished child for operation, particularly if the blood count is below 4,000,000. There may be a lowered level of plasma protein which augurs for poor wound healing subsequent to operation. Hence, it is wise to raise the protein level by infusion of blood from a suitable donor. Blood should never be given in amounts exceeding 10 cc. per pound of body weight at any one time. Transfusions in cases of pyloric stenosis are but rarely needed, and for the most part should be reserved for the poorer risk type of patient. They can be limited to about 5 per cent of the cases.

Feedings.—While the child is being thus prepared over a period of one to three days, it is well to continue the oral feedings. The infant may vomit most of this material, but a small amount of it does go through the pylorus and is absorbed from the intestinal tract. The feeding may be thickened with small amounts of cooked cereal in the proportion of 1 part of cereal to 15 or 20 parts of the formula. The addition of cereal thickens the fluid to such an extent that more of it is squeezed through the pylorus.

Drugs.—The use of *atropine,* either by the subcutaneous route or else incorporated in the feeding in borderline cases, may be of some value, but it has little advantage in the typical case of pyloric stenosis. If the child is fussy and hypertonic, the administration of small amounts of *luminal* once or twice in each twenty-four-hour period will have a quieting and beneficial effect. These drugs, however, have a rather limited usefulness.

Vitamins.—Administration of *vitamin C* has been routinely adopted in all of our cases in the last two years, with the hope of raising the vitamin

C level in the child's plasma. This is done in an effort to promote better healing of the wound after operation. If the child is vomiting most of his formula, 25 mg. of vitamin C can be incorporated daily in one of the clyses.

OPERATIVE PROCEDURES

Before 1912 gastrojejunostomy was the surgical treatment of choice for congenital pyloric stenosis; the mortality was usually well above 50 per cent. In 1908 Fredet introduced his operation, which consisted of splitting the hypertrophied pyloric muscle in a longitudinal fashion, without opening the mucosa, and then resuturing the muscle in a transverse direction. This had the great advantage of being an aseptic technic, and the results were definitely better than were the previous ones with gastrojejunostomy. In 1912 Rammstedt described the operation which is now universally employed in treatment of this condition. It consists of splitting the hypertrophied circular muscle longitudinally, but not incising the mucosa. No attempt is made to cover the muscular defect and the mucosa is allowed to pout out into this slit in the muscle. The obstruction is thereby quickly and completely relieved.

Anesthesia.—The anesthesia of choice is *ether* administered by the drop and open-mask method. We have employed this form of anesthesia in 99 per cent of our cases, and have found is extremely satisfactory. In no case has there been a death which could possibly be attributed to the anesthetic. We are not unmindful of the fact, however, that the ether in our cases has been given by anesthetists whose work is confined wholly to childhood and infancy. It is therefore probably true that ether should not be universally recommended for this operation if the available anesthetist has not had experience in dealing with babies.

Some clinics have routinely used local *novocain* infiltration of the abdominal wall. In institutions where trained anesthetists are not available, this form of anesthesia is without doubt the preferable one. We have not chosen to adopt it, because the infiltration of the abdominal wall prolongs the operative procedure unnecessarily and it also interferes with the healing of the wound in these thin and undernourished babies. Furthermore, relaxation of the abdominal wall is not as good as that obtained with ether narcosis. Straining of the baby at an inopportune moment may force the intestines out of the abdominal cavity and create shock. In two babies we employed *avertin* (100 mg. per pound of body weight) in conjunction with novocain infiltration of the abdominal wall, and the anesthesia was decidedly satisfactory. In both cases, this was employed because of a recent respiratory infection which made it unwise to administer ether. In one case *cyclopropane* anesthesia was tried, when we were studying its possibilities in abdominal surgery of infancy. The anesthesia was satisfactory, but the explosive hazards of this gas make it undesirable for such cases.

Preparation for Operation.—*Conservation of the body heat* during operation, so important in infants, may be done by wrapping the arms and legs with several layers of sheet wadding. At the wrists and ankles this sheet wadding may be pinned down to the operating table so that the extremities will not move into the operative field. A hot-water bottle slipped under the baby's back serves the dual purpose of arching it forward to give a better operative exposure, and of providing a supply of heat to the patient during operation.

Skin preparation may consist of washing with ether followed by application of half-strength tincture of iodine. A No. 10 or 12 French urethral catheter is passed through the nose, down the esophagus, and into the stomach before operation. If the stomach contains fluid material, this is rapidly washed out with bicarbonate solution. The catheter is left in place during the entire operative procedure, because through it any gas which may appear in the stomach may be expressed by the operator.

Operative Technic.—The abdominal *incision* is about 2 inches in length, is to the right of the umbilicus, and runs from the costal margin downward (Fig. 6). As the incision is developed through subcutaneous tissues, very careful *hemostasis* must be employed, and all bleeding vessels must be ligated with fine silk or with very fine plain catgut (000 or 0000 size). The rectus muscle is split. On entering the abdomen, the antrum of the stomach or the pylorus itself will present and can be easily drawn up into the wound just above the level of the skin. In order to exteriorize the pylorus in this manner, it may be necessary to twist it so that it runs almost parallel to the cutaneous incision.

Examination of the thickened pylorus will now show it to be of firm consistency. The main *blood supply* of the pylorus comes from its inferior border, and the vessels on the anterior surface of the pylorus are larger and longer than those on the posterior; so one finds the superior anterior surface to be the least vascular part of the entire pyloric ring. It is in this zone of least vascularity that the constricting muscle should be incised.

With the scalpel, a *longitudinal cut* ⅝ or ¾ inch in length is made, passing through the serosa and superficial bits of the musculature. From this stage onward the remainder of the muscle may be cut with the scalpel if desired, but it is better to use a dull handle of the scalpel. Such a blunt instrument will readily divide all the gristly and friable fibers of the muscular coat; but it will not cut into the submucosa, so there is less danger of entering the lumen of the gut. The muscle should be separated well up toward the gastric antrum and must be completely divided along

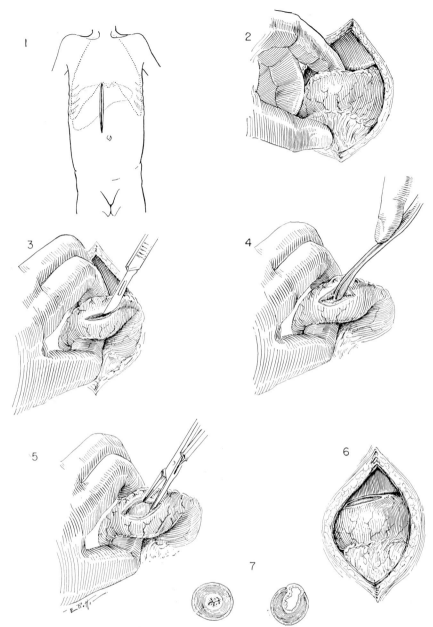

Fig. 6.—Steps in operative treatment of congenital hypertrophic pyloric stenosis. *1*, Position of the skin incision. Right rectus, muscle-splitting incision. *2*, Delivery of the pylorus up into the operative wound. *3*, Pylorus held between two fingers, and rotated downward so that incision can be made along its superior surface where the vascularity is minimal. Incision carried through only the serosa and superficial muscle fibers. *4*, Division of the deeper muscle fibers with a blunt instrument. A rounded handle of the scalpel serves best for this step. *5*, Separating the edges of the muscular coat with a hemostat, so that the mucosa is exposed and is allowed to bulge up into the muscular defect. *6*, Pylorus dropped back into the abdomen, showing the pyloromyotomy on its superior surface. *7*, Cross section of hypertrophied pylorus before operation (*left*) and after operation (*right*). Following operation the mucosa pouts up through the muscular slit to the level of the preexisting serosa.

its duodenal end. The presenting ends of the split muscle are now separated from each other by introducing a half-length or hemostatic snap between them and then separating the blades of the instrument. If this is properly done, the muscle will be opened so that a large V-shaped defect presents, but at the same time there will be no tear of the underlying submucosa and mucosa. This separation of the muscular ends is continued until the mucosa pouts up to the level of the serosa. It is necessary to have the mucosa thus pout up into the muscular defect to insure an adequate lumen for the pylorus and to prevent the severed ends of the muscle from uniting.

This procedure is practically bloodless. If there is any oozing from the cut serosa or muscular ends, it can usually be controlled by the application of a warm saline pack for a few minutes. If *bleeding* still persists, it may be necessary to ligate one or two small vessels with fine silk or catgut. In about three quarters of the cases no ligatures are necessary.

When the operator has satisfied himself that all bleeding is controlled, the pylorus is dropped back into the abdomen. No attempt is made to cover the pyloric defect with serosa or omental fat.

Complications.—The one danger in this operative procedure is the possible *perforation* of the mucosa—an accident which is most likely to occur at the duodenal end of the pyloric incision. This is due to the fact that the lumen of the gut gradually diminishes in size on the gastric end of the pylorus, but balloons out quite rapidly as it expands into the duodenum (Fig. 1). If the operator hopes to sever all of the muscle in one or two sweeps of the scalpel, he may easily cut into the duodenum where the musculature ends abruptly. Hence, great care must be exercised when working at the duodenal end of the incision. Once the duodenum has been accidentally opened, prompt recognition of the error is highly important, because an unchecked escape of duodenal contents will lead to *peritonitis*. A small opening can be closed with one or two sutures to invert the pouting mucosa and bring together the serosa over this area. If the defect is thus simply treated, most of the patients survive. In fourteen cases in which we have thus accidentally opened the duodenum and immediately closed it, there were eleven survivals and three deaths, but only one of these deaths was due to peritonitis.

Closing the Abdomen.—The abdomen must be closed with *extreme care,* if subsequent troubles with the wound are to be avoided. The abdominal wall in most of these patients is only ⅛ or 3/16 inch thick, and hence delicate sutures are necessary and delicate grasps of tissue must be taken. We have almost completely abandoned the use of *catgut* in these wounds, because the stiffness of this material may make a loop or portion of a knot protrude outward through the wound edges and thus delay healing or lead to infection. The peritoneum and posterior rectus fascia are brought to-

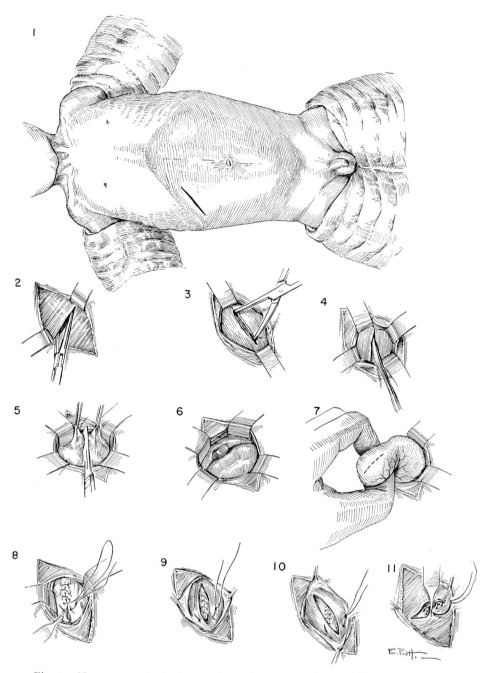

Fig. 7.—Alternate method of exposing pylorus through a gridiron incision. *1*, Position of the skin incision below the costal margin. Legs and arms are wrapped with sheet wadding to prevent heat loss during operation. *2*, Division of external oblique muscle along the direction of its fibers. *3*, Division of internal oblique muscle (or fascia). *4*, Separation of fibers of transversalis muscle. *5*, Opening of peritoneum. If the layers

gether with a continuous suture; and particular effort is made not to fray the filmlike peritoneum with unduly large forceps. Furthermore, it is important not to draw the suture up too tightly, for this may cut through the delicate tissues. A few interrupted *silk* sutures approximate the muscle, and then the anterior rectus fascia is also brought together with interrupted silk sutures. Usually the subcutaneous fat is so deficient that it is not possible to approximate this layer. The skin is brought together with interrupted sutures, with great care to gain good approximation of the skin edges which are so apt to turn inward.

The Gridiron Incision.—The routine careful closure with silk has proved more satisfactory than that with catgut; but even with silk there has been an occasional failure of wound healing in the extremely emaciated infants. We have therefore recently adopted the gridiron incision as recommended by Dr. Robertson, of Toronto. An incision about 2 inches long is made in the skin extending outward from the lateral border of the right rectus muscle and ½ inch below and parallel to the costal border (Fig. 7). The external oblique muscle is divided in the direction of its fibers, exposing the internal oblique. The fibers of this are separated in a similar manner, exposing the transversalis. The fibers of this muscle are in turn separated and the peritoneum opened. The pylorus is delivered into the wound and the operation continued as already described. In repairing this wound the peritoneum is first closed with a running suture of silk, and each muscle layer in turn is sutured with interrupted silk stitches. We have used this incision a number of times and in every instance the wound has healed per primam with a firm scar. It is slightly more difficult to deliver the pylorus through this incision, which is its only apparent disadvantage.

POSTOPERATIVE CARE

Standard Feeding Regimen.—Considerable variation is possible in the treatment after operation. In an institution where such cases are frequently seen, it is best to adopt a standard form of postoperative feeding in order that interns, nurses, and ward attendants may know what is expected in the aftercare. Therefore, we uniformly employ the following feeding regimen. As soon after operation as the patient is conscious, a feeding schedule is instituted whereby the child gets 1 ounce of fluid every two hours. This is divided as follows:

---

are thin, it is preferable to open the peritoneum and transversalis simultaneously. *6,* Abdominal exposure showing edge of liver, gallbladder, and hepatic flexure of colon. *7,* Pylorus delivered into the wound. Pyloromyotomy to be performed along the dotted line. *8,* Closure of peritoneum. *9,* Suturing of transversalis. *10,* Closure of internal oblique muscle (or fascia). *11,* Closure of external oblique muscle.

2 feedings of sterile water.

4 feedings of whey.

4 feedings ½ whey and ½ breast milk.

4 feedings, in each of which the whey is decreased by 1 dram and the breast milk is increased by 1 dram. (Thus, by the end of this time the child will be getting 1 ounce of whole breast milk.)

4 feedings of breast milk, increasing the amount by 1 dram at each feeding. (Thus, at the end of this regime the child will have 1½ ounces of breast milk every two hours.)

This total of eighteen feedings will require thirty-six hours and will automatically care for the feedings until the night of the second postoperative day. After this time the amount of milk can be gradually increased to fulfill the fluid and caloric requirements roughly of 3 ounces and 50 calories per pound daily. At the same time that the amount of feeding is increased, the interval is stretched to three hours. It is well not to increase the interval to four hours until eight to ten days have elapsed. After operation there may be occasional vomiting. The feeding regimen, however, is maintained, and it will usually be found that in two or three days' time all vomiting or regurgitation will have ceased. If breast milk is not available, a suitable formula can be substituted in the above schedule. The postoperative feedings are better tolerated, for the first four or five days, if the bottle is given while the child is still reclining in bed. After the feeding has been taken, the baby can be picked up and held in an upright position to allow eructation of any collected gas.

Parenteral Fluids.—It is obvious that the above regimen gives an inadequate amount of fluid for the first thirty-six or forty-eight hours. Hence, the oral intake must be supplemented by parenteral fluids. Two ounces of 5 per cent glucose are instilled into the rectum as soon as the patient returns from the operating room, and this is repeated in four hours. Customarily two sets of parenteral fluids (intravenous infusion and hypodermoclysis) are given on the first and possibly the second postoperative day. The postoperative administration of fluids should be continued as long as the baby shows signs of any dehydration, but they may ordinarily be discontinued after forty-eight hours. This routine has proved eminently satisfactory, but occasionally it has to be slightly altered to meet individual requirements.

RESULTS OF THERAPY

Advance in the treatment of this condition may be appreciated when one recalls that twenty-five years ago the *mortality* often ranged above 50 per cent, whereas today there are several published series in which the mortality is reduced to 1 or 2 per cent. There is no other field of surgical endeavor in which the mortality during this period has been so strikingly diminished. Table 1 lists our mortality rates with the operations in various periods from 1915 through 1939.

TABLE 1

Summary of Results in 765 Cases of Pyloric Stenosis

Years (Inclusive)	Number of Cases	Deaths	Mortality, Per Cent
1915–1922	125	13	10.4
1923–1928	150	11	7.3
1929–1931	151	3	2.0
1932–1935	162	8	4.9
1936–1939	177	1	0.56

The mortality in the last 177 cases was 0.56 per cent. These operations have been performed by the senior staff, junior staff, resident surgeon, and house officers. The patients who have recovered from the operative procedure have had excellent and lasting relief of their symptoms. Our average postoperative hospitalization has been 12.5 days. In the first portion of the series there were two infants in whom the division of the pyloric muscle was incomplete and a secondary operation had to be resorted to. In no case in the past ten years has a secondary operation been necessary, and in all cases the signs of pyloric obstruction have completely disappeared. Some of these individuals have been followed for more than twenty years and none shows any detrimental effect from having the pyloric muscle divided.

A critical review of all cases during the last eight years discloses that there have been 339 cases and nine deaths. One death was due to a Staphylococcus aureus wound infection and peritonitis, which obviously must have come from improperly prepared skin or a break in operative technic. Two children died as a result of postoperative aspiration of vomitus. Seven children had evisceration or partial disruption of the wound in the first week after operation which necessitated resuture. Six of these survived and one died of peritonitis. Two patients died of acute nutritional disturbances and uncontrollable diarrhea after operation. One died of pneumonia and two died of unexplained causes on the first and seventh postoperative days, respectively. In short, 97.3 per cent of 339 patients have survived operation and have been completely relieved of their symptoms.

BIBLIOGRAPHY

1. Donovan, E. J.: Congenital Hypertrophic Pyloric Stenosis in Infancy. J. A. M. A., *109:* 558, 1937.
2. Lamson, O. F.: Congenital Hypertrophic Pyloric Stenosis. Treatment of Accidental Perforation of Mucosa during Rammstedt Operation. Surg., Gynec. and Obst., *57:* 398, 1933.

3. Lanman, T. H., and Mahoney, P. J.: Congenital Hypertrophic Stenosis of the Pylorus. A Study of 425 Cases Treated by Pyloromyotomy. Surg., Gynec. and Obst., *56:* 205, 1933.
4. Maizels, M., and McArthur, C. B.: Cell and Plasma Chloride in the Pyloric Stenosis of Infants. Am. J. Dis. Child., *41:* 35, 1931.
5. Schnohr, E.: Chemical Changes in Blood and Tissues in Congenital Hypertrophic Pyloric Stenosis. Acta Paediat., *14:* 49, 1932.
6. Wyatt, O. S.: Hypertrophic Pyloric Stenosis; A Review of 100 Cases. Journal-Lancet, *59:* 233, 1939.

CHAPTER II

PEPTIC ULCER. GASTROSTOMY

PEPTIC ULCER

Incidence.—Ulcers of the stomach and duodenum, while admittedly rare, are the cause of serious illness in occasional children. They can appear at any age and they have been described in stillborn or even premature infants. In a three-week-old baby—who died because of another condition— we have found a duodenal ulcer which by histologic examination showed evidence of chronicity suggesting that it had been present before birth.

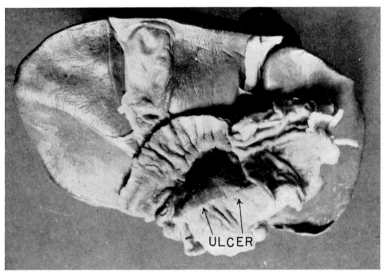

Fig. 8.—Photograph of a duodenal ulcer from a three-month-old baby who died because of exsanguinating hemorrhage.

Peptic ulcers appear to be somewhat more numerous in infancy than in childhood. As a whole they tend to run a more acute course than they do in adult life, presumably because the more bland diet and the more active regenerative processes of children promote faster healing.

Symptoms.—An ulcer is relatively asymptomatic in a high percentage of cases, and frequently the lesion is unsuspected until the time of an autopsy examination. It is barely possible that some of the vague abdominal pains and the recurrent alimentary disturbances, which are so frequent in child-

19

hood, may be due to ulcer more often than is now believed. While a "silent" clinical course is the general rule in infancy, the symptoms after the first year or two are usually quite similar to those observed in adult life.

Epigastric distress which is relieved by eating should suggest the correct diagnosis. *Pain* during the night is particularly common. *Pain* and *vomiting* which appear an hour or two after ingestion of food can result from pylorospasm or from actual mechanical block from scar formation.

Peptic ulcers in the young may give rise to: (1) malnutrition and repeated gastric upsets; (2) exsanguinating and even fatal hemorrhage (Fig. 8); (3) perforation into the general abdominal cavity; and (4) mechanical

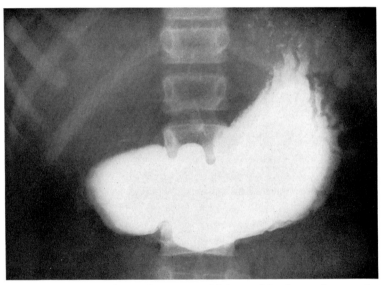

Fig. 9.—Roentgenogram from eleven-year-old boy with obstruction at the pylorus from a cicatrizing duodenal ulcer. No barium could be forced through the pylorus. (There was a 50 per cent gastric residue in subsequent eighteen-hour films.) Successful treatment by posterior gastro-enterostomy.

obstruction from cicatricial tissue near the pylorus. In general, the treatment for each of these various conditions should be much the same as that for older patients.

Medical Treatment.—When there are no complications, a cure can be effected in most cases by bed rest, a *Sippy regimen* with bland diet and neutralizing powders, frequent small feedings, and tincture of belladonna with or just before meals.

Hemorrhage is apt to be tolerated poorly and while *transfusions* should not be given too frequently or in too large amounts, the reports of fatalities from bleeding would imply that blood should be administered sooner and more liberally than is the custom with adults.

Surgical Treatment.—*Perforation* carries a very high mortality, and the one hope for survival rests in *surgical closure* of the hole. Plication of the ulcer or excision of the ulcer should never be done because these procedures are almost certain to contract and obstruct the gut and require a gastro-enterostomy—a combination which is productive of great shock in an already seriously ill child. It is better, and it is sufficient, to take three or four sutures which grasp opposite margins of the perforation and then lay a piece of omental fat (free or attached) over the opening. This fat is held in place by the sutures, which are now tied over it. This operation can be quickly completed; it does not constrict the duodenum (or stomach) ; and it effectively and permanently plugs the hole.

Mechanical obstruction is best treated by a *posterior gastrojejunostomy*. The surgeon should not be tempted to perform any type of resection, for while these have a definite place in the treatment of some adult cases, they are unnecessary in the young. On two occasions we have estab-

TABLE 2

TYPE OF ULCER IN VARIOUS AGE GROUPS
(From Bird, Limper, and Mayer[1])

Age	Stenosing Type	Perforated Type	Bleeding Type	Persistently Painful Type, Etc.	Totals
0– 2 years	9	33	45	7	94
2– 7 "	2	3	10	5	20
7–12 "	18	15	8	16	57
12–15 "	31	26	3	12	72
Totals..........	60	77	66	40	243

lished a gastro-enterostomy for obstructing duodenal ulcer in children. These were both followed by alleviation of pain, by termination of vomiting, and by very satisfactory gains in weight. The first patient was an eleven-month-old male baby who has been progressing well for seven years since operation, and the other was an eleven-year-old boy (Fig. 9) who has done extremely well during the two years since operation.

Results of Surgical Treatment.—Bird, Limper, and Mayer[1] have summarized the literature on surgery for peptic ulcers in infants and children. The data given in Table 2 are drawn from their review of 119 cases in which operation was performed and 124 representative cases in which no operation was carried out, but in which the diagnosis was reasonably certain.

These figures indicate that: ulcers are more common in infancy than in other periods of childhood; ulcers are least common from the ages of two to seven years; ulcers in infancy are apt to have serious bleeding or

2

perforation, whereas ulcers in later childhood are more apt to be perforating or stenosing. Duodenal ulcers were found to be about three times as common as gastric ones; males were affected with somewhat greater frequency than females. In the cases treated surgically in the first two years of life the mortality was 70 per cent—a rate dependent, not only upon the very young age of the patients, but also upon the more serious forms of the complications (hemorrhage and perforation). In the older children—after the second year of life—the total mortality following operation was 5 per cent. Bird, Limper, and Mayer reported the youngest case with successful operation—a 34½-hour-old baby with perforation of a duodenal ulcer.

GASTROSTOMY

Indications.—Gastrostomy is an operation which must be occasionally performed on infants and children, the indications usually being some form of mechanical obstruction above the cardia of the stomach. *Mediastinal tumors* or *cysts* may compress and obstruct the esophagus so that the nutrition of the individual must be reestablished before the thoracic lesion can be safely attacked.

The most common esophageal obstruction in childhood is that resulting from *lye burns.* The great majority of these can be adequately treated by dilatation from above, the dilator being passed along a string guide. In the more severe burns, the esophageal scarring interferes greatly with the child's nutrition and the lumen of the esophagus may be so small that dilatation cannot be safely performed when one is working solely through the mouth. In such instances a gastrostomy has a definite place in the therapeutic regimen; first, to provide a route by which adequate food can be given; second, to establish an avenue for retrograde dilatation of the esophagus.

Operative Technic.—A number of methods for constructing a gastrostomy have been previously described. By the *Stamm technic,* an opening is made in the anterior surface of the stomach and a catheter is thrust into it, which is then held in place by a circular silk suture which infolds the gastric wall. When this suture has been tightened, another is taken to turn the wall in further. A third or even fourth purse-string suture is used to fold in sufficient tissue around the catheter. In general, a Stamm gastrostomy is more apt to leak than is the Witzel type. Furthermore, the Stamm gastrostomy is not as satisfactory in children or infants as it is in the adult, because the infolding appreciably distorts and diminishes the size of the small stomach of a young individual.

A *Janeway gastrostomy,* and all modifications of it, should not be used for children. By this technic a flap is cut out on three sides and left attached to the stomach on its fourth. This flap is then fashioned into a tubelike

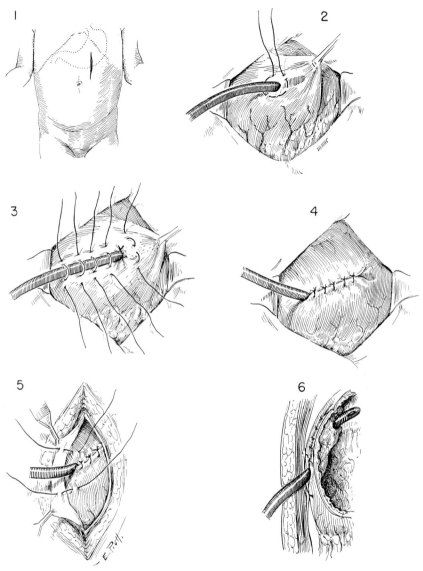

Fig. 10.—Satisfactory method of performing a gastrostomy by the Witzel technic. *1*, Position of the left rectus muscle-splitting incision. *2*, Stomach exposed and held up with an Allis clamp. Catheter thrust in through gastric wall and the opening is being closed with a purse-string suture. *3*, Purse-string suture tied. Additional sutures of silk placed in gastric wall to form an oblique channel for the catheter. *4*, Channel sutures tied, with the catheter imbedded in the gastric wall. *5*, Stomach being anchored to the peritoneum so that it will not pull away from the abdominal wall. *6*, Parasagittal view of completed operation, showing the oblique implantation of the catheter in the stomach and abdominal walls.

channel which is led to the abdominal wall and the defect in the gastric wall is suitably closed. While the principle of a side channel or valvelike side arm is presumably good, such forms of gastrostomy occasionally lead to a fatal peritonitis because of sloughing of the flap which has been raised.

The Witzel Procedure.—There is occasionally some leakage of gastric fluids through any gastrostomy, with subsequent erosion of the abdominal wall. Several forms of gastrostomy have been devised with the idea of reducing or preventing such seepage. After clinical trials of various types of gastrostomy, we have abandoned all of them except the Witzel procedure illustrated in Fig. 10. This has been satisfactory in the great majority of cases; it can be safely performed, and leakage is minimal. It can be used as a temporary gastrostomy because withdrawal of the catheter will permit the long oblique tract to close spontaneously. Likewise, it can be kept open for long periods of time if the catheter is left in place and is removed only for purposes of cleansing.

BIBLIOGRAPHY

1. Bird, C. E., Limper, M. A., and Mayer, J. M.: Surgery in Peptic Ulceration of Stomach and Duodenum in Infants and Children. Ann. Surg. (to be published).
2. Bloch, L., and Serby, A. M.: Peptic Ulcer in Children: Follow-Up Study of Cases Reported Previously and Report of Additional Cases. Am. J. of Digest. Dis. and Nutrition, *4:* 15, 1937.
3. Brockington, C. F., and Lightwood, R.: Duodenal Ulceration in Infants. An Account of Two Cases. Lancet, *2:* 1209, 1932.
4. Hunter, W., and Dryerre, H. W.: Duodenal Ulceration in Newborn. Brit. M. J., *2:* 15, 1939.
5. Kunstadter, R. H., and Gettelman, E.: Gastric Ulcer with Fatal Hemorrhage in New-Born. J. A. M. A., *106:* 207, 1936.
6. Palmer, D. W.: Duodenal Ulcer in Infancy. Ann. Surg., *73:* 545, 1921.
7. Tashiro, K., and Kobayashi, N.: Duodenal Ulcer in Infancy and Childhood. Am. J. Surg., *29:* 379, 1935.
8. Theile, P.: Beitrag zur Kenntnis der Geschwürsbildungen des Magens und Duodenum im Kindesalter. Deutsche Ztschr. f. Chir., *150:* 275, 1919.

CHAPTER III

CONGENITAL ATRESIA OF THE INTESTINE AND COLON

Congenital atresia of the intestine and colon is an uncommon malformation in which there is complete obstruction of the alimentary tract. This condition rapidly produces severe *dehydration* because of persistent vomiting, while dilatation of the blind intestine may lead to its *rupture*. These two factors are the most important causes of the extremely high mortality rate which is associated with the condition. If no surgical relief is instituted, death supervenes in most cases in the first week of life, but a few patients have lived to the age of ten or twelve days. Surgical therapy is followed by a high mortality, but an increasing number of successfully treated cases are appearing in the literature. Prompt recognition of the obstruction and immediate operation give the best hope of successful issue, and doubtless the earlier diagnosis of this anomaly in the future will improve the operative results.

EMBRYOLOGY

Most of the relevant embryologic events take place between the fifth and tenth weeks of fetal life. Prior to the fifth week the intestine presents a well defined lumen lined with epithelium. Soon after this the epithelium rapidly proliferates, and the lumen of the intestine from the pylorus to the ileocecal valve becomes obliterated by epithelial concrescences. Thus, the formerly patent intestine passes through a *solid stage* for a short period (Fig. 11). Later, vacuoles appear among these epithelial cells and a coalescence of these cystic spaces reestablishes the intestinal lumen by the twelfth week. It is well known that such a solid stage normally exists in the human intestine, but there is some question concerning the presence, extent, and duration of a solid stage in the colon.

An arrest in development during the second or third month of fetal life results in either atresia or stenosis of the intestine. An atresia, of course, is due to a persistence of one or more of the septa, while a stenosis is due to a remaining but partially perforated septum.

PATHOLOGY

Intestinal atresia may be found in two forms. In the first—and less common—variety, there is an internal diaphragm or *veil* which completely blocks the lumen (Fig. 21). In the other form, the intestine ends as a *blind*

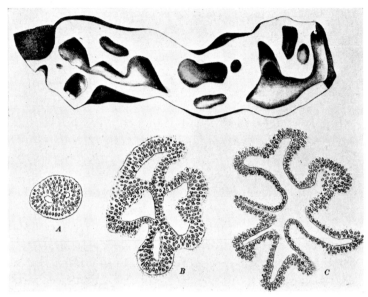

Fig. 11.—Sketches of the duodenum from the normal embryo illustrating the solid stage which normally exists in embryos between the 7 mm. and 30 mm. stages (after Keibal and Mall). *Above,* Longitudinal section of intestine showing coalescence of the walls and the formation of multiple cystic spaces. *Below: A,* Solid stage showing concrescence of epithelial surfaces. *B,* Later stage with development of isolated pockets. *C,* Final attainment of a continuous intestinal lumen.

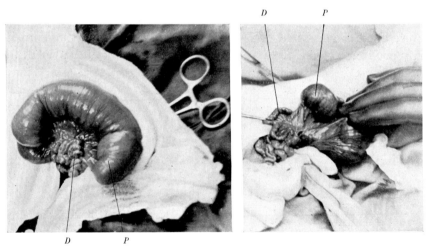

Fig. 12.—Photographs from two cases of *jejunal* atresia taken at the operating table. *P,* Proximal dilated blind intestine. *D,* Distal collapsed portion of intestine.

sac and there is a discontinuity of the bowel (Figs. 12 and 22). In the latter form the proximal distended bowel is not attached to the distal collapsed portion, or else it is connected by only a threadlike fibrous band. In some cases there may be several atresias; and the isolated, blind segments of intestine joined to one another by tiny threads give the appearance of a miniature string of sausages.

Distal to the obstruction, the intestine is very small, contains no gas, and has within its lumen only small amounts of mucus and cells which have been cast off from the lower intestinal mucosa. This collapsed intestine usually measures no more than 4 to 6 mm. in diameter and a collapsed colon is not much larger. *Proximal* to the obstruction, the intestine is very tensely dilated and the obstructed loops may be 3 or 4 cm. in diameter. This degree of distention in a newly born baby greatly thins the intestinal

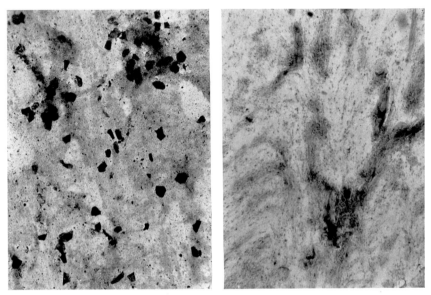

Fig. 13.—*Left,* Photomicrograph of normal child's meconium (stained with gentian violet) showing many cornified squamous epithelial cells. *Right,* Photomicrograph of meconium of a baby with atresia of the intestine (stained by same method) showing absence of cornified cells.

wall and leads to local ischemia. Necrosis and perforation of the bowel are therefore imminent dangers in any baby with intestinal atresia which has not been relieved by the third day of life.

The Meconium in Intestinal Atresia.—The meconium stool in a normal child is composed of: (1) dead cells from the intestinal lining; (2) various secretions from the stomach, intestine, liver, and pancreas; and (3) material from the amniotic fluid which is swallowed by the baby in utero. One of the constituents of amniotic fluid is the *vernix caseosa*—squamous epithelial cells desquamated from the fetus's skin. The meconium of a normal baby, therefore, contains many of these cornified cells which have passed through its intestinal tract. It is obvious that an atresia of the intestine or colon will not allow them to pass beyond the obstructed point.

Farber's Test.—Farber[5] first called attention to the above facts and devised a simple test whereby the meconium of a baby can be quickly examined and the presence or absence of swallowed vernix cells can be rapidly determined. A specimen of meconium is obtained—care being taken that it comes from the center of the stool—and is smeared on a glass slide. This is gently washed for about one minute with ether to extract the fat, is allowed to dry, and then is stained for one minute with Sterling's gentian violet. It is washed with running water and decolorized with acid alcohol. This decoloration removes the dye from all of the specimen except the cornified epithelial cells. In any newly born child with intestinal obstruction, the absence of cornified epithelial cells in the meconium is presumptive evidence that an intestinal or colonic atresia exists (Fig. 13), whereas the finding of such cells in appreciable numbers suggests that the obstruction is only partial (intestinal stenosis, or else obstruction from extrinsic pressure). If care is used to insure that the specimen studied comes from a representative (central) portion of the stool, this test is of considerable aid in establishing the correct preoperative diagnosis.

CLINICAL FINDINGS

Babies with intestinal or colonic atresia always have symptoms on the first day of life. During or after nursing there is *vomiting* which becomes progressively more frequent and more intense as subsequent feedings are taken. Atresias above the papilla of Vater are very rare; hence the vomitus in these patients almost always contains bile. The character of the vomitus will depend somewhat upon the level of the obstruction, for if the obstruction is high the vomitus will be curdled milk or thin yellowish fluid, whereas a low obstruction will produce vomitus which is malodorous and which is fecal in appearance. Persistent vomiting is usually the symptom which leads to hospitalization. Any child who continues to vomit during the first day or two of life while being fed a normal amount of breast milk or a reasonable formula should be investigated by roentgenography for intestinal obstruction.

The character and size of the *stools* are of some importance in making the diagnosis of intestinal atresia in a newly born child, but they may be misleading. Usually the stools are smaller in amount, drier in consistency, and grayish green in color rather than the tarry appearance of normal meconium. However, in some instances the stools may resemble normal meconium very closely; then the failure to find cornified epithelial cells in the first forty-eight hours of life (or the failure to find milk curds at a later date) is of great significance.

Abdominal distention may or may not be present, depending upon the level of the atresia and the length of time the patient has gone untreated. If the atresia is duodenal, distention will be limited to the epigastrium or may be absent if the stomach has been emptied by repeated vomiting. If the atresia is in the jejunum or at a lower level, abdominal distention may be marked and generalized. The time at which abdominal distention appears is variable. In some cases it has been noticed by the obstetrician at birth, the baby presumably having swallowed enough amniotic fluid in utero to dilate the intestine to the point of obstruction. In other cases the distention does not appear until the child is twenty-four or forty-eight hours old—depending upon how much milk has been ingested and how effective vomiting has been in emptying the alimentary tract. In the duodenal ob-

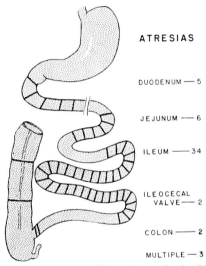

ATRESIAS

DUODENUM — 5

JEJUNUM — 6

ILEUM — 34

ILEOCECAL VALVE — 2

COLON — 2

MULTIPLE — 3

Fig. 14.—Diagram showing position of atresias in fifty-two cases.

structions, peristaltic (gastric) waves may be seen crossing the epigastrium from left to right or they (duodenal) may course down and be limited to the right side of the abdomen. If the obstruction is jejunal, ileal, or colonic, intestinal patterning may be seen over any portion of the abdominal wall.

Fever is a not uncommon finding. Some degree of it can be caused by dehydration alone. If the temperature is above 102° or 103° F., the possibility of intestinal rupture and peritonitis must be thought of.

ROENTGENOLOGIC EXAMINATION

If these babies are carefully observed during the first twenty-four or forty-eight hours of life, the clinical findings are usually sufficient to make a correct diagnosis. However, roentgenologic studies will give additional confirmatory evidence of obstruction, and in some cases will help to localize the site of the lesion. *Films* of the abdomen, without the use of contrast media, will give all the important information in most cases. A dilated duodenum or distended loops of small intestine are usually sufficient to make a correct diagnosis. If the clinical course and the x-ray findings combine to suggest strongly a diagnosis of obstruction, operation should be undertaken without further attempt to localize the actual level of obstruction.

Barium.—The administration of barium to these babies is not without danger, because the barium might clog the intestinal tract at a subsequent time but principally because of the possibility of aspirating any barium which might be vomited. If barium is given, a thin mixture should be employed.

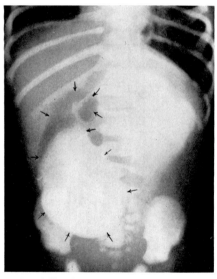

Fig. 15.—Roentgenogram following barium administration in a five-day-old child with atresia of the *lower duodenum*. Arrows outline the greatly dilated, obstructed duodenum. No barium passes beyond the point of obstruction.

If, for any reason, barium has been administered *by mouth* for roentgenologic examination, a gastric tube (small urethral catheter) should be immediately inserted into the stomach and as much barium as possible be removed by gastric lavage.

In Fig. 15 the findings are well illustrated from a case of atresia in the *third portion of the duodenum*. Here the ballooned-out duodenum is almost as large as the stomach and no barium or gas bubbles are seen in the intestines beyond. If the obstruction is lower in the intestinal tract and only two or three loops of distended bowel are seen, as in Fig. 16, atresia of the *jejunum* can be suspected. If multiple dilated loops are encountered, as in Fig. 17 or 18, an atresia of the *ileum* is suggested, but it is impossible

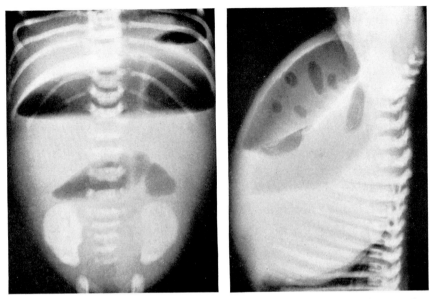

Fig. 16.—Roentgenograms of a six-day-old baby with atresia of the *jejunum* who was subsequently successfully treated by lateral anastomosis. *Left,* Film taken of the child in the head-up position. *Right,* Lateral film with the child in the inverted position to show the extent of the dilated loops.

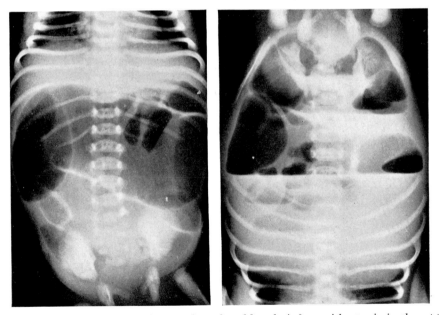

Fig. 17.—Roentgenograms from a three-day-old male infant with atresia in the *upper ileum,* showing diffuse, marked distention of the intestinal loops. *Left,* Film taken with the child in a prone position. *Right,* Film taken with the child in a head-down position showing the stair-step fluid levels and the gas-filled loops extending well into the pelvis.

to differentiate between a low ileal and a colonic obstruction by x-ray films. It is desirable to examine these babies in an upright position and also in

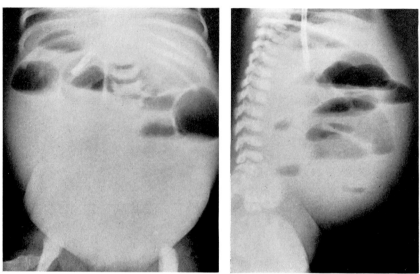

Fig. 18.—Roentgenograms of a ten-hour-old female with atresia of *midileum* which was later successfully treated by lateral ileo-ileostomy. Diffusely dilated loops of bowel may be seen in the anteroposterior and lateral films.

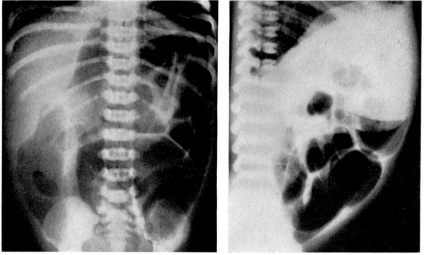

Fig. 19.—Roentgenograms of a four-day-old male with atresia of the *ascending colon* which was found to be gangrenous at operation. Anterior and lateral films showed diffuse gas distention of loops without showing the location of the blind pouch.

an inverted position. Films taken in an anteroposterior or lateral direction with the baby in head-up and in head-down positions will better show the extent of the gas-filled and fluid-filled intestinal loops.

Because of the marked distention in most of these subjects (as is indicated in Figs. 17, 18, and 19), the administration of a barium enema to determine the *patency of the colon* only adds to the great discomfort and distress of the baby. Even if an obstruction in the colon were demonstrated by this means, it would not alter the operative exposure in any way; hence this examination should never be employed.

If the child has been treated with an ileostomy and the abdomen thus decompressed, a *barium-enema* examination may give valuable information without distress in determining the size and continuity of the colon. If the lower bowel is thus found to be normal but small, the ileostomy may be

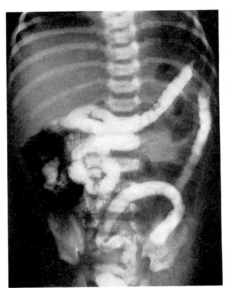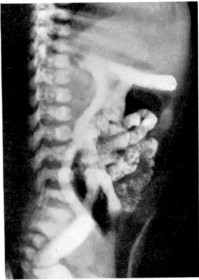

Fig. 20.—Barium-enema examination in a one-month-old child who had been previously treated with ileostomy for atresia of the *ileum*. The pencillike, small caliber of the colon and distal ileum can be readily appreciated from these films.

closed and an anastomotic procedure established with a feeling of certainty that the bowel is patent below the anastomosis.

The *presence of fluid* within the abdominal cavity can be suspected from the x-ray films in some individuals. In Figs. 18 and 19 there are opaque areas between adjacent loops of bowel which are suggestive of intraperitoneal fluid. Such findings do not necessarily mean perforation and peritonitis, because a large amount of fluid may accumulate solely from obstruction of the gut.

TREATMENT

Individuals with atresia of the intestinal tract will die if left untreated; they rarely survive for more than a week without surgical relief. Usually perforation and fatal peritonitis will supervene if the intestine is not decompressed by the third or fourth day. However, some infants who are not operated upon until the sixth day will have only impending necrosis without actual perforation of the intestine.

The mortality for operative procedures is extremely high, and successfully treated cases are still rarities in the medical literature. However, it is becoming evident that with earlier establishment of a diagnosis, the surgical

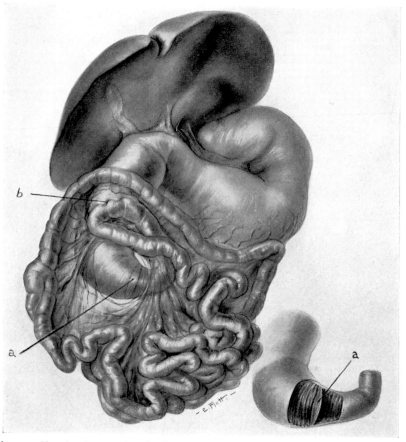

Fig. 21.—Sketch of operative findings and treatment in a case of atresia of the *third part of the duodenum*. There is a septum across the intestinal lumen as shown at *a*. The duodenum is dilated down to the point of obstruction. The jejunum, ileum, and colon are quite collapsed. Treatment by retrocolic duodenojejunostomy at *b*.

treatment is meeting with increasing success. This type of therapy should be undertaken in every case, no matter how critical the condition of the child may be.

Preoperative Measures.—Prior to operation, an *inlying gastric tube* should be inserted. A No. 8 F. or 10 F. soft-rubber urethral catheter with extra holes cut in it makes a satisfactory gastric tube. It is important to use gastric suction to avoid aspiration of vomitus and subsequent pneumonia, which is a not infrequent cause of death in these babies.

Preoperative treatment includes liberal administration of *parenteral fluids* which may be given as 10 per cent glucose intravenously (10 cc. per pound of body weight) and as physiologic saline subcutaneously (15 cc. per pound of body weight). If there has been any suggestion of hemorrhagic disease of the newborn, a small *transfusion* of approximately 5 cc. of blood per pound of body weight will reduce the dangers of hemorrhage during or following operation.

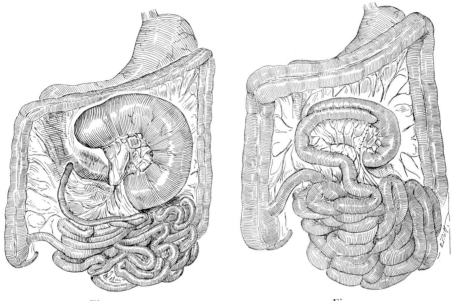

Fig. 22.   Fig. 23.

Fig. 22.—Operative findings in a case with *lower jejunal* atresia. The jejunum ends blindly and is not connected with the lower segment of bowel. Jejunum greatly distended; ileum and colon collapsed.

Fig. 23.—Surgical treatment for the case of jejunal atresia shown in Fig. 22. Lateral jejuno-ileostomy performed, as shown. Ileal loops and colon distend in a few days after establishment of this anastomosis.

When placed on the operating table, the baby's arms and legs should be wrapped with sheet wadding to *conserve body heat,* and a hot-water bottle should be placed under the back to supply heat and reduce subsequent shock.

Operative Technic.—Some operators have employed *local anesthesia* for the abdominal wall, but we have routinely used drop *ether* with an open mask, feeling that this gives better relaxation and exposure.

Exposure of Intestine.—A long right rectus-muscle splitting or retracting *incision,* with its midpoint opposite the umbilicus, will give exposure to any part of the intestinal tract. The incision should be 3 or 4 inches in length. On opening the abdomen there is always some free peritoneal fluid which has been produced by the obstructed intestine. As much as several hundred cc. of this clear yellowish fluid may be found. If the fluid is cloudy or malodorous, a perforation of the gut must be at once suspected and sought for.

The intestines proximal to the point of obstruction will be found greatly dilated and will usually extrude themselves through the abdominal wound. These loops may be as much as 3 or 4 cm. in diameter; they are very tense and they must be carefully handled for fear of rupture. The intestines below the obstruction are collapsed, and are somewhat smaller than an average lead pencil—that is, 4 to 5 mm. in diameter. They contain no gas and by the time operation is performed usually little or no meconium can be palpated within their lumina.

Establishment of a Direct Side-to-Side Anastomosis.—If the proximal loop is *perforated* or *gangrenous,* it should be resected and the end of the intestine turned in. A side-to-side type of anastomosis is now established between the proximal and distal loops. This should be done without the application of clamps to the tiny collapsed distal bowel, but a small intestinal clamp may be used on the upper segment to prevent soiling. As the suture of the intestines of such diminutive size cannot be completed by the end-to-end method, a side-to-side anastomosis is always used in these small infants. Furthermore, the use of aseptic types of anastomoses—such as the Parker-Kerr technic—is not practical with intestines this small. Mikulicz procedures have little to offer. While the aseptic aspects of this latter operation have much merit, it is doubtful if the fluid loss from the enterostomy could be controlled before the two loops could be joined by a crushing clamp.

Type of Sutures.—A lateral anastomosis is preferably made in two layers (Fig. 24); a continuous, very fine *silk* suture on a small atraumatic needle is best suited for the external layer. The inner layer may be performed with a *oooo chromic catgut* on an atraumatic needle, the type used for ureteral sutures serving well for this purpose. The inner catgut layer is taken as an over-and-over stitch on the posterior row, and is continued anteriorly as a *Connell* stitch. In some cases the distal intestine is so small that only one layer of sutures can be placed. When this is so the Connell type of suture should be employed throughout. Great delicacy must be used in the suture of such intestines, because the distal loop is extremely small and the proximal loop is apt to be thin and friable. Very small forceps must be used; a small hemostat probably serves best for a needle-holder.

The great disparity in the size of the loops which are anastomosed adds to the difficulties of operation. If the proximal loop is very distended it is

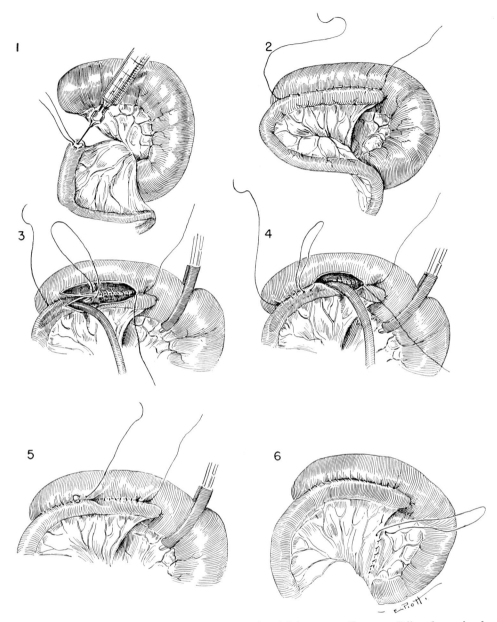

Fig. 24.—Side-to-side anastomosis for atresia of *jejunum* or *ileum*. *1*, Dilated proximal and collapsed distal loops end blindly. The latter is being distended with mineral oil and air. *2*, Primary line of suture with fine silk on an atraumatic needle (such as an eye suture or blood-vessel suture). *3*, Rubber-covered clamp on proximal loop to prevent peristaltic rushes. Loops opened. Continuous over-and-over stitch of fine atraumatic silk or chromic catgut (oooo). Catheter in distal loop to help define the edge and to prevent constriction of tiny intestine when corner is rounded with inner layer of suture. *4*, Inner suture being continued anteriorly as a Connell stitch. *5*, Inner row complete. Outer continuous row being placed. *6*, Anastomosis completed. Mesenteric defect closure.

best to aspirate it with a needle, and turn in this part of the bowel with a *figure-of-8* or a *circular* stitch. The small distal loop can be increased in size if necessary by puncturing it with a needle and injecting air or fluid. In many cases it is helpful to insert a small urethral catheter into the distal loop after it is opened because the edges of the tiny intestine can be better identified when placing the sutures.

The hole in the mesentery is now closed so that no bowel can prolapse through the defect.

Relief of Obstruction of Distal Bowel.—Since the small size of the distal intestine and colon leads to partial obstruction after the anastomosis has been performed, every effort should be made to distend the distal bowel. While this can be subsequently partly done by administration of enemata after operation, it has been our practice to inject salt solution or small amounts of mineral oil into the distal loop before completing the anastomosis.

Multiple Atresias.—Great care must be taken during operation to make sure that multiple atresias do not exist. If several atresias are found, a point for the anastomosis must be selected in the distal loop which is beyond the lowermost atresia. If there are several isolated, collapsed, sausagelike bits of bowel, these may be resected, but it is probably better treatment to leave them in place and to remove them subsequently (for fear of cyst formation) if the child should survive.

Ileostomy Is Contraindicated.—To one inexperienced in this field, it would appear that ileostomy would be the procedure of choice in order to relieve the abdominal distention, the respiratory embarrassment, and the intestinal obstruction. However, there is adequate proof that ileostomy is a poor surgical procedure. In the twenty cases in which we have performed it there have been no survivals. To our knowledge there has been no case in the literature which has been successful with enterostomy alone. The use of an enterostomy in a newly born child always leads to *extreme dehydration* which cannot be combated, even with vigorous administration of parenteral fluids and blood. Intravenous injections of water, hemoglobin, plasma, glucose, and sodium chloride will support the child, but are insufficient to maintain life. It is obvious that some other important substance is lost from the intestinal stoma.

Ileostomy Preliminary to Anastomosis.—While the results with ileostomy have been uniformly disappointing, it is pertinent to mention two patients who were first treated by ileostomy and who lived for three and four weeks respectively, at which times anastomosis of the proximal and distal loops was undertaken. Both of these children died, but it is important to recognize that they were temporarily relieved of their obstruction and might have been cured if the anastomosis had been attempted at an earlier date. It is, therefore, reasonable to suggest that in the future therapeutic attempts should be made to establish aseptically an ileostomy (when the obstruction is below the jejunum) and then proceed with the anastomosis in two or three days' time. In this way the bowel will have been decompressed, the baby will have improved its respiratory and circulatory apparatus, and possibly not too much fluid will have been lost. Furthermore, in the second stage of the procedure the peritoneal cavity would probably stand infection better than it would if anastomosis and soiling had been done at the first operation. This is only a suggestion, and its value should be established or disproved by future trial.

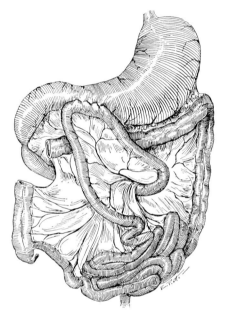

Fig. 25.—Method of surgical treatment in a case of *duodenal* atresia with obstruction just proximal to the papilla of Vater. Obstruction is at the indented portion of the duodenum. Sketch made from a 4-pound baby who was successfully treated by anterior gastro-jejunostomy. (A portion of the hepatic flexure of the colon has been omitted to show the duodenum.)

Duodenal and Jejunal Atresias.—It is obvious that any form of treatment other than direct anastomosis will carry a high mortality rate when applied to duodenal or jejunal atresias. To exteriorize the blind pouch in such cases would immediately lead to uncontrollable loss of fluid and electrolytes. In the cases with duodenal atresia above the level of the papilla of Vater (Fig. 25), a *gastrojejunostomy* is the procedure of choice. With duodenal atresias below the papilla of Vater, antecolic or preferably retrocolic *duodenojejunostomy* is the most efficacious operation. In atresias of the jejunum, ileum, or colon, anastomosis should be made between those parts of the alimentary tract immediately above and below the obstructing point.

Postoperative Treatment.—Treatment following operation demands a great deal of patience, attention, and supportive care. The stomach should be repeatedly washed out or aspirated by constant suction, as long as there is any tendency to vomiting. The colon should be dilated with saline enemas two or three times per day. *Feedings* must be instituted with extreme care and should be started only when there is evidence that the vomiting is diminishing in frequency and amount. *Parenteral fluids* two or three times per twenty-four hours must be given to maintain the fluid balance. A *transfusion* of citrated blood will be required immediately after operation to prevent shock and bleeding caused by hemorrhagic disease of the newborn. Transfusions thereafter should be given as often as is necessary to maintain the red blood count and the plasma protein at normal levels.

RESULTS OF THERAPY

To review the operative results and treatment of these cases is extremely discouraging. It is necessary, however, to study the results of various forms of therapy in order to obtain what value there is in past experiences. Until three decades ago no successful case of treatment for this condition had ever been recorded. The continued attempts by surgical means have gradually led to reports of successful cases.

Sites of Atresia and Types of Operation.—A summary of the findings in fifty-two cases treated by surgery at the Children's Hospital is given in Table 3. The sites of atresia and the types of operation in the respective cases are here summarized. Four patients with *duodenal* atresia were all treated by duodenojejunostomy and there were no recoveries. One patient with a duodenal atresia proximal to the ampulla of Vater was successfully treated by an anterior gastrojejunostomy. Six patients with *jejunal* atresia were all treated by primary anastomosis and there were three recoveries. Thirty-four patients with atresia of the *ileum* were treated by various procedures, but the three successful cases all had primary anastomoses. Many of the patients with ileal atresia who were treated by ileostomy were in the earlier part of our series and because of the uniformly fatal results with that operation we have completely abandoned the use of ileostomies. Atresias of the *ileocecal valve* or *colon* are rare and we have encountered only four of them. All of the patients with these have died, in spite of treatment by either ileostomy or anastomosis, and it is assumed that the drier form and the higher bacterial count of the intestinal content at these levels leads to greater mortality because of spreading infection and disruption of the anastomoses.

Causes of Death.—The causes of death in this series of patients were varied. In some babies there were other abnormalities, such as congenital heart disease, or esophageal atresia. When the deaths followed ileostomy, there were usually profound dehydration, inanition, and gradual wasting which was followed by a terminal pulmonary infection. When death followed primary anastomosis it was usually because of a spreading peritonitis resulting from disruption of the friable bowel at the site of anastomosis. Since most of these cases were treated before the advent of chemotherapy, the results in the future will probably be improved with the use of drugs designed to combat peritonitis and pneumonia.

TABLE 3

RESULTS OF OPERATIVE TREATMENT IN FIFTY-TWO CASES OF INTESTINAL OR COLONIC ATRESIA

Site of Atresia	Operation	Results	
		Deaths	Recoveries
Duodenum (5 cases)	Duodenojejunostomy	4	0
	Gastrojejunostomy	0	1
Jejunum (6 cases)	Duodenojejunostomy	1	0
	Jejuno-ileostomy (1 with resection)	2	3
Ileum (34 cases)	Ileostomy (2 with resection)	20	0
	Ileostomy; later ileocolostomy	2	0
	Ileostomy, with ileo-ileostomy	2	1
	Ileo-ileostomy or ileocolostomy	7	2
Ileocecal valve (2 cases)	Ileostomy	1	0
	Ileostomy and ileosigmoidostomy	1	0
Ascending colon (2 cases)	Ileocolostomy (1 with resection)	2	0
Multiple (3 cases)	Miscellaneous procedures	3	0
Totals		45	7

Relief of Symptoms.—In those seven individuals who have survived operation, there has been complete relief of intestinal symptoms, and general development has proceeded normally. In one child with a midileac atresia, considerable bowel had to be resected because of gangrene and impending perforation. This child, who is now five years of age, has had a refractile type of rickets which is presumably due to the removal of a part of the intestinal tract concerned with the absorption of calcium. The mineral deficiency in this patient can be combated only with the continuous administration of large amounts of vitamin D, but with this treatment the blood calcium level has been kept normal and rickets has been controlled.

END RESULTS IN INTRINSIC CONGENITAL INTESTINAL OBSTRUCTION
(BOTH ATRESIA AND STENOSIS)

In those subjects with a congenital obstruction of the jejunum, ileum, or colon, there is usually no difficulty in determining at the operating table whether a partial or a complete blockage exists. If the obstruction is in the duodenum, however, it may be extremely difficult or even impossible to tell whether a stenosis or an atresia is present. Should the intestine below the duodenal obstruction contain any gas, the lesion obviously must be a stenosis. If a stenosed duodenum has only a pinhole-sized lumen, the gut beyond it may be quite collapsed and the operator be led to believe that the obstruction is complete. We have made this mistake in some cases, and have found at subsequent autopsy that a small opening was actually present. There is, therefore, some justification for not making too sharp a line of

TABLE 4

Operative Results in Seventy-four Cases with Intrinsic Obstruction (Atresia or Stenosis) of the Intestine or Colon

Site of Atresia or Stenosis	Number of Cases Treated	Results	
		Deaths	Recoveries
Duodenum....................	16	8	8
Jejunum.....................	8	4	4
Ileum.......................	41	36	5
Ileocecal valve..............	3	3	0
Colon.......................	3	3	0
Multiple lesions.............	3	3	0
Totals..................	74	57	17

demarcation in discussing atresias and stenoses. Indeed, it is probably better to group the two conditions as *intrinsic obstruction* of the intestine. Table 4 lists the end results in our seventy-four cases of intrinsic obstruction, which include the atresias considered in this chapter and the stenoses considered in the following chapter.

BIBLIOGRAPHY

1. Bolling, R. W.: Complete Congenital Obstruction of the Duodenum, Duodenojejunostomy at Nine Days. Ann. Surg., *83:* 543, 1926.
2. Demmer, F.: Atresia Ilei. Resectio ileocoecalis Heilung. Arch. f. Klin. Chir., *147:* 471, 1927.
3. Donovan, E. J.: Congenital Atresia of the Duodenum in the Newborn. Ann. Surg., *103:* 455, 1936.
4. Ernst, N. P.: A Case of Congenital Atresia of the Duodenum Treated Successfully by Operation. Brit. Med. J., *1:* 644, 1916.
5. Farber, S.: Congenital Atresia of the Alimentary Tract: Diagnosis by Microscopic Examination of Meconium. J. A. M. A., *100:* 1753, 1933.

6. Fockens, P.: Ein operativ geheilter Fall von kongenitaler Dünndarmatresie. Zentralbl. f. Chir., *38:* 532, 1911.

7. Ladd, W. E.: Congenital Obstruction of the Duodenum in Children. New England J. Med., *206:* 277, 1932.

8. Ladd, W. E.: Congenital Obstruction of the Small Intestine. J. A. M. A., *101:* 1453, 1933.

9. Ladd, W. E.: Surgical Diseases of the Alimentary Tract in Infants. New England J. Med., *215:* 705, 1936.

10. Ladd, W. E.: Congenital Duodenal Obstruction. Surgery, *1:* 878, 1937.

11. McIntosh, R. and Donovan, E. J.: Disturbances of Rotation of the Intestinal Tract; Clinical Picture Based on Observations in 20 Cases. Am. J. Dis. Child., *57:* 116, 1939.

12. Miller, E. M.: Bowel Obstruction in the New Born. Ann. Surg., *110:* 587, 1939.

13. Morton, J. J., and Jones, T. B.: Obstructions about the Mesentery in Infants. Ann. Surg., *104:* 864, 1936.

14. Sweet, G. B., and Robertson, C.: A Case of Congenital Atresia of the Jejunum (with Recovery). Arch. Dis. Childhood, *2:* 186, 1927.

15. Webb, C. H., and Wangensteen, O. H.: Congenital Intestinal Atresia. Am. J. Dis. Child., *41:* 262, 1931.

16. Weeks, A., and Delprat, G. D.: Congenital Intestinal Obstruction: Atresia of Jejunum. Report of Two Cases. Surg. Clin. North America, *7:* 1193, 1927.

CHAPTER IV

CONGENITAL STENOSIS OF THE INTESTINE AND COLON

Many of the remarks in the last chapter on intestinal atresias may also be applied to stenoses of the intestine and colon. There are, however, some differences in the symptomatology, methods of treatment, and prognosis in the two conditions which make it desirable to present these two abnormalities separately. Many reports in the literature give rise to a confusion because authors have not carefully differentiated between intestinal atresia and intestinal stenosis. A close scrutiny of some published cases of "successfully treated atresias" makes plain the fact that what is listed as atresia is often actually stenosis.

EMBRYOLOGY

In the chapter on atresias of the intestine it was noted that the intestinal tube passes through *a solid stage* at one time during embryologic development. The epithelial concrescences which give rise to this solid form subsequently disappear in the normal embryo. If, however, there is an

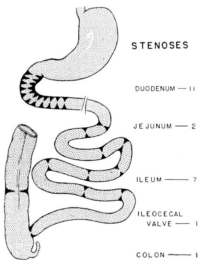

STENOSES

DUODENUM — 11

JEJUNUM — 2

ILEUM ——— 7

ILEOCECAL VALVE — 1

COLON ——— 1

Fig. 26.—Diagram showing positions of stenoses of alimentary tract in twenty-two patients.

incomplete reduction from the solid stage, a diaphragm of tissue remains within the intestinal lumen, which may be perforated in only one small point. Such an obstructing lesion may appear at any level from the pylorus to the rectum. These stenoses are much more common in the duodenum than elsewhere; about half of our patients had a duodenal obstruction while one third of them had an ileal lesion (Fig. 26).

PATHOLOGY

The intestinal lumen at the *narrowed zone* is of variable size. In many cases the opening is little more than 2 or 3 mm. in diameter, and will barely admit a probe. The aperture may be larger, and in a few specimens there is only a slight constriction of the bowel. *Microscopic examination* of the narrowed zone shows heaped-up mucosa and submucosal tissues which

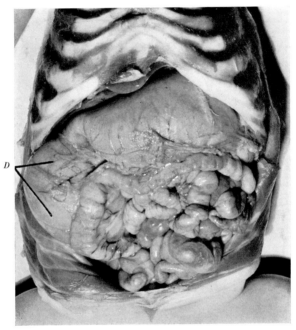

Fig. 27.—Postmortem photograph of an eight-month-old child with *duodenal* stenosis. The duodenum (*D*) proximal to the obstruction is greatly dilated. Same patient as in Fig. 29.

may be supported by accessory smooth muscle and irregularly distributed connective tissue. In those stenoses with only a slight narrowing of the intestinal tube, microscopic examination of a longitudinal section may show little more than increased fibrous tissue in the submucosa or muscularis.

Above the obstruction the intestinal tube is always dilated to some degree (Fig. 27). If the stenosed area has a very small diameter, the proximal intestine is markedly distended. When the stenosis is in the second or third part of the duodenum, the duodenum above this may be almost as large as the stomach, and the pylorus may be quite patulous. While the distention in some of these cases may be marked, we have never encountered rupture of the gut such as is frequently seen in cases of atresia.

In our experience, no case has had more than one stenosis, which is in contrast to the findings in cases of atresia, where more than one obstruction is sometimes found.

SYMPTOMS AND SIGNS

Symptoms in Early, Severe Cases.—About half of these individuals (ten out of twenty-two cases) had clinical findings which were difficult or impossible to distinguish from those of intestinal atresia, because the patients had the signs of obstruction during the first week of life.

The most marked symptom is *persistent vomiting,* which usually follows the ingestion of milk. In one case the vomitus did not contain bile, and the stenosis was subsequently found just above the ampulla of Vater. In all other patients the vomitus was colored green. *Abdominal distention* is present if the obstruction is low, but it is limited to the epigastrium when the obstruction is in the jejunum or duodenum. *Loss of weight* or failure to gain weight is common. The *stools* are diminished in number and size in most cases, but in a few individuals there is passage of some milk curds which indicates an incomplete type of obstruction. The finding of cornified epithelial cells on microscopic examination of the *meconium* during the first two or three days of life is further evidence that the obstruction is incomplete.

Symptoms in Late Cases.—While the symptoms in the above-described group are severe enough to bring the babies to the hospital in the first week of life, the remaining half of the patients with intestinal stenosis do not appear until a later age. A small group are first seen in the second or third week of life, and in these the frequency of *vomiting* and the degree of *dehydration* are not as great as in those babies who are hospitalized earlier. The *stools* in these older babies may be scanty, and of course they do contain some milk curds. These older infants are more apt to be brought in to the medical service for "regulation of feeding," or for other study to determine the nature of their trouble, which is seldom apparent at first examination.

Four of our twenty-two patients with stenosis were initially hospitalized after the first year of life. In other words, the symptoms were so mild that the individuals had gone for many months or years with only occasional vomiting, possibly intermittent abdominal pain, or retarded gain in weight. These older patients are apt to have symptoms which are vague and hence they are often treated for long periods by changing of diets, administration of laxatives, or by use of atropine compounds before it is evident that an organic abnormality is present. The ages at which our twenty-two patients were hospitalized were as follows:

First week of life .... 11 cases
Second week 4   "
Third week 3   "
14 months .... 1 case
18 months 1   "
5 years 1   "
9 years 1   "

Physical Findings.—The physical findings in these individuals vary with the age of the individual and with the degree of obstruction. If the obstruction is high, *distention* of the epigastrium or of the right upper quadrant may be obvious, and indeed, a dilated duodenum can usually be palpated if it has not been deflated by repeated vomiting. *Peristaltic waves* may pass downward in the right upper quadrant. When the obstruction is in the lower jejunum or ileum, large dilated loops may give a rather general distention and visible peristalsis may be observed. In babies coming to the physician's attention in the first week of life, the obstructions are usually of a severe grade, the physical findings are more striking, and dehydration is advanced. This is in contrast to those patients who have their initial symptoms in later months or years and in whom the physical findings are apt to be minimal.

ROENTGENOLOGIC EXAMINATION

In almost all cases there is roentgenologic evidence of dilated intestine above the point of obstruction. A *film* of the abdomen without the use of contrast media may give all the information which is required. Thus, in

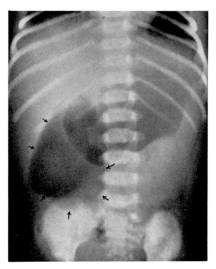

Fig. 28.—Roentgenogram of five-day-old female infant with stenosis in the *terminal portion of the duodenum*. Arrows outline the distended duodenum. Patient successfully treated by retrocolic duodenojejunostomy.

Fig. 28, the stomach is filled with gas and the duodenum is greatly dilated. If such observations are made, no further roentgenologic examination need be done and operation can be proceeded with at once.

Barium.—If there is any question about the presence of obstruction, a thin barium mixture can be administered. The findings in such a case are illustrated in Fig. 29; the duodenum can be seen to be greatly distended and only a few flecks of barium have passed into the intestine beyond. The administration of barium in these cases is not without danger and indeed one of our patients suddenly died twelve hours after such a barium examination. The postmortem examination in this case showed no demonstrable

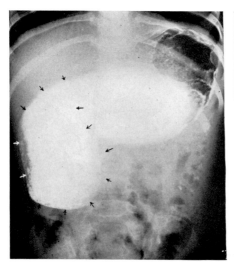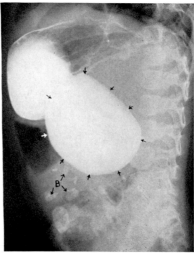

Fig. 29.—Roentgenograms with barium meal in an eight-month-old infant with *duodenal* stenosis. Dilated portion of the duodenum is outlined with arrows. In the lateral view a few flecks of barium (*B*) indicate that the obstruction is not complete. Child died twelve hours after administration of barium. Autopsy showed a stenosis just proximal to the papilla of Vater.

cause of death. There was no evidence of aspiration. Presumably, the greatly dilated stomach and duodenum either pressed on the inferior vena cava, or else set up reflex mechanisms which in some way disturbed the cardiovascular apparatus.

TREATMENT

Dehydration should be adequately combated before operation is started. The upper intestinal tract should be deflated to facilitate the operative procedure and to prevent vomiting and aspiration.

Operative Technic.—*Exposure of the Intestine.*—In a baby under one month of age a *right paramedian incision* opposite to and above the umbilicus will give an adequate exposure. In older children, the incision must be placed according to the site of obstruction as previously determined by roentgenologic examination.

Dilatation of the Stenotic Region.—Two methods are available for the surgical treatment of stenoses. The intestine may be opened below or above the site of obstruction and a dilating instrument, such as a hemostat or half-length snap, introduced into the intestinal lumen to stretch the stenotic area. We gave this procedure several trials, but it was never as successful as we anticipated that it would be.

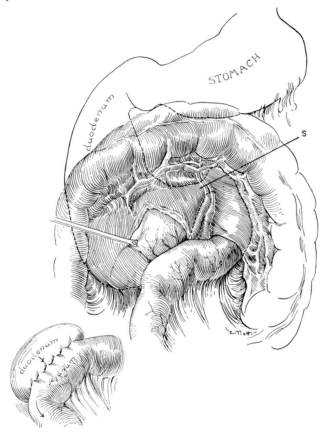

Fig. 30.—Sketch of preferred method in treatment of stenosis (S) of the *second or third part of the duodenum* by retrocolic duodenojejunostomy. Antiperistaltic unions have given as satisfactory results as isoperistaltic anastomoses.

While dilatation of the stenosis is tempting because of its simplicity, three *complications* militate against its use: (1) If the intestine is opened below the stenosis, this collapsed bowel may be so small that it is subsequently closed with difficulty. (2) If the bowel is opened above the obstruction it may be found that the obstruction is not completely relieved and the line of intestinal suture above a remaining obstruction may subsequently leak. (3) Dilatation of the stenotic region is often difficult and incomplete, because fibrous tissue within the wall of the intestine may be unyielding, and the intestine may tear. It is therefore preferable to avoid

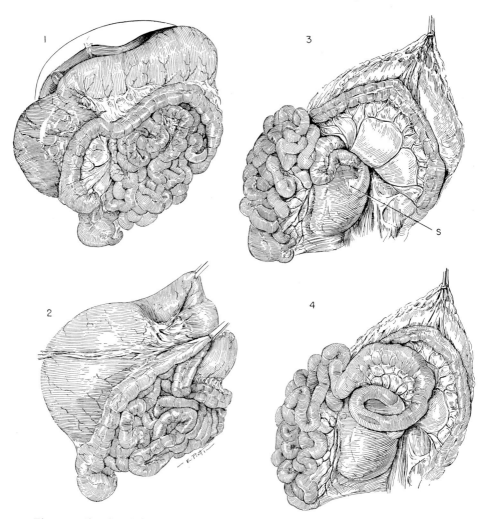

Fig. 31.—Sketch of findings and treatment in a case with stenosis of the *upper jejunum. 1,* View obtained on opening the abdomen. The duodenum below the pylorus is greatly dilated. *2,* Exposure of duodenum gained when the stomach and hepatic flexure of the colon are pulled toward the midline. *3,* View obtained when the transverse colon is elevated and the intestines are pulled to the patient's right. Stenosis at *S,* with greatly dilated jejunum proximal to this point. *4,* Treatment by anastomosis to left of mesentery, with isoperistaltic jejunojejunostomy.

dilating or cutting an obstructing diaphragm, because it is technically quicker and more satisfactory to perform a short-circuiting anastomosis.

Establishment of a Primary Anastomosis.—Anastomosis of a *side-to-side type* can be rapidly done by bringing together portions of bowel immediately above and below the stenosis. If duodenal obstruction exists above the papilla of Vater (which is a rare finding) a *gastrojejunostomy* is preferable, but in all other types of duodenal obstruction, a *duodenojejunostomy* gives better drainage of the duodenal loop. In one of our cases a gastroenterostomy was performed for an obstruction in the third part of the duodenum, but the child had loss of appetite and subsequent roentgenologic examination showed barium churning in the obstructed duodenum and then being regurgitated back into the stomach. In this patient a duodenojejunostomy was secondarily established with successful issue. In most cases a duodenojejunostomy can be made behind the colon by piercing the transverse mesocolon; if for any technical reason an *antecolic* duodenojejunostomy seems easier, it is an acceptable procedure, as is demonstrated by reported cases. When short-circuiting anastomoses are done, they are ordinarily made isoperistaltic, but an antiperistaltic union rarely gives any untoward symptoms or complications.

The anastomoses in these subjects usually offer little or no technical difficulty; the distal bowel, while somewhat collapsed, is always larger than the distal intestine in cases of atresia. Therefore, two layers of sutures can always be placed. It has been our practice to employ an external continuous layer of silk and an internal layer of continuous ooo or oooo catgut suture with an over-and-over stitch posteriorly and a Connell stitch anteriorly.

There has been sufficient experience to show that *enterostomy* in these cases is a uniformly fatal procedure, even when established for a low ileac or a colonic obstruction. It is therefore imperative to establish a primary anastomosis if success is to be hoped for.

Postoperative Treatment.—The postoperative treatment includes an immediate *transfusion* if much blood has been lost during the operative procedure. For several days the stomach and duodenum should be kept deflated by an *inlying tube* in order to diminish the tension on the suture line and to reduce peristaltic activity. *Feedings* should be withheld for three or four days to permit healing of the anastomosis. Fluid and caloric requirement can easily be met by parenteral routes.

RESULTS OF TREATMENT

In our series of twenty-two patients with stenoses of various parts of the intestinal tract, twelve died and ten recovered. In the first portion of this series several patients were treated by enterostomy or colostomy, which we have now completely abandoned. The operative results in later years, therefore, are better than the above figures would indicate. Some of the statistics are summarized in Table 5.

TABLE 5

RESULTS OF OPERATIVE TREATMENT IN TWENTY-TWO CASES OF INTESTINAL OR COLONIC STENOSIS

Site of Stenosis	Operation	Results	
		Deaths	Recoveries
Duodenum (11 cases)	Jejunostomy (for feeding)	1	0
	Gastro-enterostomy	1	1
	Gastro-enterostomy; later duodenojejunostomy	0	1
	Duodenojejunostomy	2	5
Jejunum (2 cases)	Jejunojejunostomy	1	0
	Duodenojejunostomy	0	1
Ileum (7 cases)	Ileostomy	3	0
	Resection and ileo-ileostomy	2	1
	Ileocolostomy	0	1
Ileocecal Valve (1 case)	Ileosigmoidostomy and ileostomy	1	0
Ascending colon (1 case)	Colostomy	1	0
	Totals	12	10

The *site* of stenosis has considerable prognostic importance. The higher the obstruction, the better the outlook. Of eleven cases with duodenal stenosis, seven recovered. In two cases with jejunal stenosis, one recovered. In seven cases with ileal stenosis, two recovered. In patients with stenosis at the ileocecal valve or at the colon there was a uniformly fatal result.

BIBLIOGRAPHY

1. Cannon, P. R., and Halpert, B.: Congenital Stenosis of the Third Portion of the Duodenum with Acute Occlusion and Rupture of the Stomach. Arch. Path., 8: 611, 1929.
2. Cautley, E.: Duodenal Stenosis. Brit. J. Child. Dis., 16: 65, 1919.
3. Garvin, J. A.: Congenital Occlusion of the Duodenum. Am. J. Dis. Child., 35: 109, 1928.
4. Kuliga, P.: Zur Genese der congenitalen Dünndarmstenosen und Atresien. Beitr. z. path. Anat. u. z. allg. Path., 33: 481, 1903.
5. Ladd, W. E.: Congenital Obstruction of the Small Intestine, J.A.M.A., 101: 1453, 1933.
6. Ladd, W. E.: Congenital Duodenal Obstruction. Surgery, 1: 878, 1937.
7. Webb, C. H., and Wangensteen, O. H.: Congenital Intestinal Atresia. Am. J. Dis. Child., 41: 262, 1931.

CHAPTER V

INTESTINAL OBSTRUCTION RESULTING FROM MALROTATION OF THE INTESTINES AND COLON

Of particular interest to the surgeon who must deal with intestinal obstruction in children is the condition of *incomplete rotation* of the intestine. As will be subsequently described, improper rotation (which is almost always an incomplete rotation) produces characteristic findings of high intestinal obstruction resulting from external pressure on the second or third portions of the duodenum. Our operative experience in this field has been largely concerned with incomplete rotations of the intestine and midgut volvulus, which are the only ones considered in this chapter.

There have been well over two hundred reports in the literature describing this condition. Most of these are of autopsy findings and quite a few of them represent postmortem studies following unsuccessful abdominal explorations. This same state of affairs characterized the observations and treatments in the first part of our series many years ago. After a number of fatalities with these anomalies, repeated study at the autopsy table showed that an apparently complicated lesion could be easily treated by rather simple means. With the institution of this suggested therapy in subsequent cases a striking improvement in results has been obtained. If the surgeon has not familiarized himself with this condition, he will be confused on opening the abdomen of a newly born baby with such an anomaly. Conversely, if he recognizes the abnormality immediately he can easily institute measures which give high promise of successful issue.

EMBRYOLOGY

The pathologic condition described in this chapter is wholly concerned with the development and position of the *midgut,* which includes that portion of the alimentary tube from the duodenum to the midpart of the transverse colon. The midgut is comprised of two segments: (1) the *prearterial* portion, which is included between the duodenum and the vitelline duct (or Meckel's diverticulum) ; and (2) the *postarterial* portion, or that portion from the vitelline duct (or Meckel's diverticulum) downward to the midtransverse colon.

Normal Rotations and Attachments of Intestinal Tract.—From the sixth to the tenth weeks of embryonic life, the alimentary tube grows at a faster rate than does the celomic cavity, and a portion of the midgut protrudes out into the base of the umbilical cord (Fig. 32) . At about the tenth week

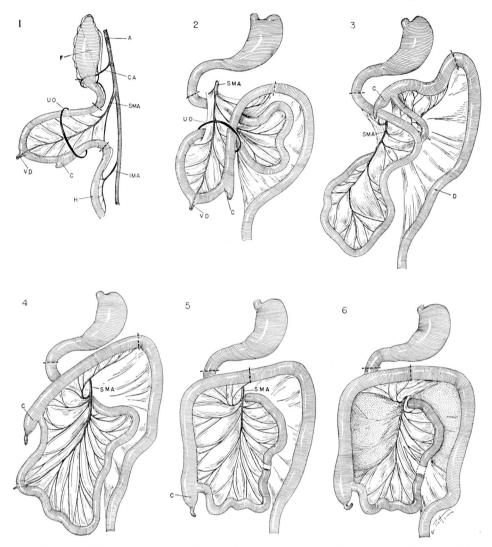

Fig. 32.—Schematic drawing of normal development, rotation, and attachment of the midgut. The midgut in each sketch is that part included between the dotted lines and represents that portion of the alimentary tract from duodenum to midtransverse colon which is supplied by the superior mesenteric artery.

A, Aorta	*H*, Hindgut
C, Cecum	*IMA*, Inferior Mesenteric Artery
CA, Coeliac Axis	*SMA*, Superior Mesenteric Artery
D, Descending Colon	*UO*, Umbilical Orifice
F, Foregut	*VD*, Vitelline Duct

1, Fifth week of fetal life—lateral view. The foregut, midgut, and hindgut with their respective blood supplies are indicated. Most of the midgut is extruded into the base of the umbilical cord where it normally resides from about the fifth to the tenth week.

2, Tenth week of fetal life—anterior view. The intestine is elongating and the hindgut is displaced to the left side of the abdomen. The developing, intra-abdominal intestines the peritoneal cavity grows at a greater rate and the midgut is withdrawn into it. As this recedes into the abdomen it *rotates* in a counterclockwise direction (as one faces the fetus). It is therefore evident that the post-arterial portion of the midgut, which includes the terminal ileum, cecum, ascending colon, and transverse colon, lies wholly in the left side of the abdomen. The anticlockwise rotation continues until the cecum comes to lie in the superior part of the abdomen. Thus, in the eleventh week of fetal life, the cecum and first portion of the colon are in the epigastrium. As the rotation continues, the cecum passes into the right upper quadrant and then finally ends its migration in the right lower quadrant.

After this rotation is completed, the cecum and ascending colon attain peritoneal reflections and attachments in the right side of the abdomen, and the mesentery of the small bowel likewise becomes attached to the posterior abdominal wall from the duodenojejunal junction obliquely downward toward the cecum.

Malrotations.—Most of the clinical findings in malrotations of the intestinal tract can be understood if this normal embryology is borne in mind. Arrests in development during the tenth or eleventh week of fetal life will give rise to anomalies which are characterized by: (1) an incompletely rotated cecum; (2) a lack of attachment of the mesentery along the posterior abdominal wall; or (3) a completely rotated cecum which is mobile and unattached.

PATHOLOGY

Obstruction of the Descending Duodenum.—With incomplete rotation of the cecum one commonly finds this organ just below the distal half of the stomach and bands of reflected peritoneum running from it (or the ascending colon) to the right posterolateral part of the abdominal wall (Figs. 37, 39, and 40). These bands or folds therefore lie directly across the descending portion of the duodenum and partly obstruct this viscus by external

---

come to lie behind the superior mesenteric artery. A portion of the midgut still protrudes through the umbilical orifice into the base of the cord.

3, Eleventh week of fetal life. All of the alimentary tract is withdrawn into the abdomen. The cecum lies in the epigastrium, beneath the stomach.

4, Late in eleventh week of fetal life. The colon is rotating, so that the cecum lies in the right upper quadrant of the abdomen.

5, Rotation of the colon is complete, and the cecum lies in a normal position. There is a common mesentery—the mesocolon of the ascending colon being continuous with the mesentery of the ileum. There is no posterior attachment of this common mesentery except at the origin of the superior mesenteric artery.

6, Final stage in attachment of the mesenteries. The stippled portions become fused and anchored to the posterior abdominal wall, so that the ascending and descending parts of the colon are anchored and the mesentery of the jejunum and ileum have a posterior attachment from the origin of the superior mesenteric artery obliquely downward to the cecum.

pressure. In a smaller number of cases the cecum has proceeded farther but is yet incompletely rotated, so that it lies directly over the duodenum and obstructs it by external pressure.

Volvulus of Midgut.—In association with these abnormal positions of the cecum, the mesentery of the small intestine lacks its normal fixation, so that it has only a short rudimentary attachment just below the origin of the superior mesenteric artery. When the intestine from the duodenojejunal junction to the transverse colon is thus supported by an incompletely anchored mesentery, there may be a volvulus of the entire midgut. This rotation takes place around the high and rudimentary attachment of the mesentery (Fig. 39), the volvulus usually being in a clockwise direction. The mesentery and intestines may be twisted a full 360 degrees or more; indeed, one of our cases had a twist of four complete turns. When volvulus takes place, a coil of intestine wraps itself around the base of the mesentery and at first glance gives the impression that there is a herniation of bowel through a hole in the mesentery. However, this is an illusion, because untwisting of the volvulus shows that there is no hole in the mesentery.

Effects of Volvulus.—When such a volvulus takes place, two serious conditions are at once established. First, the twisting of structures around the small attachment of the mesentery angulates and obstructs the intestine at the duodenojejunal junction and in the transverse colon. Second, the torsion gives rise to partial or complete occlusion of the superior mesenteric vessels. Hence, *infarction* of the entire midgut may supervene.

On opening the abdomen, this anomaly may be recognized by the fact that one immediately sees small intestinal loops without seeing the ascending or transverse colon (Fig. 39). Hence, if the right half of the colon is hidden by small intestines (particularly if presenting loops are bluish or discolored by congestion), the operator should immediately suspect that he is dealing with an unattached mesentery and a volvulus of the midgut.

From the above descriptions, it is obvious that there are really two separate lesions in these cases. One is concerned with the *obstruction of the descending duodenum* by an overlying cecum or peritoneal band. The other is concerned with the *volvulus of the midgut*. It is important to appreciate the fact that these two conditions can coexist, because so many operators have merely reduced the volvulus and have subsequently had the patient die from unrelieved duodenal obstruction which was caused by the abnormally placed cecum.

One may deduce that obstructions in this type of abnormality will bring about *dilatation* of certain portions of the gastro-intestinal tract. In the usual case the duodenum is considerably dilated in its upper half (Figs. 33 and 34). If there is a volvulus of the midgut, the jejunum and ileum may be quite collapsed at first because duodenal contents cannot enter this

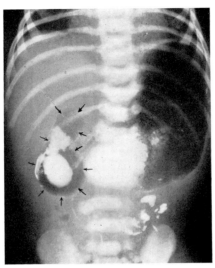

Fig. 33.—Roentgenogram with barium meal in a ten-day-old female who had vomited since the first day of life. The duodenum, outlined by arrows, is dilated. Little barium has passed beyond the duodenum. At operation an incompletely rotated cecum lay across and obstructed the duodenum by extrinsic pressure. Release of the cecum toward the patient's left led to recovery.

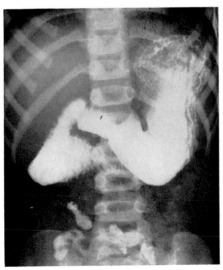

Fig. 34.—Roentgenogram from a three-year-old boy with intermittent vomiting since birth. At operation the third portion of the duodenum was found obstructed by transduodenal bands which ran over to a cecum which lay beneath the gastric antrum. Division of these bands completely relieved the vomiting spells.

obstructed segment. However, if the volvulus is present for some time, gas collects in this isolated midgut because of local bacterial growth. Hence, the jejunum, ileum, and ascending colon may become greatly distended (Fig. 36).

Normally Placed, Unattached Cecum.—In the majority of cases which have come to our attention, there has been an incomplete rotation of the cecum, and a lack of normal attachment of the small bowel to the posterior abdominal wall. There are, however, minor degrees of this same condition. In other words, one may have: (1) a normally placed, unattached cecum with an unattached mesentery of the small intestine, or (2) a normally placed, unattached cecum with a partially attached ileal mesentery. It is important to bear in mind that an unattached, mobile cecum and an incompletely attached mesentery are closely related conditions. Hence, if one of these is found at operation the other should be sought for.

Partly Attached Great Omentum.—An additional finding in some of these cases, which has little clinical significance, is related to the attachment of the great omentum. Normally, this structure arises from the stomach and then later overlies the transverse colon to which it becomes fused. In some patients with incomplete rotation of the colon, the stomach and colon are not connected with each other, and the omentum hangs only from the stomach.

SYMPTOMS AND SIGNS

The majority of these individuals have clinical findings which bring them to the physician's attention in the newly born period. Symptoms may not appear until later, or else they may be so mild that hospitalization is not sought until later childhood or even adult life. Twenty-six of our forty-four patients entered the hospital within three weeks after birth. It must be remembered, however, that many of the older individuals in the remaining eighteen cases had been having symptoms for months or even years. The ages at operation for this whole group were as follows:

1st week	9 cases		4th year	1 case
2nd week	9 "		5th year	2 cases
3rd week	8 "		6th year	1 case
4th week	2 "		7th year	1 "
2nd month	3 "		9th year	2 cases
3rd month	2 "		10th year	1 case
9th month	1 case		12th year	1 "
11th month	1 "			

Clinical Picture in Infancy.—Obstruction of the duodenum causes *vomiting,* and this is the outstanding complaint. Since the obstruction is low in the duodenum, the vomitus usually contains bile, but the peritoneal bands are on rare occasions above the papilla of Vater and the vomitus is not greenish. Vomiting is usually persistent and occurs after most of the feedings. Inasmuch as the obstruction is usually partial, there may be some passage of curd-containing stools.

Abdominal distention usually appears, but at first it is limited to the epigastrium, because only the stomach and duodenum are dilated. Careful inspection may show peristaltic waves passing downward in the right side of the epigastrium. If the patient has not been treated with parenteral fluids, *dehydration* of severe degree rapidly occurs because there is loss of pancreatic juices, bile, and gastric secretions in large amounts. If dehydration is severe, a *fever* of moderate or high degree may be encountered.

If the patient is untreated for a few days, the abdominal distention may become generalized because of an associated midgut volvulus which entraps gas in the jejunum and ileum. The temperature may reach 105° F. or more. Such fever may arise from either dehydration or from volvulus and infarction of a large part of the intestinal tract. In cases with generalized abdominal distention the *stools* are usually scanty and there are poor returns from enemata, because the volvulus of the midgut has obstructed the colon as well as the duodenum.

Laboratory data will usually show concentration of urine and there may be an elevation in the red blood count. Hemoconcentration may also give rise to a slightly elevated white blood count, but a marked *leukocytosis* should immediately arouse suspicion of an infarcted intestine.

Of the forty-four cases which we have surgically treated for incomplete rotation of the colon with resulting intestinal obstruction, nine patients were under one week of age. In this small group, the clinical picture might be confused with that of *intestinal atresia* or *stenosis*. It is not important to determine which of these three conditions exists, for in any case it is only necessary to establish the diagnosis of intestinal obstruction and explore the abdomen on this basis.

Clinical Picture in Older Children.—When the condition is found in older children, there is usually a history of long-continued or recurring attacks of *abdominal pain, nausea,* and *vomiting,* which have been glossed over as "food poisonings," "intestinal grippe," etc. These individuals may have only recurring minor abdominal complaints, or else they may have a superimposed alarming episode (from volvulus) which immediately brings them for surgical treatment.

Patients with Coeliac Syndrome.—Of increasing importance is a group of individuals with a clinical picture simulating coeliac disease. These children have persistent or recurrent abdominal distention and pain, poor absorption of food, intolerance to certain substances, and either constipation or diarrhea. These complaints are presumably brought about by twisting of the midgut in such a way that the terminal ileum is temporarily obstructed. It is therefore important to examine roentgenologically (barium enema) all individuals with a coeliac syndrome to detect any unrotated cecum or mobile cecum, because surgical correction of such abnormalities may completely relieve the patient's symptoms.

ROENTGENOLOGIC EXAMINATION

The clinical history and physical findings will usually suggest the correct diagnosis, but this should be confirmed by proper roentgenologic investigation. A *film* of the abdomen without the use of contrast media usually shows a gas-filled, dilated stomach and duodenum. In a few cases vomiting has been so effective that the duodenum and stomach are empty and no evidence of high intestinal obstruction is gained from this simple study. If a baby is seen in the first week of life, there may be only a few small bubbles of air in the intestinal tract below the level of the duodenum (Fig. 35). In marked contrast to this there may be an enormous distention of the entire jejunum and ileum (Fig. 36).

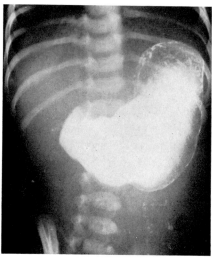

Fig. 35.—Roentgenogram from a three-week-old infant with persistent vomiting since birth. Retention of most of the barium in the stomach at four hours. There are, however, a few flecks of barium in the left lower quadrant, indicating that the obstruction is not complete. Patient had an incompletely rotated cecum (pressing on the first part of the duodenum) and a volvulus of the entire midgut.

Barium.—A *barium meal* almost always gives additional information, but it must be used with caution because the material may become inspissated and difficult to eliminate. More important, however, is the fact that barium may be vomited and aspirated, and thus give rise to pulmonary pathology. If barium is to be employed, only a thin mixture and a small amount should be used. The stomach is usually larger than normal and the duodenum is distinctly dilated. Barium can be seen passing down to the point of obstruction, and *fluoroscopically* may be observed to churn up and down in the enlarged duodenum. Only a small amount of the barium will pass beyond this region.

If additional studies are desired, a *barium enema* will show the cecum in the epigastrium and in an incompletely rotated position. In a few cases the transverse colon appears in a normal position as far backward as the hepatic flexure, but then the ascending colon and cecum are sharply angulated and doubled up underneath the transverse colon.

In most cases it is not necessary to examine the individual with contrast media by mouth or by enemata. As soon as clinical study and x-ray investigation from plain films show that some obstruction exists, it is best to proceed with operation and not carry out further roentgenologic studies.

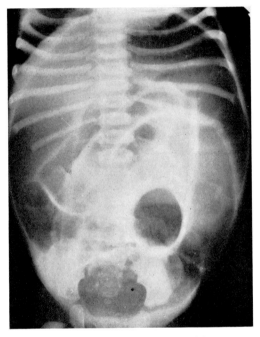

Fig. 36.—Roentgenogram of three-month-old baby with symptoms and signs of acute intestinal obstruction for thirty-six hours. Abdomen greatly distended. Intestinal loops diffusely dilated in the film. Findings at operation—unattached cecum and mesentery with a volvulus of the midgut.

Study of Older Children.—While the suggestions laid down in the preceding paragraph have been found valuable for newly born infants, they are not applicable to older children. Extensive investigation in the older individual is without danger and may be necessary to make certain that there is an abnormality of some part of the intestine or colon which is responsible for the patient's symptoms. It is therefore advisable to study the stomach, duodenum, and intestines thoroughly with a barium meal and also to visualize the colon with a barium enema. It is well to bear in mind that abnormal positions of the cecum and ascending colon may be the only roentgenologic finding and no evidence of intestinal obstruction may be forthcoming if the patient is not having an attack at the time.

TREATMENT

A review of the literature on this subject indicates that the surgical treatment has been extremely discouraging and that the mortality rates have been extraordinarily high. In contrast, a review of our own material gives a much better outlook. An improvement in results may be attributed to better preoperative care, adoption of an operation which completely relieves obstruction, shorter operating-time (because the existing condition is promptly recognized), and proper supportive treatment during the early postoperative days.

Preoperative Treatment.—The majority of these patients present acute surgical emergencies, are dehydrated, and are in rather poor general condition. Fluids and electrolytes should be restored by the administration of subcutaneous *physiologic saline* and by the intravenous administration of 10 per cent *glucose*. A small catheter should be introduced through one nostril, and led down into the stomach for aspiration of fluid and gas which has collected there. In small infants a No. 8 or 10 soft-rubber urethral catheter serves admirably for this purpose, if several holes are cut in the end which lies in the stomach. *Deflation of the stomach* is important for two reasons. First, reduction of its size will greatly facilitate the intra-abdominal manipulations. Second, the danger of vomiting and aspiration after operation will be lessened.

Operative Technic.—*Anesthesia.*—The anesthesia in all of these cases should be general narcosis, preferably with *ether*. Great relaxation of the abdominal wall will be necessary to explore the abdomen completely and to deliver the loops of intestine as subsequently described. It is essential to have an anesthetic which will completely abolish pain when the intestines are delivered and the mesentery is pulled upon. Local anesthesia is therefore unsatisfactory.

Exposure of the Intestine.—In exploring one of these patients it is necessary to have a generous exposure. A *long paramedian incision* running from the xiphoid process downward well below the umbilicus will be found essential. In the presence of such intestinal obstruction some abdominal fluid is always encountered which can be rapidly sucked away.

On inspection of the abdominal viscera one of two conditions is found: (1) The cecum lies in the right upper quadrant and the ascending and transverse colon are readily visible. (2) The small intestine is the presenting part of the alimentary tract and the ascending colon is hidden from view.

1. *When the Ascending and Transverse Colon Presents* (*Duodenal*

Obstruction).—Here, the obstruction in the duodenum results from direct pressure by the overlying cecum or by peritoneal bands which cross over to the colon or cecum (Fig. 37). This duodenal obstruction is relieved by a comparatively simple operation devised by one of the writers (Ladd) some years ago. The posterior parietal peritoneum is incised just to the right of the cecum, which permits clearing of the anterior surface of the duodenum until the latter is exposed throughout its whole length (Fig. 38). In doing this the cecum is transferred to the left and all pressure is taken off the duodenum. No attempt is made to restore the normal anatomic position of the cecum, which is not only unimportant, but is apt to

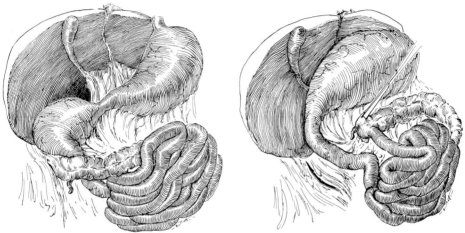

Fig. 37.   Fig. 38.

Fig. 37.—Appearance of abdominal viscera in a newly born child who had acute intestinal obstruction since the first day of life. An incompletely rotated cecum lies across the third part of the duodenum and obstructs it by extrinsic pressure (see Fig. 38 for treatment of this).

Fig. 38.—Method of surgical treatment in the case shown in Fig. 37. The peritoneal reflection which had anchored the cecum across the duodenum has been cut and the cecum is allowed to slide toward the midline of the abdomen, where it is left. This completely relieves the duodenal obstruction.

be unsuccessful in relieving the patient's symptoms. This operation affords lasting relief, is aseptic, and is far superior to any of the short-circuiting anastomoses which have sometimes been employed for this condition.

2. *When the Small Intestine Presents (Midgut Volvulus)*.—When, on opening the abdomen, the surgeon sees only a bluish, discolored small intestine, and the right half of the colon is not visible, he should at once suspect a midgut volvulus (Fig. 39). To one who is unfamiliar with this picture, it may be extremely puzzling. There is difficulty in finding the cecum or ascending colon and it often appears that loops of ileum are herniating through the mesentery of another portion of the intestine. If

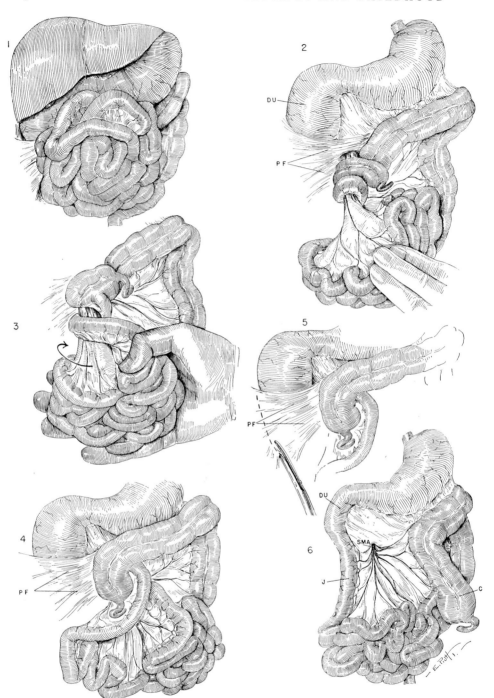

Fig. 39.—Operative treatment of acute intestinal obstruction arising from incompletely rotated cecum associated with volvulus of the midgut.

C, Cecum. DU, Duodenum. *J,* Jejunum. *PF,* Peritoneal Folds. *SMA,* Superior Mesenteric Artery.

the surgeon attempts to evaluate the findings without delivering all the intestines outside the abdomen, he will become hopelessly confused, waste valuable time, and usually not find out what he is dealing with. The whole midgut must be *pulled out* onto the abdominal wall. This can be done readily and with little shock in these patients, who have only a rudimentary mesenteric attachment.

After the intestines have been delivered, the volvulus can be recognized. It has usually taken place in a clockwise direction and may go through an arc of 360 degrees, or, as in one of our patients, through four complete turns. The volvulus is reduced by turning the mass in the appropriate direction. When this is accomplished, a normal color returns to the intestines and the surgeon might be led to believe that the operation has been completed. This is a grave error which frequently leads to a fatality. The *cecum* and *ascending colon,* which now lie in the right upper quadrant, *must be freed and transferred to the left.* This can be rapidly done by merely incising the peritoneum to the right of the ascending colon. When this peritoneal fold has been slit, the duodenum will be seen coursing downward in the right paravertebral gutter to join the jejunum. The entire colon will lie in the left side of the abdomen.

These descriptions of the treatment for intestinal obstruction due to malrotation of the colon and to midgut volvulus give the main principles which are essential for the treatment of such conditions. If they are adhered to with slight changes to suit the individual case most gratifying results will be obtained in relieving the patient's symptoms.

1, Appearance of viscera on opening abdominal cavity. The small intestines are seen at once and appear to hide the right half of the colon.

2, The intestinal mass is delivered out of the wound and pulled downward, showing the base of the mesentery. Coils of intestine or ascending colon are wrapped around the root of an incompletely anchored mesentery. The volvulus has taken place in a clockwise direction. The descending duodenum is dilated because of extrinsic pressure from the peritoneal folds which cross it and run to the colon.

3, The volvulus is reduced by taking the entire intestinal mass in the hand and rotating it in an anticlockwise direction (in most cases).

4, The volvulus is now completely reduced and the cecum lies in the right paravertebral gutter. The peritoneal folds over the cecum can now be seen as they press on the duodenum. The duodenum is still obstructed by these folds.

5, Method of releasing the duodenal obstruction by cutting the peritoneal folds which compress the second or third part of the duodenum. The folds are cut along the dotted line. These folds do not carry any blood supply to the intestine or colon.

6, Appearance of the intestines and ascending colon at the end of the operative procedure. The duodenum descends along the right paravertebral gutter to join the jejunum. The small intestines lie on the right side of the abdomen, while the cecum and ascending colon slide to the midline or left side of the abdomen. All obstruction is relieved by this procedure. The superior mesenteric artery and its branches are left exposed as shown.

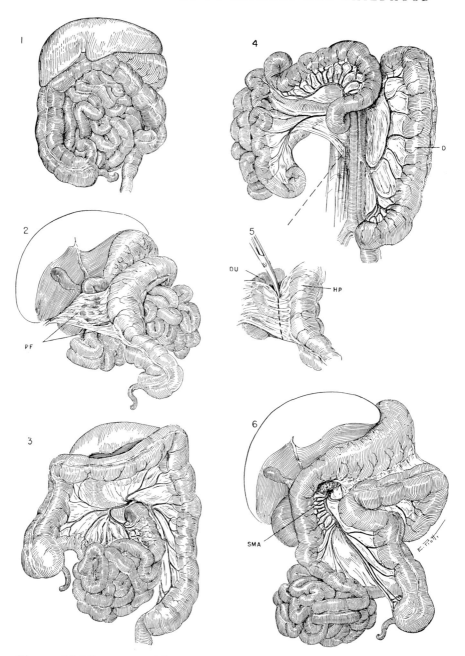

Fig. 40.—Mobile cecum and incompletely attached mesentery. Operative findings and treatment as carried out in a nine-year-old boy who had had intermittent attacks of abdominal pain, vomiting, and distention for several years. Child operated upon in interval between attacks.

DU, Duodenum. *HP*, Hepatic Flexure. *PF*, Peritoneal Folds. *SMA*, Superior Mesenteric Artery.

1, Normal position and appearance of the viscera on opening the abdominal cavity.

Symptomless Cases.—All children with an incompletely rotated colon are not necessarily candidates for surgery. We have followed a few individuals who are known to have an incompletely rotated cecum but who have never had symptoms from it. This group is relatively small when compared to the number of persons who do have complaints from an abnormally placed intestine or colon.

Mobile Cecum.—In an occasional child there are symptoms from a mobile cecum which lacks a normal posterior attachment. Such individuals may be treated in two ways: (1) If there is a normal oblique attachment of the mesentery, then the mobile cecum can be tacked down posteriorly with suitably placed sutures. (2) If, in addition, the mesentery does not have a normal posterior attachment (Fig. 40), then it is technically easier, safer, and quicker to slit the peritoneum at the right of the hepatic flexure, so that the entire right half of the colon shifts over into the left side of the abdomen.

RESULTS OF TREATMENT

On summarizing the literature as a whole, one finds *mortality* figures which are unwarrantably high in the treatment of these cases. A review of the material at the Children's Hospital (Table 6) shows that thirty-five cases have been operated upon according to principles which are set forth above. In eight of these, death has followed from supervening pneumonia, shock, or as a result of other severe congenital anomalies, such as cardiac malformation. All of the remaining twenty-seven patients have survived and have been relieved of their complaints. In no case has there been a recurrence of the obstruction or volvulus.

2, Findings when the cecum and ascending colon are drawn to the left. The cecum and ascending colon are mobile and are unattached posteriorly. There are peritoneal folds running from beneath the liver over to the hepatic flexure of the colon.

3, View obtained when the intestines are drawn downward. The mesentery of the ascending colon is directly continuous with the mesentery of the small intestine.

4, View obtained when the intestines are drawn upward and to the right. The mesentery has only a rudimentary attachment high on the abdominal wall. It is lacking its normal posterior anchorage, which should extend along the dotted line. The previous attacks in this boy were due to recurring volvulus of the entire midgut, the volvulus taking place around this high and small mesenteric attachment.

5, Method of treatment in such a case. The peritoneal folds crossing the duodenum to the hepatic flexure of the colon are cut along the dotted line.

6, Position of the viscera at the end of the operative procedure. Duodenum runs downward in the right paravertebral gutter to join the jejunum. The ascending colon has been allowed to slip to the left side of the abdomen. The entire superior mesenteric artery and its branches are thus exposed. This completely relieves attacks, because it widens structures from duodenum to hepatic flexure of the colon and thereby prevents subsequent volvulus. Furthermore, if subsequent minor twists should take place, they will not angulate and obstruct the intestine at the duodenojejunal junction.

TABLE 6

RESULTS OF OPERATIVE TREATMENT IN FORTY-FOUR CASES OF CONGENITAL, EXTRINSIC, INTESTINAL
OBSTRUCTION

Operation	Results	
	Deaths	Recoveries
Reduction of volvulus	4	0
Anterior gastro-enterostomy	1	0
Miscellaneous procedures	4	0
Ladd's operation	8	27
(As shown in Figs. 38 and 39)		
Totals	17	27

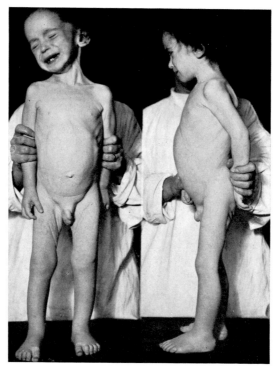

Fig. 41.—Photograph of twenty-one-month-old boy who had been treated for several
months as a case of coeliac disease. There had been recurrent attacks of abdominal swelling, associated with vomiting or diarrhea. The above lateral view shows the prominence
of the abdomen during one of these seizures. Barium enema showed an incompletely
rotated cecum. At operation the distention was found to be due to a volvulus of the
entire midgut without infarction of the bowel. Successful treatment by reduction of
volvulus and release of the cecum toward the midline. The child has had no attacks since
operation.

While most of the patients in the present series were one to three weeks of age, and were critically ill with acute intestinal obstruction, there were a few older individuals with recurrent abdominal pain and vomiting, resulting from minor degrees of incomplete rotation of the alimentary tract. Under such circumstances the finding of an incompletely rotated cecum by barium-enema examination led to successful surgical treatment of intermittent intestinal obstruction.

There have also been some gratifying results in older children who had clinical pictures suggestive of coeliac disease and roentgenologic findings of an incompletely rotated cecum. In these cases a release of the cecum toward the left side of the abdomen has produced clinical improvement. It is therefore evident that all subjects with symptoms suggestive of coeliac disease should be roentgenologically examined by barium enema to detect any unusual position or mobility of the cecum and ascending colon which might be corrected by surgery.

Bibliography

1. Dott, N. M.: Anomalies of Intestinal Rotation: Their Embryology and Surgical Aspects, with report of Five Cases. Brit. J. Surg., *11:* 251, 1923.
2. Frazer, J. E., and Robbins, R. H.: On the Factors Concerned in Causing Rotation of the Intestine in Man. J. Anat. and Physiol., *50:* 75, 1915.
3. Gardner, C. E., Jr., and Hart, D.: Anomalies of Intestinal Rotation as a Cause of Intestinal Obstruction; Report of Two Personal Observations; Review of One Hundred and Three Reported Cases. Arch. Surg., *29:* 942, 1934.
4. Raymond, H. E., and Dragstedt, L. R.: Anomalies of Intestinal Rotation: A Review of the Literature with Report of Two Cases. Surg., Gynec. and Obst., *53:* 316, 1931.
5. Hecker, P., Grünwald, E., and Kuhlmann, C. J.: Les anomalies congénitales de forme et de position du gros intestin et leur importance chirurgicale. Rev. de chir., *64:* 661, 1926.
6. Jones, T. B., and Morton, J. J.: Congenital Malformations of the Intestine in Children. Am. J. Surg., *39:* 382, 1938.
7. King, E. S. J.: Two Uncommon Forms of Intestinal Obstruction Occurring Consecutively: Compound Volvulus and Retroposition of the Transverse Colon. Brit. J. Surg., *24:* 817, 1937.
8. Koszler, V.: Zur Klinik des Mesenterium commune. Arch. f. Kinderh., *110:* 166, 1937.
9. Ladd, W. E.: Congenital Obstruction of the Small Intestine. J. A. M. A., *101:* 1453, 1933.
10. Ladd, W. E.: Surgical Diseases of the Alimentary Tract in Infants. New England J. Med., *215:* 705, 1936.
11. McIntosh, R., and Donovan, E. J.: Disturbances of Rotation of the Intestinal Tract; Clinical Picture Based on Observations in Twenty Cases. Am. J. Dis. Child., *57:* 116, 1939.
12. Miller, R., and Gage, H. C.: Gastromegaly and Chronic Duodenal Ileus in Children. Arch. Dis. Childhood, *5:* 83, 1930.
13. Mole, R. H.: Congenital Non-Rotation of the Intestine. Brit. J. Surg., *17:* 670, 1930.
14. Morton, J. J., and Jones, T. B.: Obstructions About the Mesentery in Infants. Ann. Surg., *104:* 864, 1936.

5

15. Reisman, H. A.: Congenital Obstruction of the Alimentary Tract. J. Pediat., *10:* 622, 1937.

16. Rubin, E. L.: Radiological Aspects of Anomalies of Intestinal Rotation. Lancet, *2:* 1222, 1935.

17. Wakefield, E. G., and Mayo, C. W.: Intestinal Obstruction Produced by Mesenteric Bands in Association with Failure of Intestinal Rotation. Arch. Surg., *33:* 47, 1936.

18. Waugh, G. E.: Congenital Malformations of the Mesentery: A Clinical Entity. Brit. J. Surg., *15:* 438, 1928.

CHAPTER VI

MECKEL'S DIVERTICULUM

Meckel's diverticulum is said to occur in 2 or 3 per cent of all individuals coming to autopsy examination. This outpocketing from the ileum does not often give rise to important pathology, but when it does so the resulting lesion may be a serious one. The vagaries of Meckel's diverticu-

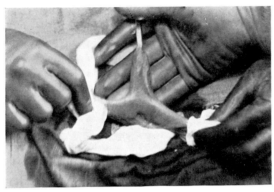

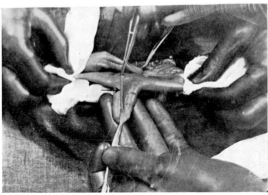

Fig. 42.—Photographs of Meckel's diverticulum taken at the operating table. *Above,* Diverticulum held upward. *Below,* Diverticulum turned downward to show the band representing the vitello-intestinal artery, which is indicated by an arrow.

lum are well known to surgeons who have had any breadth of experience in abdominal surgery, particularly if they have done much children's work. Our material includes seventy-three patients with symptoms arising from the diverticulum or one of its complications.

71

EMBRYOLOGY

During early embryonic life the intestine has a wide anterior communication with the yolk sac. This opening is gradually narrowed to form the tubelike vitello-intestinal duct. The yolk sac remains within the cord and the vitelline duct becomes reduced to the long, slender yolk stalk which then loses its connection with the intestine at about the 7 mm. stage.

Meckel's diverticulum represents that portion of the vitelline duct which had opened into the ileum. This small pouch is usually disconnected from the umbilicus, but a cord of tissue, the remnant of the primitive yolk stalk, may join the terminal ileum to the inner aspect of the umbilicus. If a longer portion of the vitelline duct remains patent, the intestine may attain an external opening at the navel.

PATHOLOGY

Meckel's diverticulum arises from the ileum 18 inches to 3 feet above the ileocecal valve. It opens on the antimesenteric side of the intestine, but may curve around and lie against the side of the gut, to which it becomes adherent. Rarely the diverticulum swings over against the mesentery and acquires a filmy covering which gives it the appearance of having an intramesenteric position.

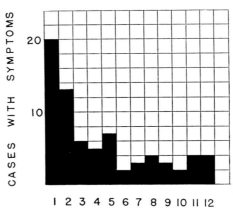

Fig. 43.—Chart showing age at which seventy-three patients developed symptoms from a Meckel's diverticulum or its complications.

The diverticulum is a fingerlike outpocketing, which usually has a diameter somewhat less than that of the adjacent bowel and a length varying from ½ inch up to 2 or 3 inches. One of our specimens was a large orange-sized cyst which had only a small communication with the intestine. Several writers have described examples of "jejunum duplex," "ileum duplex," or "giant diverticula," which are tubelike structures a foot or more

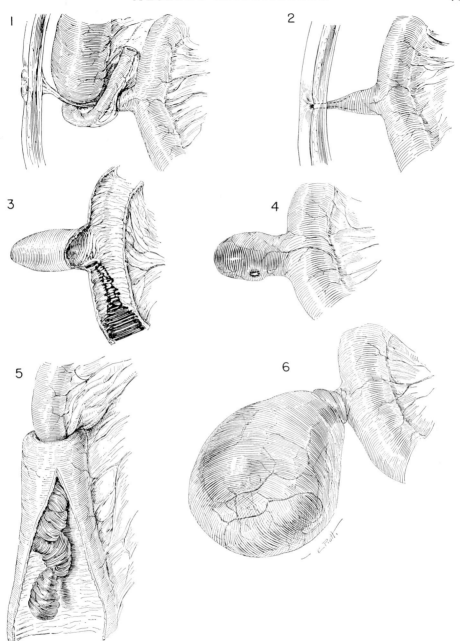

Fig. 44.—Sketches showing some of the ways in which Meckel's diverticulum gave rise to pathology in seventy-three cases: *1*, Intestinal obstruction caused by a band running from the diverticulum to the inner side of the umbilicus—six cases. *2*, Fistula at umbilicus—one case. *3*, Ulceration in the diverticulum giving rise to intestinal hemorrhage —twenty-six cases. *4*, Diverticulitis with or without perforation—ten cases. *5*, Diverticulum as a leading point of intussusception—seventeen cases. *6*, Twisting and infarction of diverticulum—one case. In twelve additional patients there was abdominal pain, presumably originating from the diverticulum, but without demonstrable pathology in the diverticulum.

long, lying on the mesenteric border of the bowel. These have been thought to originate from Meckel's diverticula, but we do not agree with this view. Accumulated evidence favors classifying these with the "duplications" (Chapter VII), which can occur anywhere along the alimentary tract from the tongue to anus.

The *lining* of a Meckel's diverticulum does not necessarily correspond to that of the ileum, to which it is attached. In seventy-three diverticula the histologic findings in the mucosa were as follows:

```
Gastric and ileal mucosa ........................... 40 cases
Ileal only ......................................... 24  "
Duodenal and ileal ................................. 4   "
Colonic and ileal .................................. 4   "
Pancreatic tissue and ileal ........................ 1 case
```

Important *pathologic complications* may arise from a Meckel's diverticulum in many ways (Fig. 44). In seventy-three patients we have removed this structure because of the following conditions:

```
1. Hemorrhage ..................................... 26 cases
2. Leading point of intussusception .............. 17  "
3. Abdominal pain ................................ 12  "
4. Inflammation, with or without perforation ..... 10  "
5. Obstruction from band (to umbilicus) .......... 6   "
6. Umbilical fistula ............................. 1 case
7. Volvulus and infarction of diverticulum ....... 1   "
```

Hemorrhage from a diverticulum almost invariably arises from a small peptic ulcer at the neck of the pouch or in the near-by intestine, which is presumably due to local digestion of the mucous membrane by the action of hydrochloric acid and pepsin which are secreted from aberrant gastric mucosa lining the diverticulum. Such a supposed relationship is substantiated by the fact that in twenty-six patients with massive bleeding from a Meckel's diverticulum, pathologic examination disclosed gastric mucosa in twenty-five of the specimens.

It is not uncommon for a diverticulum, particularly if it is broad and short, to become inverted; and when it does so it may be the *starting point of an intussusception*. When once this process has started the intussusceptum will be progressively dragged along into the terminal ileum or colon.

Inflammation of the diverticulum was found ten times in our series, and in six of these there was progression of the disease to actual *rupture* and contamination of the abdominal cavity with intestinal contents. This condition is particularly dangerous, because the migratory nature of the diverticulum and the absence of a protecting omentum in young children makes free perforation a rapidly spreading and often fatal type of infection. While microscopic examination shows significant bacterial growth and inflammation, the finding of gastric mucosa in some specimens suggests the possibility that digestive ferments may have initiated the erosion in these cases.

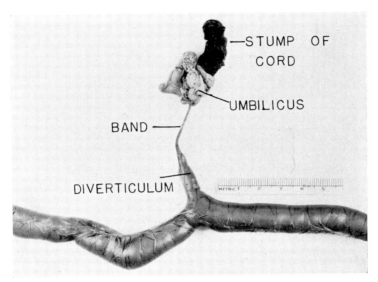

Fig. 45.—Specimen taken from autopsy examination of a three-day-old infant showing a band running from the Meckel's diverticulum to the inner surface of the umbilicus.

A vestigial band connecting the ileum to the inner side of the umbilicus may produce *intestinal obstruction* if a loop of gut is pulled tightly

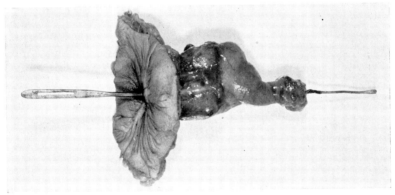

Fig. 46.—Surgical specimen from a ten-year-old boy with an intermittently discharging umbilical fecal fistula. Portion of skin at left side of specimen. A probe pierces the sinus tract.

over it. If the tip of a diverticulum becomes adherent to near-by intestine or mesentery, a pocket is formed through which coils of gut can prolapse and become obstructed.

Tuberculosis and *neoplasms* in Meckel's diverticula have been described, but we have not encountered either of these in our series.

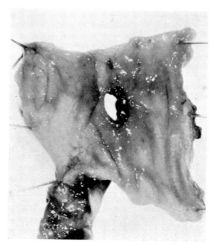

Fig. 47.—Photograph of an opened Meckel's diverticulum showing a central perforation. Removed from a six-month-old boy with peritonitis.

Meckel's diverticula appear to be somewhat more common in males than in females, the proportion being 70 per cent and 30 per cent, respectively, in our patients.

CLINICAL FINDINGS

Meckel's diverticulum may manifest itself at any age. If, however, complications do arise, they are more apt to do so early in life (Fig. 43). Approximately half (45 per cent) of all patients came to the hospital within the first two years of life. The youngest was five hours of age; the oldest was twelve years.

Hemorrhage.—Massive hemorrhage was the chief symptom in twenty-six children, 80 per cent of whom were under two years of age. The principal and alarming symptom is usually the sudden passage of a *bloody stool* in a young child in whom there have been no previous symptoms. This bleeding is apt to be copious and while the first stool might be dark or black in color, subsequent ones are almost invariably bright red. The extent of bleeding may be judged from the fact that the red count sometimes drops to 1,500,000 or 2,000,000. The massiveness of the bleeding is in contrast to the spotting of blood which occurs with anal fissures or rectal polyps. Bleeding from a Meckel's diverticulum is unattended by pain, or else there is only mild discomfort, which is in sharp contrast to the agonizing pain which accompanies the bleeding of intussusception. Though several of our patients had one to three previous episodes of melena, it is more common to have a single attack of bleeding which is severe enough to bring the child quickly to a physician's attention. With such hemorrhage, *lethargy, collapse, pallor* and *increased pulse rate* are frequently concomitant findings.

Intussusception.—When intussusception is started by a diverticulum, there are no features to distinguish it from the idiopathic type of intussusception which is common in childhood and for which no anatomic abnormality can be found. The clinical picture, therefore, is one of *intermittent abdominal pain* which recurs at intervals of fifteen to twenty minutes. In the early hours of the illness the child will double over, cry out in distress, turn pale, and vomit during the momentary paroxysms of pain. Between seizures he will be relaxed, comparatively comfortable, and even playful. As the condition progresses he will give evidence of *shock and collapse* in these interims. Abdominal pain and symptoms of intestinal obstruction may exist for many hours before melena appears.

Appendicitis Simulated.—The clinical course of a Meckel's diverticulitis may simulate that of acute appendicitis and indeed may be indistinguishable from it. The sequence of periumbilical pain, nausea, vomiting, fever, and leukocytosis is common to both conditions. If appendicitis is of some hours' standing there may be shift of pain and maximal tenderness to the right lower quadrant. In diverticulitis, however, there is no such shift, or else the shift is to some other part of the abdomen in which the diverticulum happens to lie for the moment.

Obstruction.—Constriction of intestinal loops which are caught over an omphalomesenteric cord have no symptoms to distinguish them from other forms of acute intestinal obstruction.

Umbilical Sinus.—An umbilical sinus from which there is a repeated discharge of mucus or other fluid should at once arouse suspicion of a Meckel's diverticulum communicating with the navel. Insertion of a small catheter into the fistula, instillation of a bit of lipiodol, and roentgenologic study may give important information concerning a communication with the intestine and thus rule out a patent urachus, which would connect with the urinary bladder. If *fecal material* exudes from the umbilicus—and there has been no previous operative procedure or disease of the abdomen to cause an intestinal fistula—one can make the proper diagnosis with great certainty. In one of our patients a mucoid discharge was found to contain both hydrochloric acid and pepsin; and examination of the subsequently removed diverticulum showed it to contain gastric mucosa.

Rare Cases with Symptoms Simulating Peritonitis.—In one patient with a twisted and infarcted diverticulum (Fig. 49), the clinical findings were those of generalized abdominal pain, diffuse tenderness and marked rigidity. The extent of this peritoneal irritation gave rise to the impression that a peritonitis was present, but at subsequent operation the peritoneal fluid was found to be sterile.

Vague Symptoms without Demonstrable Pathology.—In a small number of children abdominal pain of a vague and nagging sort can apparently

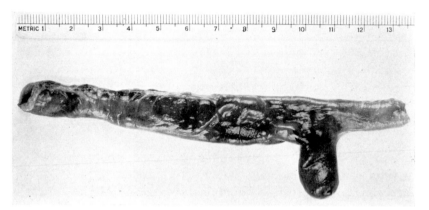

Fig. 48.—Surgical specimen consisting of portion of ileum and a Meckel's diverticulum. The diverticulum had been the leading point of an intussusception. Gut resected because of necrosis.

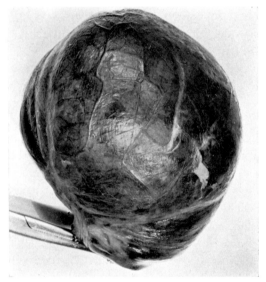

Fig. 49.—Orange-sized Meckel's diverticulum which had become twisted and infarcted. Specimen from a ten-year-old boy.

originate from a Meckel's diverticulum. The pain may be periumbilical or poorly localized; it is usually unattended by vomiting; and it may recur at irregular intervals. Physical examination may reveal no abdominal abnormality. When the diverticulum is exposed at operation there may be no inflammation, kinking, or intestinal obstruction, and it is not clear just why the structure should give rise to symptoms. It is possible that there is some interference with the proper peristaltic activity of the intestine when the diverticulum is present. In most of these cases the concurrent removal of the appendix makes it difficult to tell which of the two caused the pain. However, in a sufficient number of cases relief has been obtained from diverticulectomy alone to prove that symptoms can originate from a diverticulum which on pathologic examination shows nothing remarkable.

ROENTGENOLOGIC EXAMINATION

Roentgenologic examinations are practically useless in attempting to visualize a Meckel's diverticulum. We have conducted many gastro-intestinal series with contrast media in patients who were subsequently found to have a diverticulum at operation. In only one child did some of the barium collect in a small area which presumably represented the pouch. Our disappointing experiences have led us to abandon roentgenography as a means of detecting the presence of this congenital anomaly.

TREATMENT

Diverticulectomy: Practical Considerations.—*Excision and Suture.*—Some practical points in the treatment of Meckel's diverticula might be suggested. After removing these diverticula, the remaining stumps should not be turned in with a purse-string suture for fear of unduly constricting the gut. Removal of the pouch should be done by first placing two clamps (half-lengths or Kocher clamps) obliquely across its base to prevent spillage, and then cutting between these with the actual *cautery* (Fig. 50). If handled gently, the seared edges will stick together and can be turned in (without opening the intestine) by continuous fine chromic or silk suture which grasps all layers except the mucosa. This is then further reinforced with a second running stitch or, better still, with interrupted Halsted stitches. This method of diverticulectomy is practically aseptic and is superior to the operation in which the intestine is opened longitudinally and sutured transversely. If an oblique line of resection and intestinal suture has been done, the closure will not unduly constrict or angulate the gut.

Diverticulum with Thickened Base.—Most of these diverticula have a thin enough base so that the above-described method of removal can be carried out. In some cases, however, the base of the diverticulum is thickened because of edematous gastric mucosa, aberrant pancreatic tissue, or inflammatory disease. In such cases it is impossible to get a satisfactory turn-in of the intestinal coats and it is preferable to make a large, *wedge-shaped excision* of the diverticular base followed by repair of the intestine. If this procedure is not possible because of very extensive thickening

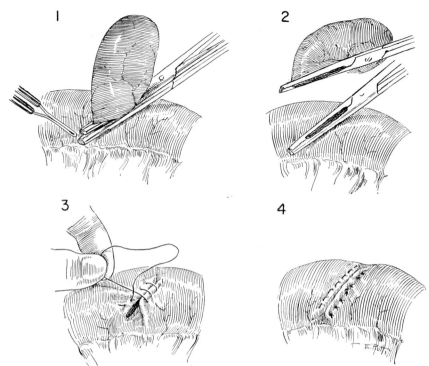

Fig. 50.—Recommended method of surgical removal of a Meckel's diverticulum: *1*, Cautery cutting away diverticulum between double Kocher clamps. The clamps are placed at an angle of 45 degrees with the intestinal tube. *2*, Diverticulum has been cut away. Position of the remaining clamps is shown. *3*, Without opening the intestinal lumen, stump is inverted with a continuous suture which penetrates all layers except the mucosa. *4*, Reinforcing line of Halsted mattress sutures. This type of removal prevents obstruction from constriction or angulation of the gut.

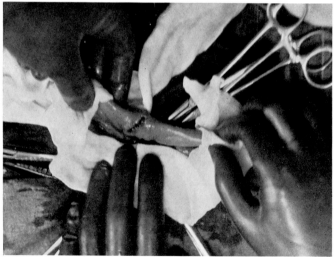

Fig. 51.—Photograph taken at operating table showing oblique line of closure following removal of a Meckel's diverticulum. There is no constriction or angulation of the intestine.

around the base, it may be necessary to resect the diverticulum with a small piece of bowel and then perform a *side-to-side anastomosis*.

Diverticulum Which Is Leading Point of Intussusception.—When a diverticulum has been the leading point of an intussusception, the intussusception should be reduced (if possible) and the diverticulum everted. If the child is in satisfactory condition and the circulation in the intestinal wall has been well preserved, the diverticulum may be removed. If, however, there is considerable damage to diverticular or intestinal wall without actual necrosis, or if the child is in poor condition, it is best to leave the excision of the diverticulum until a second operation, because immediate removal is too apt to induce fatal shock or produce peritonitis from soiling of the devitalized gut and peritoneal surfaces.

Symptomless Cases.—A diverticulum which has not given rise to symptoms, but which is discovered during the course of laparotomy for some other lesion, should be excised if the condition of the patient is satisfactory. A Meckel's diverticulum is always a potential source of future trouble and should be eliminated if it is possible to do so without appreciable risk.

RESULTS OF THERAPY

Employing the above-outlined methods of treatment in seventy-three patients, the mortality figures given in Table 7 have obtained.

TABLE 7

RESULTS OF OPERATIVE TREATMENT IN SEVENTY-THREE CASES OF MECKEL'S DIVERTICULUM

Presenting Complication of Meckel's Diverticulum	Recovered	Died
Hemorrhage	24	2
Leading point of intussusception	10	7
Abdominal pain	12	0
Inflammation, with or without perforation	4	6
Obstruction from band	6	0
Umbilical fistula	0	1
Twist and infarction of diverticulum	1	0
Totals	57	16

Reviewing our material with the purpose of finding ways in which the operative mortality can be reduced, we come to the following conclusions:

1. In those patients with *massive hemorrhage,* transfusion and operation should be performed immediately to prevent death from exsanguination.

2. When resection must be employed for a *gangrenous diverticulum* or intestine following an *intussusception,* it is preferable to use aseptic methods because of the great danger of a spreading peritonitis. This is best

executed by the Mikulicz procedure, which exteriorizes the bowel and closes the abdominal wall before cutting off the damaged intestine.

3. When *inflammatory conditions* of the diverticulum are suspected, operation should be instituted immediately, in order to prevent free perforation into the general peritoneal cavity and its attendant high mortality rate.

With the application of these principles the survival statistics in the future will undoubtedly be improved.

BIBLIOGRAPHY

1. Christie, A.: Meckel's Diverticulum. A Pathologic Study of Sixty-three Cases. Am. J. Dis. Child., *42:* 544, 1931.
2. Collins, D. C., Collins, F. K., and Andrews, V. L.: Ulcerating Carcinoid Tumor of Meckel's Diverticulum. Am. J. Surg., *40:* 454, 1938.
3. Faust, L. S., and Walters, W.: Fibrosarcoma of Meckel's Diverticulum Producing Intestinal Hemorrhage. Minnesota Med., *14:* 233, 1931.
4. Gray, H. K., and Kernohan, J. W.: Meckel's Diverticulum Associated with Intussusception and Adenocarcinoma of Ectopic Gastric Mucosa; Report of Case. J. A. M. A., *108:* 1480, 1937.
5. Halstead, A. E.: Intestinal Obstruction from Meckel's Diverticulum. Ann. Surg., *35:* 471, 1902.
6. Hudson, H. W., Jr.: Meckel's Diverticulum in Children; Second Clinical and Pathological Study with a Report of Thirteen Additional Cases. New England J. Med., *208:* 525, 1933.
7. Lindau, A., and Wulff, H.: The Peptic Genesis of Gastric and Duodenal Ulcer, Especially in the Light of Ulcers of Meckel's Diverticulum and the Postoperative Ulcers in the Jejunum. Surg., Gynec. and Obst., *53:* 621, 1931.
8. Michael, P.: Tuberculosis of Meckel's Diverticulum. Arch. Surg., *25:* 1152, 1932.
9. Poate, H. R. G.: Volvulus of Meckel's Diverticulum. Australian and New Zealand J. Surg., *7:* 351, 1938.
10. Skinner, I. C., and Walters, W.: Leiomyosarcoma of Meckel's Diverticulum, with Roentgenologic Demonstration of Diverticulum. Proc. Staff Meet., Mayo Clinic, *14:* 102, 1939.
11. Womack, N. A., and Siegert, R. B.: Surgical Aspects of Lesions of Meckel's Diverticulum. Ann. Surg., *108:* 221, 1938.

CHAPTER VII

DUPLICATIONS OF THE ALIMENTARY TRACT

Duplications are spherical or elongated hollow structures which possess a coat of smooth muscle, which are lined by a mucous membrane, and which are intimately attached to some portion of the alimentary tube. They may appear at any level from the base of the tongue to the anus. They are more commonly found in relation to the small intestine than to any other part of the gastro-intestinal tract.

Terminology.—These lesions have been described in the literature under various names, including "enterogenous cysts," "enteric cysts," "ileum duplex," "giant diverticula," "inclusion cysts," and "duplications of the alimentary tract." Many of these terms are quite descriptive of the individual specimens, but they do not call attention to the fact that they all have a common embryologic derivation and should therefore be grouped together as similar abnormalities. The terms "enteric cysts" and "enterogenous cysts" call attention to the close relationship of the lesions to the intestinal tract, but they can hardly be applied to the long tubular structures which course through the mesentery alongside of the gut. Likewise, "giant diverticula" is unsuitable because a great majority of the specimens do not possess a communication with the alimentary tube which this name suggests. "Ileum duplex" has been used to designate some specimens, but does not adequately describe the condition when seen in the jejunum, duodenum, stomach, or colon. "Inclusion cysts" conveys the idea that the structure is largely embedded within the intestinal wall; this is true in a few cases, but is certainly not characteristic of the group as a whole.

It is proper, we believe, to employ an all-inclusive name for these malformations which have appeared in divers locations and which have many shapes and sizes. We have therefore chosen to group them as "duplications of the alimentary tract," because they are a replica of some portion of the alimentary tract, though not necessarily of that portion to which they are contiguous. It is logical to assume that they are all due to the same kind of developmental aberration.

PATHOLOGY

A number of these lesions have been previously described in the literature, but the following summary has been largely based upon the study of surgical and autopsy specimens by Dr. Sidney Farber at the Boston Children's Hospital.

Duplications of the alimentary tract present a great variety of gross findings, some of which are portrayed in the figures of this chapter. There are three characteristics which are common to all of them: (1) each is contiguous with and strongly adherent to some part of the alimentary tube; (2) each has a smooth muscle coat, usually of two layers; (3) each is lined with a mucosa or epithelium similar to that of some part of the stomach, intestine, or colon.

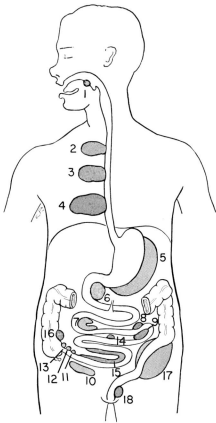

Fig. 52.—Sketch showing distribution of eighteen duplications of the alimentary tract. The number beside each lesion indicates the patient as listed in Table 8, p. 96.

Sites of Occurrence.—The sites at which duplications have been observed in our series of eighteen cases were as follows: base of the tongue in one; esophagus in three; stomach in one; duodenum in one; jejunum in two; ileum in seven; cecum in one; sigmoid in one; rectum in one. This experience coincides with the reports of others and shows that the condition is most frequently encountered along the small intestine. The cystic structure may or may not communicate with the adjacent intestinal lumen. In two of our cases there was such a communication, but in the remaining sixteen there was no such opening.

Firm Union with Intestine.—The adherence of a duplication to the intestine (stomach, esophagus, or colon) is an important point in recognition of one of these lesions at the operating table. There may be a slight furrow between the duplication and the intestine, but attempts to dissect the lesion away will show that a firm union exists and there is no plane of cleavage between them. In short, the muscular coat of the duplication is intimately fused with the muscularis of the alimentary tract. This feature is best appreciated by a microscopic study, which shows that the two muscular coats really form a common layer (Fig. 56).

Types of Epithelial Lining.—The type of epithelium which lines a duplication always resembles that of some part of the alimentary tract, but it

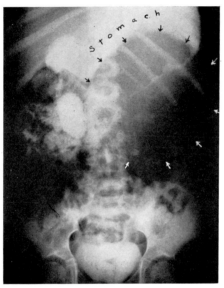

Fig. 53 (Case 5).—Roentgenogram of a patient with a large duplication of the stomach which is outlined by arrows. The stomach is filled with barium and is indented along the greater curvature by the duplication. (See Fig. 54.)

does not necessarily correspond to the mucosa at the level at which the duplication is found. Thus, a cyst of the tongue was found to be lined by colonic mucosa and a cyst of the rectum was partially lined by gastric epithelium. Indeed, in some of the specimens two or even three types of alimentary tract mucosa have been found. For the most part the epithelial lining is well preserved and it can be readily identified by microscopic study, but in occasional specimens the lining has been partially destroyed by pressure necrosis from entrapped fluid.

Types of Fluid.—The type of fluid within a duplication depends upon several factors. In the majority of cases it is a clear, colorless, mucoid substance which has been secreted by its own membrane. In occasional speci-

6

mens the pressure of the secreted and entrapped fluid is so high that there is necrosis and sloughing of the lining membrane. The fluid may then become hemorrhagic or murky colored. If there is an opening into the bowel the duplication contents are similar to those of the adjacent alimentary tract.

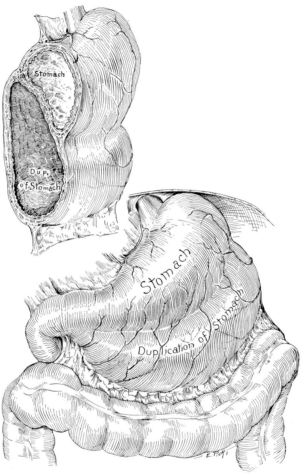

Fig. 54 (Case 5).—Drawing of a large gastric duplication as found at operation. The cystic structure is attached along the greater curvature of the stomach from the pylorus almost to the cardia. Insert shows a cross section of the stomach and its duplication at the level of the gastric incisura.

Variations in Size.—Duplications vary greatly in size. In some positions, such as the duodenal curvature or along the rectal wall, small cysts will attract early attention. Conversely, the ileum or sigmoid can give rise to enormous duplications with relatively minor symptoms. Some of the spherical cysts are smaller than a golf ball; others are larger than a grapefruit. One duplication which arose from the posterior surface and greater curvature of the stomach in a six-year-old girl was almost as large as the normal stomach itself. A few of the specimens have been sausage-shaped and lay along the mesenteric border of the intestine to form a double-barreled structure (Figs. 58 and 61). In Case 15 this tube was about 2 cm. in diameter and 38 cm. in length; it was contiguous to the terminal ileum.

Differentiation from Mesenteric Cysts.—It is highly important for the surgeon to recognize the pathologic difference between duplications and

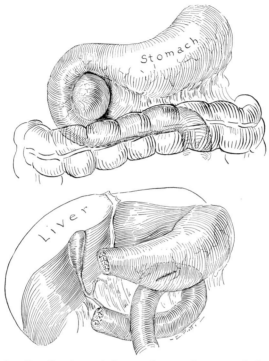

Fig. 55 (Case 6).—Duplication of first and second parts of duodenum in a five-week-old baby. Successful treatment by excision and establishment of a posterior gastrojejunostomy.

mesenteric cysts. The latter are lymphatic in origin, have a thin wall, and can be readily peeled away from adjacent viscera. In contrast to these findings, the duplication has a thicker, muscular wall which can rarely be dissected away from the intestine without opening the duplication or the intestine. It is therefore evident that the mesenteric cyst can usually be removed without disturbing the intestine, but that in removing a duplication a portion of the intestine must usually be resected as well.

EMBRYOLOGY

Several theories have been put forth to explain the origin of duplications. Those arising from some portion of the ileum were previously thought to represent aberrations in development of a *Meckel's diverticulum*. For several reasons this theory is scarcely plausible, and in any event it does not explain the origin of duplications in the upper and lower portions of the alimentary tract. *Sequestration,* or a pinching off of a group of cells from the primordial intestinal tube, could easily account for the development of near-by cysts which attain all of the histologic elements of an alimentary-tract wall.

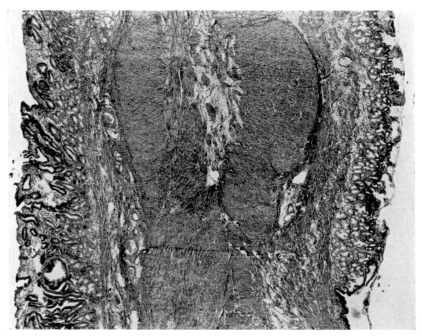

Fig. 56 (Case 6).—Photomicrograph of the common wall between the duodenum and the duodenal duplication. Duodenal mucosa appears at the left; duplication mucosa is shown at the right. Between them are the intermixed, smooth muscle coats without a plane of cleavage between them.

The most probable theory is that advanced by Lewis and Thyng,[7] who frequently found diverticula in various portions of fetal alimentary tracts of pigs, rabbits, cats, sheep, and man. These outpocketings are most often seen in the ileum, a fact which corresponds to the greater frequency of duplications in the ileum. These small outpocketings in the intestinal wall—which are not related to Meckel's diverticulum—normally regress, but if one of them is pinched off the structure could easily give rise to an adjacent duplication.

CLINICAL SYMPTOMS AND SIGNS

Duplications are usually observed in childhood ages but they may be found at any time in later life. The nature of the process is one which attracts attention in early years. Our youngest patient was two weeks old and the oldest was nine years of age. The various symptoms produced by these abnormalities may be roughly grouped under three categories: (1) The cyst or tubelike structure may become so dilated that it encroaches upon the adjacent intestine and partially *obstructs* it. (2) The lining membrane may produce such a large amount of fluid that internal pressure is high and *pain* is produced by distention of the structure. (3) The duplication, lying as it does within the leaves of the mesentery, may press upon the mesenteric blood vessels and produce *necrosis, sloughing,* and *bleeding* of the adjacent intestine.

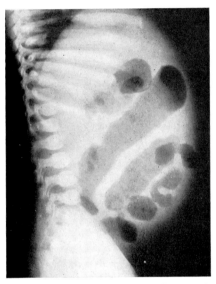

Fig. 57 (Case 7).—Lateral roentgenogram of abdomen showing dilated intestinal loops, accumulation of fluid between the loops, and marked abdominal distention. The findings are indicative of obstruction which was subsequently found to be caused by a duplication of the lower part of the jejunum (Fig. 58).

In the duplication of the stomach, Case 5, the large lesion did not give rise to mechanical obstruction of the stomach and the primary complaints were those of *epigastric fullness* and discomfort. The majority of duplications of the duodenum, jejunum, and ileum produced partial intestinal obstruction with *colicky pain, vomiting, visible peristalsis,* and possibly signs of *dehydration.* The long tubular duplication of the terminal ileum (Fig. 61) led to severe, painless, and repeated *hemorrhage* from the lower intestinal tract, because of sloughing and ulceration of the ileal mucosa. A small cyst of the cecum, near the ileocecal valve, was the leading point of an *intussusception.* The cyst of the rectal wall (Figs. 63 and 64) encroached on the rectal lumen, and led to *constipation* and abdominal distention.

Physical Findings.—By physical examination the mass can usually be felt in some portion of the abdomen. A rounded, smooth, usually nontender

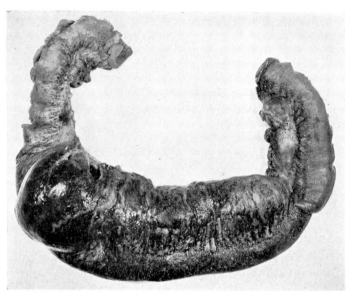

Fig. 58 (Case 7).—Surgical specimen of duplication of the jejunum. The intestinal tract appears at the periphery of the specimen. The sausage-shaped duplication is very adherent to the mesenteric side of the intestine, and it was impossible to dissect it away from the jejunum.

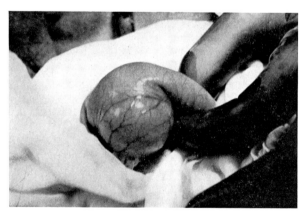

Fig. 59 (Case 8).—Operating-room photograph showing golf-ball-sized duplication of the lower jejunum in a two-week-old child. The overlying adjacent intestine is compressed on one surface of the cystic structure. The mesenteric blood vessels running to the intestine can be seen coursing over the surface of the cyst. Successful result following resection of cyst and intestine, and lateral anastomosis of the same.

lump can be palpated and is often freely movable. The duplication of the stomach was of such a large size that it could be easily felt and was first thought to be a distended stomach or transverse colon. However, it per-

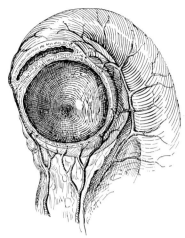

Fig. 60.—Drawing of the surgically removed specimen shown in Fig. 59. The duplication lies within the mesentery, is intimately attached to the intestine, and partially obstructs the latter by compression. The mesenteric arteries and veins course over the surface of the cyst.

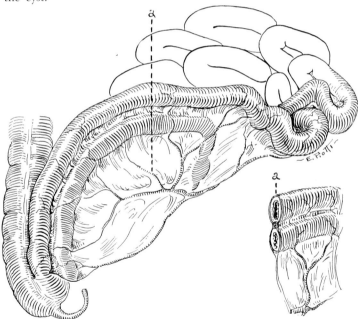

Fig. 61 (Case 15).—Drawing of a long tubular duplication of the lower ileum, which communicated with the intestine near the ileocecal valve. Duplication 38 cm. long. Insert A shows cross section of the double-barreled structure and relation of duplication to the mesentery and the intestine.

sisted after lavage and cleansing of the stomach and colon. Except for the gastric duplication, most of the lesions exhibited signs of partial intestinal obstruction, including *visible peristalsis,* slight or moderate *abdominal dis-*

tention, and *increased audible peristaltic activity.* The tubelike ileal duplication of Case 15 could not be felt through the abdominal wall, and there were no physical signs of obstruction. The only positive findings in this boy were marked *anemia* and severe *melena.* The cyst of the sigmoid, Case 17, was freely movable, elastic, nontender, and without signs of colonic obstruction. The duplication of the posterior rectal wall could be easily felt with an examining finger in the rectum.

ROENTGENOLOGIC DATA

In the girl with a duplication of the *stomach,* x-ray studies aided in showing the size of the lesion and determining its position with relation to the other abdominal viscera (Fig. 53). A gastro-intestinal series indicated the mass to be behind and below the stomach, with a smooth bulge into the gastric lumen along the greater curvature. Barium enema visualized the transverse colon displaced downward and not obstructed.

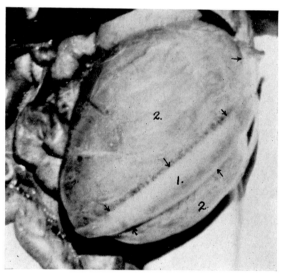

Fig. 62.—Autopsy photograph showing cystic duplication (12 by 10 by 8 cm.) of the sigmoid in a two-week-old infant. Arrows indicate the flattened sigmoid (*1*) as it courses over the surface of the duplication (*2*).

The *duodenal* cyst (Fig. 55) compressed the first and second portions of the duodenum and exhibited definite evidence of duodenal obstruction when studies were performed with a barium series. Dilated intestine was found above some but not all of the jejunal and ileal lesions. Not infrequently, as much could be learned from films in the postero-anterior and lateral directions without contrast media as could be determined with the use of a barium series. Distention of intestinal loops (Fig. 57), particularly if localized to one part of the abdomen, indicated obstruction and often gave some idea of the level at which the lesion existed.

The large duplication of the *sigmoid* in a two-week-old baby showed a rounded area of rather uniform density with peripheral displacement of gas-filled viscera. Barium-enema studies were not made in this case, but undoubtedly they would have shown the sigmoid to course over the surface of the mass.

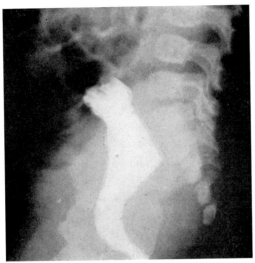

Fig. 63.—Lateral roentgenogram of patient with duplication of the rectum. Barium shows the rectum displaced forward by a mass in the hollow of the sacrum.

Roentgenograms of the *rectal* duplication (Fig. 63) were important because they outlined the superior extent of the lesion and because the absence of bony defect in the lumbar and sacral vertebrae made us certain that the pelvic mass was not an anterior meningocele.

TREATMENT

Pathologic Considerations.—These lesions cannot be treated by any means other than surgical attack. Two points must be borne in mind which again stress the importance of pathology with relation to operative procedure. First, the cystic structure and intestine have a common wall at one point and usually the two cannot be separated from one another without injuring the bowel. Second, the arteries and veins of the contiguous portion of the alimentary tract usually course over the surface of the cyst and hence attempts to resect this alone may so interrupt the blood vessels that the intestine will become necrotic.

Operative Technic.—In the majority of cases the treatment of choice is *resection* of the duplication and its adjacent gut and then reestablishment of intestinal continuity by a *side-to-side anastomosis*. There are, however, certain locations which prohibit this form of treatment because of the anatomic peculiarities of the region.

Examples of these problems might be mentioned in more detail as follows: The duplication of the *stomach* (Fig. 54) might have been treated by total gastrectomy and establishment of an esophagojejunostomy. This undertaking appeared to be rather hazardous and hence was avoided. It might have been treated by the injection of necrotizing fluids to sclerose its mucous membrane. As an alternative, the cyst was opened, a portion of it resected and the remainder marsupialized to the anterior abdominal wall so that it could be tightly packed with gauze to destroy its lining. With-

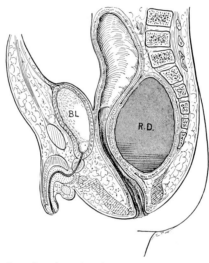

Fig. 64.—Reconstruction drawing showing duplication anterior to the sacrum producing partial obstruction of the rectum.

BL, Bladder. *RD,* Rectal Duplication.

drawing the packing some days after operation allowed the cyst walls to fall together and coalesce. The cystic duplication of the duodenum (Fig. 55) was treated by *excision of the mass* and the first part of the duodenum, combined with a *posterior gastrojejunostomy*. The postoperative condition of this five-week-old baby has been very satisfactory.

Gardner and Hart[3] established a *window* between a cyst and the adjacent duodenum, with success. This simple procedure is well worth remembering whenever poor general condition of a patient demands a short operation. While this technic may adequately take care of a small duplication, it might possibly lead to troublesome symptoms if the resulting side pocket were large and not adequately drained.

The duplication of the posterior *rectal wall* (Fig. 64) was first aspirated by another physician through a posterior sacral approach. Fortunately no infection occurred, but after each aspiration the cyst again refilled in five or six days' time. Operation on this six-month-old baby was performed through a curvilinear transverse incision behind the anus, with dissection up in front of the sacrum to expose the mass. Little difficulty was encountered in freeing the cyst along its posterior, superior, and lateral sur-

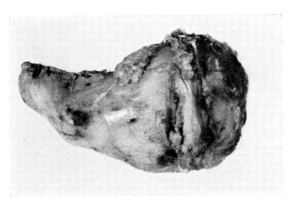

Fig. 65 (Case 18).—Photograph of duplication of the rectum which was successfully excised.

faces where there were good planes of cleavage. However, in the further course of the dissection a large opening was made in the posterior portion of the rectum. This was repaired by folding the edges inward with three layers of interrupted, fine chromic catgut sutures. The rectal wall healed per primam, there was no suppuration in the perirectal spaces, and the child quickly recovered.

RESULTS OF TREATMENT

There have not been a sufficient number of these cases to permit a definite statement of the percentage of cures which might be expected. Of the eighteen duplications we have observed in various parts of the alimentary tract, fourteen occurred within the abdomen (Table 8). Eleven of these abdominal lesions have been operated upon, and eight of the patients have recovered and are completely free of symptoms. The three deaths occurred in the earlier part of the series. In one case there was rupture and peritonitis prior to hospitalization; in the second there was a volvulus and extensive infarction of intestine; the third died of operative shock. These fatalities point out the serious nature of duplications, but a review of the more recent cases, which have been treated by the methods outlined above, shows conclusively that the great majority of these patients can be treated with an insignificant mortality.

TABLE 8

ANALYSIS OF EIGHTEEN CASES WITH DUPLICATIONS OF THE ALIMENTARY TRACT

Case	Age	Position of Cyst	Size of Duplication—Type of Mucous Membrane	Treatment	Result
1	..	Base of tongue	1 cm. in diameter Colonic	Excision	Recovered
2	11 months	Right pleural cavity	4 to 5 cm. in diameter Gastric	Excision	Recovered
3	2 years	Mediastinum	10 by 6 by 5 cm. Gastric	Excision	Recovered
4	7 months	Right pleural cavity	8 by 5 by 4 cm. Gastric	Excision	Died
5	7 years	Along stomach	Large as stomach itself Necrotic	Partial excision Marsupialization	Recovered
6	5 weeks	Duodenum	4.5 by 3.5 by 3.5 cm. Duodenal	Resection. Gastro-enterostomy	Recovered
7	6 months	Jejunum	22 by 6 by 6 cm. Gastric	Mikulicz resection	Died
8	2 weeks	Jejunum	4 cm. in diameter Jejunal	Resection and anastomosis	Recovered
9	3 months	Ileum	7 by 4 by 4 cm. Gastric	None	Died
10	19 months	Terminal ileum	15.5 by 4 by 5 cm. Columnar epithelium	Excision	Recovered
11	12 days	Terminal ileum	1.5 cm. in diameter Ileal	Resection and anastomosis	Recovered
12	9 years	Terminal ileum	1.2 cm. in diameter (?)	Not yet treated*	
13	2 months	Terminal ileum	2 cm. in diameter Ileal	Resection and anastomosis	Recovered
14	6 years	Ileum	3 cm. in diameter Ileal	Resection and anastomosis	Recovered
15	2 years	Ileum	38 cm. long, 2 cm. in diameter Gastric	Resection and anastomosis	Died
16	3 months	Cecum	4 cm. in diameter Colonic	Resection and anastomosis	Died
17	2 weeks	Sigmoid	12 by 10 by 8 cm. Ileal and colonic	Not treated	Died
18	6 months	Rectum	5 by 2.5 by 2.5 cm. Mixed	Excision. Rectum repaired	Recovered

* This cyst was discovered during operation for acute appendicitis and has not yet been removed.

BIBLIOGRAPHY

1. Basman, J.: Enterogenous Cyst of the Duodenum Simulating Pyloric Stenosis. J. Pediat., *12:* 363, 1938.
2. Black, R. A., and Benjamin, E. L.: Enterogenous Abnormalities: Cysts and Diverticula. Am. J. Dis. Child., *51:* 1126, 1936.
3. Gardner, C. E., Jr., and Hart, D.: Enterogenous Cysts of the Duodenum: Report of a Case and Review of the Literature. J. A. M. A., *104:* 1809, 1935.
4. Hudson, H. W., Jr.: Giant Diverticula or Reduplications of the Intestinal Tract. New England J. Med., *213:* 1123, 1935.
5. Ladd, W. E.: Duplications of the Alimentary Tract. South. M. J., *30:* 363, 1937.
6. Ladd, W. E., and Gross, R. E.: Surgical Treatment of Duplications of the Alimentary Tract: Enterogenous Cysts, Enteric Cysts, or Ileum Duplex. Surg., Gynec. and Obst., *70:* 295, 1940.
7. Lewis, F. T., and Thyng, F. W.: The Regular Occurrence of Intestinal Diverticula in Embryos of the Pig, Rabbit and Man. Am. J. Anat., *7:* 505, 1907.
8. McLanahan, S., and Stone, H. B.: Enterogenous Cysts. Surg., Gynec. and Obst., *58:* 1027, 1934.
9. Mixter, C. G., and Clifford, S. H.: Congenital Mediastinal Cysts of Gastrogenic and Bronchogenic Origin. Ann. Surg., *90:* 714, 1929.
10. Pachman, D. J.: Enterogenous Intramural Cysts of the Intestines. Am. J. Dis. Child., *58:* 485, 1939.

CHAPTER VIII

FOREIGN BODIES IN THE GASTRO-INTESTINAL TRACT

Infants and children are prone to put into their mouths nondigestible materials which are not infrequently swallowed. A wide variety of objects may enter the gastro-intestinal tract, ranging from sharp pins or nails to smooth coins or buttons and from small finger rings to moderate-sized toys of all sorts. It is almost inconceivable how some of these pointed or sharp things can course along the alimentary tube without injuring its mucous membrane or causing abdominal pain. Indeed, it is difficult to understand how some of the larger bodies pass through the esophagus, the pylorus, or the ileocecal valve at all. The great majority of them start on their way with little more than a gulp or a short fit of coughing. In fact, many are swallowed without the slightest difficulty and the accident is suspected only because of the disappearance of an object with which a child had been previously playing.

Objects Recovered.—In a series of 337 such patients at the Children's Hospital, the foreign bodies listed in Table 9 were retrieved from the alimentary tract.

TABLE 9

FOREIGN BODIES SWALLOWED BY 337 CHILDREN

Penny	77	Piece of glass	3	Rivet	1
Closed safety pin	38	Toy whistle	2	Dice	1
Open safety pin	35	Doll eye	2	Moth ball	1
Nickel coin	26	Steel nut	2	Book fastener	1
Straight pin	22	Religious charm	2	Piece of wire	1
Bobby pin	18	Wooden ball	2	Locket	1
Nail	13	Metal cap	2	Thermometer bulb	1
Ring	10	Piece of lead pencil	2	Toy watch	1
Tack	7	Pen point	2	Shoe buckle	1
Marble	7	Toy horn	2	Rubber balloon	1
Quarter coin	7	Toy pipe	1	Key ring	1
Button	6	Dental brace	1	Piece of steel	1
Screw	6	Toy spoon	1	Lead soldier	1
Campaign button	5	Paper clip	1	Toy train car	1
Needle	4	Rattle handle	1	Collar button	1
Bead	3	Tooth	1	Ball bearing	1
Key	3	Lead type	1	Toy scissors	1
Bolt	3	Small bell	1	Hair ball	1

Age Incidence.—The majority of these children were from six months to four years of age. The youngest was three months, and the oldest was fifteen years. The distributions were as follows:

Under 1 year 36
1 year 46
2 years 65
3 years 62
4 years 53
5 years 28
6 years 15
7 to 15 years 32

SYMPTOMS

Occasionally foreign bodies lodge in the esophagus and will require the services of an esophagoscopist for removal. Most objects which are swallowed pass directly into the stomach, and once they have done so it is

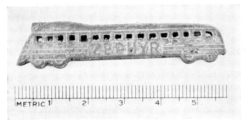

Fig. 66.—Photograph of metal toy car after it had spontaneously passed through the intestinal tract of a three-year-old girl.

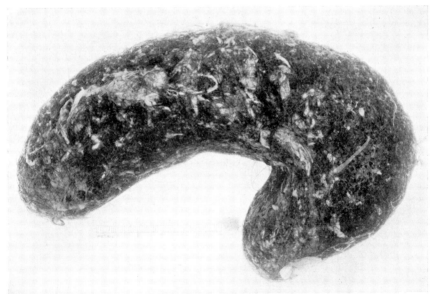

Fig. 67.—Large hair ball surgically removed from the stomach of a five-year-old girl.

uncommon for them to give rise to symptoms. Well over 95 per cent progress through the alimentary tract without discomfort of any sort and their elimination may not be recognized unless the stools are carefully examined.

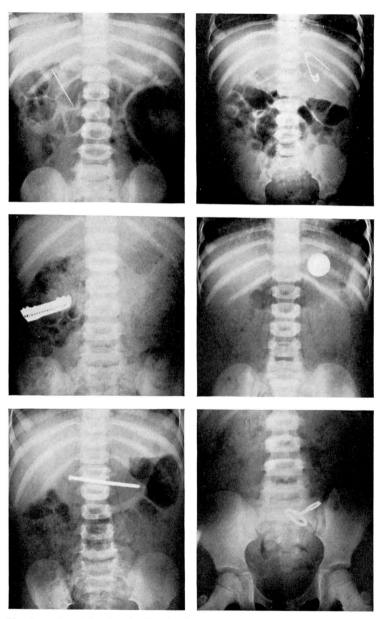

Fig. 68.—Samples of foreign bodies in the gastro-intestinal tracts of children. Needle (in the top left roentgenogram) pierced second part of duodenum and projected into the liver, necessitating surgical removal. All of the other foreign bodies, including open safety pin, toy car, five-cent piece, large nail, and a can opener, passed spontaneously through the alimentary tract.

If the bodies are unusually large in relation to the size of the patient, there may be occasional mild *abdominal cramps* and rarely *vomiting*. Jagged or irregular objects may scratch the anus and initiate minor *bleeding*. The appetite is rarely interfered with. *Perforation* of the intestine is exceedingly rare, and even if it does take place it occurs so slowly that omentum, liver, or other viscus becomes adherent to the intestine at this point to prevent escape of the sharp object or infected material into the general peritoneal cavity. Therefore, perforation is usually not attended by pain, tenderness, spasm, or fever.

Trichobezoar.—The formation of a trichobezoar is apt to be followed by poor health over a long period of time, because the gastric lumen becomes largely occluded by a dense mass which interferes with the ingestion and digestion of food. The habit of plucking and chewing hair would appear to be an innocuous one, but the gradually enlarging and matted bolus finally produces partial gastric obstruction. A history of hair-eating, poor appetite, occasional vomiting, eructations of malodorous gas, and failure to gain weight properly are highly suggestive of a trichobezoar, particularly if a mass can be palpated in the epigastrium.

ROENTGENOLOGIC EXAMINATION

Fortunately, most of the foreign bodies which are swallowed are opaque to x-rays (Fig. 68). Roentgenologic examinations are of value in determining that a missing object actually resides in the gastro-intestinal tract, and also in watching its progress or lack of progress along the enteric canal. Fluoroscopic observation or a plain film will usually give all the information which is desired, but the use of a contrasting medium is occasionally of value.

In one patient the position of a stationary needle was not clear. Studies with a barium gastro-intestinal series and a barium enema gave the impression that it was outside of the alimentary tract. This was confirmed at laparotomy, when it was found to have completely escaped from the stomach or intestine (site of perforation could not be located) and was wrapped in a wad of omentum.

TREATMENT

The treatment of foreign bodies in the gastro-intestinal tract cannot be dogmatically stated, for it will necessarily depend upon the exigencies of the individual case. In general, *conservative* treatment is all that is required, and without doubt many laparotomies can be avoided if several days' delay and patience are exercised. Of our 337 patients, 323 eliminated their foreign material normally in the stool while operation was deemed advisable in only fourteen.

7

Conservative Therapy.—With conservative therapy, the child should be kept on its *normal diet.* Large amounts of bread or porridge (with the idea of forming a protecting bolus around an open safety pin or needle) have little to recommend them. Active *catharsis* should certainly be avoided for fear of increasing the intestinal peristalsis and enhancing the possibility of intestinal irritation or perforation. If constipation has been present, small amounts of *mineral oil* may be prescribed with impunity. All of the *stools* should be collected in a suitable container so that they can be examined with a stick until the foreign body is identified. In general, there need be no haste about discontinuing a conservative regimen in favor of oper-

TABLE 10

LIST OF ALL BABIES UNDER TWENTY-FOUR MONTHS OF AGE WITH SWALLOWED FOREIGN BODIES

Spontaneous Passage in Stool (75 Patients)

Age in Months	Object	Age in Months	Object
23, 20, 19, 15, 15, 14, 12, 12, 11, 11, 11, 11, 10, 9, 9, 9, 8, 8, 8, 6, 5	Open safety pin	17, 16	Stove bolt
		14	Rivet
23, 22, 22, 22, 22, 22, 21, 20, 20, 19, 18, 17, 16, 14	Penny	15	Screen wire
		11	Rattle handle
20, 19, 19, 16, 15, 11, 11, 10, 8, 7	Closed safety pin	14	Clock key
		6, 4	Bobby pin
		11	Toy eye
20, 17, 16, 12, 11	Straight pin	18	Screw
22, 20	Nickel coin	19, 9	Button
18, 16	Marble	10, 7, 6	Tack
17	Moth ball	22	Collar button
19	Religious charm	10	Piece of lead pencil
11	Piece of glass		
14	Ring		

Surgical Removal (7 Patients)

Age in Months	Object
17, 15, 11, 11, 10, 5, 5	Open safety pin

ative treatment. Most of these objects will be eliminated within a few days, but occasionally one will require several weeks. The mere size of an object is not often a deterrent factor in its passing through the intestine, for almost any solid and rigid object which can get into the stomach (no matter how small the patient) will be eventually spontaneously eliminated in the stool.

Smooth materials, such as buttons, coins and toy whistles, may be left unoperated upon for as long as *three or four weeks* or more without danger, and indeed we have never had to remove one of these rounded or relatively smooth foreign bodies by operative means, if the intestine was normal to begin with. One child had congenital stenosis of the jejunum, at which point a nickel coin was lodged. At operation, the coin was removed, a re-section performed, and a lateral anastomosis established. *Sharp objects*, such as straight pins, open safety pins, needles, broken glass, and nails, must be regarded with some concern. All of these can be spontaneously passed in the majority of instances, but frequent checks with x-ray films are desirable to make sure that progress is being made. If a sharp object remains in one place for more than three or four days, it is well to consider surgical removal.

Operative Treatment.—The *indications for operation* in these cases were: (1) failure of progress of a needle, open safety pin, or bobby pin in eight; (2) failure of progress of a nickel coin which had stopped at a congenital stenosis of the jejunum in one; (3) perforation (or suspected perforation) by a nonprogressing pointed object in four; (4) for removal of a gastric hair ball in one.

The chances for a spontaneous passage of foreign substances through the intestinal tract of an infant or older child would presumably depend somewhat on the *size* of the object in relation to the size of the individual. In order to point out what the alimentary tract is capable of eliminating, Table 10 lists all infants under two years of age, the objects they swallowed, and whether spontaneous or surgical removal was effected. This summary indicates that any object which can be swallowed by a baby will pass about as readily as it would in an older child, and that operation need not be done merely because a patient is small or young.

Operative withdrawal of a foreign body is almost always an upper abdominal procedure. Rigid materials may catch anywhere in the intestine, but in the present series the pylorus and the duodenal curves were the only anatomic structures which arrested progress in such a way as to require operation. Whenever the foreign object passed beyond the duodenum, there was always a subsequent unimpeded course through the remainder of the alimentary tract (except for one girl with a coin caught at a congenital jejunal stenosis).

SUMMARY AND CONCLUSIONS

In summary, the treatment of most gastro-intestinal foreign bodies in infants and children should be conservative. Of the manifold substances which are swallowed, *95 per cent* will be eliminated spontaneously without symptoms and without danger of injury to the alimentary tract. A little caution is necessary when straight pins, open safety pins, bobby pins, needles, or other sharp objects are being dealt with. While 85 per cent of these will safely pass, their progress should be checked every few days with roentgenograms, and surgical intervention should be considered if lodgment occurs in one place for more than three or four days. Of the array of foreign bodies listed in Table 9, it was necessary to remove only three needles, eight open safety pins, one bobby pin, one nickel coin, and one hair ball. There were no deaths in the series, and there was no case of complicating peritonitis from intestinal perforation.

BIBLIOGRAPHY

DeBakey, M., and Ochsner, A.: Bezoars and Concretions: Comprehensive Review of the Literature with Analysis of 303 Collected Cases and Presentation of 8 Additional Cases. Surgery, *4:* 934, 1938.

Donovan, E. J.: Meckel's Diverticulum Perforated by Foreign Body. Ann. Surg., *106:* 953, 1937.

Jackson, C., and Jackson, C. L.: Foreign Bodies in Intestines. M. Rec., *140:* 285, 1934.

Johnson, C. I., and Ferguson, C. F.: Foreign Bodies in the Air and Food Passages. New England J. Med., *215:* 1054, 1936.

Lyons, C. G., and Cody, G. L.: Bezoar. Radiology, *31:* 225, 1938.

Storck, A., Rothschild, J. E., and Ochsner, A.: Intestinal Obstruction Due to Intraluminal Foreign Bodies. Ann. Surg., *109:* 844, 1939.

CHAPTER IX

INTUSSUSCEPTION

Intussusception is the telescoping of one portion of the intestine or colon into a more distal segment of the enteric tube. When an intussusceptum has been drawn into its intussuscipiens, the process is almost invariably a progressive one until death supervenes or operative relief is afforded.

Intussusception is one of the most important surgical emergencies in infancy and early childhood. The *frequency* with which this condition is encountered may be judged from the fact that 484 cases were treated at the Children's Hospital from 1908 to 1939, inclusive. During the period 1928 through 1939 there were 202 patients, an average of about twenty per year. The generally high mortality rates reported in the literature indicate the need for more widespread knowledge of the condition and its treatment. Reduction of these death rates in the future must depend not only upon the surgeon's skill in operative technic, but also upon the recognition of cases by the pediatrician and general practitioner within a period of twenty-four hours, when the prognosis is still favorable.

ETIOLOGY AND CLASSIFICATION

Intussusception in the adult is usually brought about by some mechanical abnormality, whereas in the childhood and infancy group such factors are found in only a small minority of cases. In the present series of 484 patients, demonstrable etiologic agents were found as follows: *Meckel's diverticulum* in seventeen; *intestinal polyp* in four; *duplication* in one; *lymphoma* in one. This adds up to twenty-three, or 5 per cent of the entire group. In the remaining 461 individuals no definite cause could be found for the intussusception. The fact that intussusception is so apt to occur between the ages of four and ten months strongly suggests that the change from a milk to a more solid *diet* may alter the intestinal peristalsis in such a way that intussusception is initiated. It is well recognized that intussusception occasionally makes its appearance during or shortly after *acute enteritis,* at which time the disturbed intestinal peristaltic movement may set the stage for the prolapse of one segment into another. *Allergic states* may possibly account for disturbed peristaltic activity. This has been suggested by a few cases of intussusception, but more extensive investigation of other patients has left us with little evidence regarding the culpability of allergic conditions in intussusception. In short, the etiologic agent in 90 to 95 per cent of childhood intussusception is still unknown.

Classification.—Intussusceptions are classified by compound appellations which indicate the part of the intestinal tube (intussusceptum) which tele-

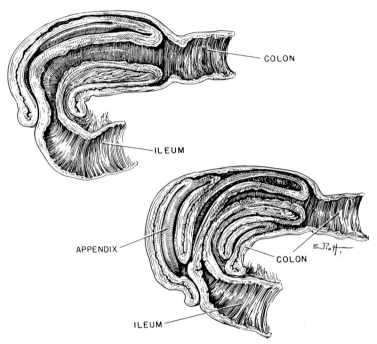

Fig. 69.—Common forms of intussusception. *Left,* Ileo-colic type in which the ileocecal valve is the leading point. *Right,* Ileo-ileo-colic type, in which ileum has progressed into ileum and colon and then another telescoping has begun at the ileocecal valve.

scopes into the intussuscipiens. The name of the most common form, the *ileo-colic,* implies that the ileum has advanced into the colon. Complex vari-

TABLE 11

TYPES OF INTUSSUSCEPTION IN 484 CASES

Type of Intussusception	Per Cent of Series
Jejuno-ileal or ileo-ileal	5
Ileo-colic	75
Ileo-ileo-colic	12
Colo-colic	2
Type not stated	5
Multiple intussusception	1
Retrograde intussusception	0.2

eties are occasionally seen, for example the *ileo-ileo-colic* (Fig. 69), in which the ileum enters the ileum and this entire mass prolapses into the colon. The percentage of occurrence of these various types is listed in Table 11.

SYMPTOMS AND SIGNS

Intussusception tends to occur within more or less definite *age groups*. Table 12, Fig. 72, and Fig. 73, point out the ages of patients in our series. The peak of incidence occurs from the third to the eleventh months, during which time 75 per cent of the cases are found. Boys are more often affected than girls: the proportion is 62 per cent males and 38 per cent females in our series.

One rarely finds intussusception in a child who is thin, undernourished, and poorly developed. On the contrary, babies with intussusception are usually very well nourished and are generally above the average in physical development. This *fat and healthy appearance* is apt to mislead the physician if he sees the baby in the early hours of illness. Thus, the first visit may result only in the impression that the parent is overanxious, whereas a return visit the next day shows that the child is desperately ill.

Clinical Symptoms.—The clinical manifestations of intussusception are almost always alarming and should immediately suggest the correct diag-

TABLE 12

INCIDENCE OF INTUSSUSCEPTION ACCORDING TO AGE (484 CASES)

Age	Cases	Age	Cases	Age	Cases	Age	Cases
1 month	1	10 months	30	19 months	7	4 to 5 years	16
2 months	10	11 months	19	20 months	4	5 to 6 years	6
3 months	15	12 months	5	21 months	2	6 to 7 years	4
4 months	39	13 months	11	22 months	5	7 to 8 years	2
5 months	61	14 months	4	23 months	2	8 to 9 years	3
6 months	57	15 months	2	24 months	3	9 to 10 years	1
7 months	59	16 months	2	2 to 3 years	22	10 to 11 years	1
8 months	37	17 months	2	3 to 4 years	14	11 to 12 years	0
9 months	32	18 months	6				

nosis. Recurrent, colicky *abdominal pain* is an almost universal finding. While these patients are usually so young that they cannot describe their complaints, the parent or attendant notices that the child intermittently becomes pale and either doubles over or draws up his legs in obvious severe pain. This ten- or fifteen-second paroxysm may be accompanied by grunting respirations and by a burst of crying. After it is past the child may resume a playful attitude and appear well, only to have a return of pain five or ten minutes later. *Vomiting* is an early symptom; it may be repeated and severe.

During the first hours of illness, the intense, recurring pain is the alarming symptom; but as the obstruction continues, *pallor, sweating, dehydration,* and *shock* appear and increase in severity as time elapses. If the condition is left untreated the individual becomes moribund at the end of two or three days. The passage of *bloody stools* occurs in about 85 per cent of the cases, but they may not be found in the first twelve to fourteen hours. After the initiation of symptoms there may be one or more normal bowel movements without melena, but after this, bright red or dark brownish bloody mucoid material is passed. The amount of bleeding varies greatly from case to case. It may only stain the diaper or it may be copious enough to induce severe shock.

Physical Findings.—The physical findings and general condition of the baby vary with the duration of symptoms. If obstruction has existed for only a few hours, the child may appear relatively well. If intussusception has

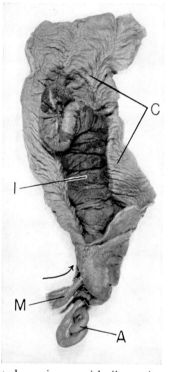

Fig. 70.—Surgically resected specimen, with ileum intussuscepted into cecum and ascending colon. The specimen is opened on its posterior surface. Arrow shows direction and point of entry of ileum into the colon.

A, Appendix. *C,* Colon. *I,* Intussusceptum. *M,* Portion of mesentery entering the intussusception.

been present for a longer period, the baby is listless and extremely ill, the body tissues are dehydrated, and the eyes are sunken or lusterless. Usually the pulse is rapid, the skin pale, and sweating marked. Even though a state of shock and partial collapse exists, there will be momentary periods during which the baby cries out, thrashes around, and is obviously in agony.

Careful *palpation* of the abdomen is most important, because a mass can be felt in about 85 per cent of the cases. While this may be only an ill-defined lump, it is more often described as a sausage-shaped structure. It is

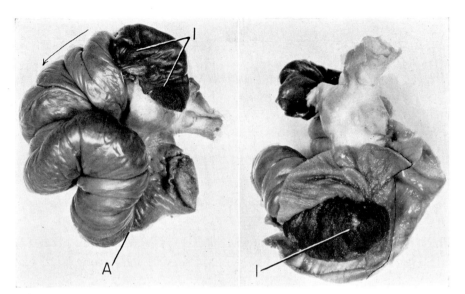

Fig. 71.—Specimen showing intussusception of ileum into ileum. *Left,* The intestine (*I*) has passed into the intussuscipiens as far as the point *A. Right,* Intussuscipiens cut open to show the hemorrhagic intussusceptum (*I*) .

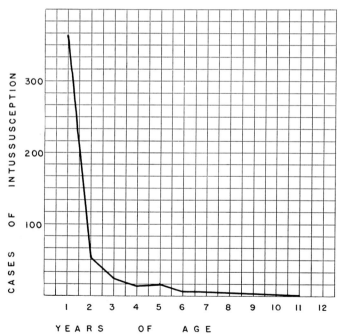

Fig. 72.—Age distribution of 484 cases of intussusception; 85 per cent of the patients are less than two years of age.

rather firm and as a rule is not tender. Occasionally it can be felt to increase in hardness if the baby is examined during a paroxysm of pain. If the intussusception has not progressed far, the mass may be situated under the edge of the liver where it evades detection. The right lower quadrant may appear to be "empty" when it is palpated (*Dance's sign*) because of invagination of the cecum up into the colon.

If no definite mass can be felt in a very fat or uncooperative child whose history is strongly suggestive of intussusception, it is advisable to palpate

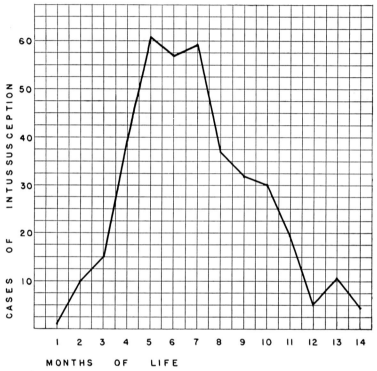

Fig. 73.—Age distribution of patients with intussusception which occurred in the first fourteen months of life. The peak incidence of this condition is between the fourth and tenth months of life.

the abdomen *under general anesthesia*. This should always be done with the operating room set up and prepared for immediate surgery if the findings of the ether examination warrant it.

By *rectal examination* blood is found in the great majority of patients. The finger may detect an advancing portion of bowel within the rectal lumen. This intussusceptum has the general shape of a cervix uteri. Even though the tip of the advancing bowel cannot be felt within the rectal lumen, bimanual examination may reveal a mass higher up in the peritoneal cavity which would be missed by abdominal palpation alone. In 122 cases (25 per cent of the series) an abdominal mass could be felt by rectal examination. In four cases the intussusceptum had proceeded so far that it protruded from the anus. The differentiation between intussusception of this type and a *prolapsed rectum* can be readily made by passing the finger into the rectum *between* the intussusceptum and the surrounding anal sphincter. In a prolapse of the rectum there is no such space to admit a

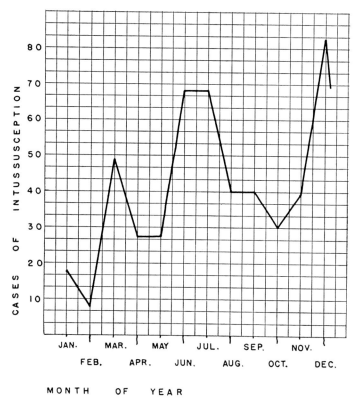

Fig. 74.—Incidence of intussusception by months of the year.

finger.* Fever is absent in the early stages of the condition, but it is usually present in those who have had symptoms long enough to become dehydrated.

* Prolapse of the rectum is a not uncommon condition in babies and young children. While it may be related to meningocele or other neurologic disorders in which there is perineal paralysis and loss of sphincter tone, it usually appears in otherwise normal subjects. The rectum may prolapse for several inches, become engorged, and bleed profusely. With adequate digital pressure by a gloved hand the mass can usually be reduced. Operative treatment is required only when the prolapse becomes gangrenous or after nonoperative measures have failed. A two- or three-week regimen of daily administration of mineral oil and keeping the buttocks strapped together with adhesive tape between defecations will almost always allow the rectum to become adherent in a normal position.

ROENTGENOLOGIC EXAMINATION

In typical cases of acute intussusception, the history and physical findings are sufficient to make a diagnosis, and roentgenologic studies are not necessary. In only twenty-five of the present 484 patients was the diagnosis sufficiently in question to require x-ray examination with a barium enema. In twenty-three of these a positive diagnosis of intussusception was made by roentgenograms and confirmed by immediate laparotomy. In two cases (ileo-ileal type) the roentgenologic findings were normal, but intussusceptions were subsequently found at operation.

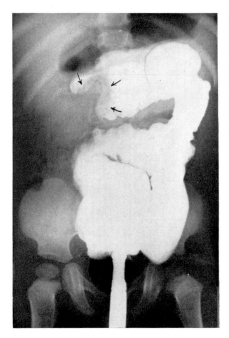 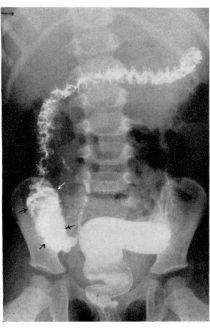

Fig. 75.—Typical roentgenographic findings with a barium enema in a case of intussusception. *Left,* The barium cannot be forced back beyond the middle of the transverse colon where there is a filling defect (outlined by arrows). *Right,* Postevacuation film showing barium remaining around an intussusceptum in the cecum. The intussusception has been partially reduced by the hydrostatic pressure of the enema.

Inasmuch as the majority of intussusceptions in this age group progress so that the intussusceptum enters the colon, certain features are found on *barium-enema examination.* These may be summarized as: (1) obstruction to the retrograde injection of barium; (2) a cupola effect or cupping in the head of the barium as it meets the intussusceptum; (3) a thin cylindrical shell of barium surrounding the intussusceptum (and inside the intussuscipiens); (4) a cylindrical shell of barium, surrounding and outlining the intussusceptum, which remains after evacuation of the enema; (5) a partial (or complete) retrogression of the intussusceptum if the barium is injected with sufficient pressure.

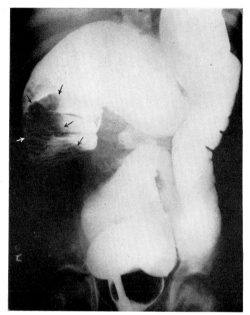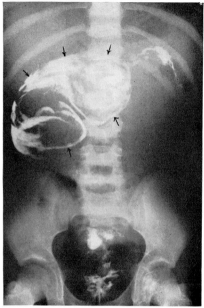

Fig. 76.—Roentgenograms with contrast enema showing features of a typical ileocolic intussusception. *Left,* Filling defect, outlined by arrows, in the ascending colon. *Right,* Postevacuation film indicating a thin sheath of barium around an intussusceptum which lies in the hepatic flexure and proximal half of the transverse colon.

TREATMENT

Nonoperative Methods.—In 1874 Hutchinson first successfully performed operative reduction of an intussusception, and since that time the treatment of this condition has progressively tended toward operative intervention. In spite of the almost universal adoption of surgical treatment there have been several reports, notably those of Hipsley[5] and Monrad,[12] favoring reduction by *colonic injection of fluids or air.* Arntzen and Helsted,[1] Retan,[16] and Stephens[21] advocated reduction with a barium enema under fluoroscopic control. Without doubt, many early ileo-colic intussusceptions can be reduced by these means. However, we are strongly opposed to treatment by colonic inflation for several reasons: (1) A considerable number of patients come to subsequent operation because of irreducibility or because the operator is uncertain that complete reduction has been effected. Operation is therefore delayed and the child has been subjected to a procedure which depletes its narrow margin of reserve. (2) Colonic inflation has a limited effectiveness above the ileocecal valve and an ileal portion of the intussusception may be left unreduced. (3) An existing polyp or

Meckel's diverticulum will be completely overlooked, whereas this additional pathologic condition could be recognized if laparotomy had been performed.

Operative Treatment.—*Short Duration of Symptoms a Factor in Favorable Results.*—By limiting ourselves to operative treatment, a simplification of therapy has been obtained which has significantly improved our results.

When one studies the published surgical mortality rates, which run as high as 45 per cent, the 100 cases treated by Hipsley[5] with hydrostatic pressure, with a mortality of 5 per cent, at first glance appear favorable. However, it is misleading to compare the results of different authors or of different methods without considering the average duration of symptoms in each series of cases. It is important to note that quicker hospitalization was obtained in Australia (Clubbe's and Hipsley's series) thirty years ago than we are able to secure in the United States today. Thus, Clubbe's cases in 1909 with an average illness of seventeen hours may be compared with the following illustrative series in America: Robbins'[17] patients had an average symptom-duration of almost forty-five hours; Peterson's and Carter's,[15] thirty-two hours; our own recent patients, thirty hours.

To the casual observer these differences of a relatively few hours may seem to be trivial, but a glance at Fig. 79 shows that the prognosis is excellent in the first twenty-four hours of the condition, whereas the mortality rises sharply after this time. Inasmuch as the average duration of symptoms in Hipsley's series was only seventeen hours, we regard his mortality of 5 per cent as unduly high, because we have had no mortality in patients with symptoms of similar duration. It is probable that Hipsley's good results were not due as much to a superior method of treatment as they were to the rapidity with which patients were referred to him. This early procurement of cases was the fruit of many years' effort on the part of Hipsley and his teacher, Clubbe, in encouraging the pediatrician and practitioner of Australia to recognize the condition and act before it was too late. Too great an estimate cannot be placed upon the educational work of these men.

Preoperative Measures.—Since intussusception is regarded as a surgical emergency, it has been our practice to expedite operation as much as possible. Yet, if shock or dehydration is marked, thirty or forty minutes can be profitably spent on administering parenteral *fluids* or giving a *transfusion* before operation. The average patient can be admitted, operated upon, and put to bed within an hour. The child's extremities should be wrapped with cotton batting *to prevent loss of heat,* and a hot-water bottle should be placed under the back to supply heat during the surgical procedure. We routinely *deflate the stomach* before operation in order to reduce to a minimum the dangers from aspirated vomitus.

Anesthesia.—Ether by the open-drop method is the anesthesia of choice.

Exposure of Intestine.—Proper placement of the *incision* facilitates the procedure. It should not be made over the presenting mass if this appears in the epigastrium or the left side of the abdomen. It should be routinely made as a right paramedian opening, with its central part opposite the umbilicus, splitting the rectus muscle or retracting it laterally. Reduction of that part of the intussusception which involves the descending or transverse colon never presents the difficulties that are to be found in the region of the ileocecal valve or the terminal ileum. Hence, an incision on the right side of the abdomen will give the maximum exposure during the most troublesome part of the operation.

Reduction of the Intussusception.—In the manipulation of an intussusception the operator must always take into account the extreme friability of the hemorrhagic and damaged intestine. Hence, *gentleness* is essential in all manipulations to avoid intestinal disruption and peritonitis. Several fingers are passed into the left side of the abdomen to locate the head of the intussusception which is then pushed backward along the colon. When it reaches the cecum or ascending colon the entire remaining intussusception mass is delivered outside of the abdomen so that it can be more easily inspected and handled. Reduction is continued with a process of milking back or *"taxis"*—the gentle compression of the intussuscipiens with the entire hand in such a way that the invaginated part is slowly squeezed out. There may be a temptation to pull out the intussusceptum, but this should be either strictly avoided or else done with the utmost delicacy. The dripping on of warm saline and continued annular pressure of the hand over the swollen intestine tends to reduce the edema and vascular engorgement. Slight stretching of the receiving ring with a blunt instrument may help in the reduction. With persistence and patience 95 per cent of intussusceptions can be manually reduced.

Small *tears* in the peritoneal coats of the gut are in themselves not particularly dangerous, but they serve as a warning to the operator that the muscularis or mucosa will soon tear if he is not careful. If these peritoneal tears are long, or if they extend into the musculature, a few quickly placed interrupted sutures will suffice to repair them.

Once the intussusception has been completely reduced, the involved portion of gut should be examined to determine its *viability*. There is always some degree of hemorrhage, swelling, edema, and discoloration, but an intestine of questionable viability will often improve in appearance within a few minutes if it is warmed and moistened with salt solution. If there is peristaltic activity over the involved portion of the gut, or if it contracts when gently pinched with smooth forceps, the intestine should not be resected.

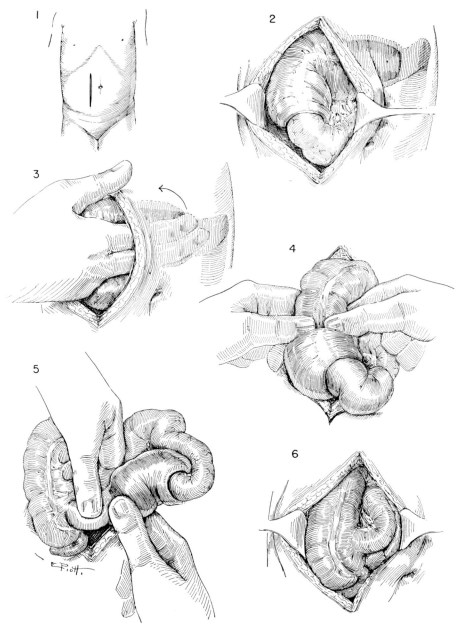

Fig. 77.—Method of operative reduction of ileo-colic intussusception. *1*, Incision is always made on right side of abdomen, regardless of position of palpable mass. *2*, Findings on opening abdomen. Ileum is intussuscepted into ascending colon. Intussusception extends almost to the splenic flexure. *3*, Portion of hand passed in to left side of abdomen so that the finger tips can push back intussusceptum in direction of arrow. *4*, Intussusception has been reduced to the ascending colon which is now delivered out of the abdomen. Squeezing over the distal end of the mass is now begun. *5*, Cecum and appendix have been delivered. Remaining intussusception in ileum is reduced by continued squeezing on the receding mass. *6*, Reduction completed and intestines returned to abdomen.

Only through experience can an operator know how long to persist in attempts at reduction in a case where complete reduction appears to be impossible. It is better to spend twenty minutes or half an hour in completing a reduction than it is to resort too soon to resection, with its higher danger of peritonitis and death. On the other hand, long-continued unsuccessful attempts at reduction may so exhaust the child that the operator is eventually forced to resection in spite of the fact that the patient cannot possibly survive this formidable procedure.

Additional Operative Procedures.—In conjunction with reduction of intussusceptions, the following procedures have been performed in our series: (1) In ten cases enterostomy was done when the intestine was of doubtful viability. (This procedure has now been abandoned because an intestine with such questionable viability should be excised.) (2) In nine cases a Meckel's diverticulum was excised. (3) In eighteen cases the appendix was removed. (4) In one case the terminal part of the ileum was sutured down to the posterior parietal peritoneum. (5) In two cases intestinal polyps were removed. Many of these additional operative procedures were done in the early part of the series. *Today our policy is to do nothing more than is absolutely necessary during operation for intussusception.* If a Meckel's diverticulum is present and is gangrenous or cannot be everted, it obviously must be removed. If an intestinal polyp is so large that it blocks the lumen of the gut, it must be excised at this time. If the appendix has been injured by being included in the intussusception mass so that its blood supply is questionable, it should be removed. However, mere engorgement and swelling of the appendix is certainly no indication for appendectomy at such a time.

Any procedure which opens the intestinal tract in one of these cases greatly increases the possibility of a peritonitis, because the injured intestine has a lowered vitality and cannot withstand infection as well as a normal intestine. Hence, the slightest soiling of the peritoneal cavity may induce a spreading infection with a high probability of fatal issue. Therefore, whenever possible it is better to defer any opening of the intestinal tract to a *second* procedure (ten days or two weeks later) when the circulation of the intestine will have returned to normal and the peritoneal cavity can better withstand the slight soiling which accompanies removal of an appendix, polyp, or Meckel's diverticulum.

Some authors have advised routine *removal of the appendix* in these cases, believing that irritation from appendicitis produced the invagination and intussusception. Little credence should be placed in this theory. The cautious operator will not remove the appendix unless it is gangrenous or its vessels are thrombosed.

Resection of the Intussusception.—In any large series of cases, there will

8

always be some individuals for whom resection of an intussusception must be employed. In babies under one year of age, this carries an extremely high mortality, averaging around 75 per cent or more. In our series forty-three resections were done. Eighteen of these were combined with anastomoses (ileo-colostomy or ileo-ileostomy) with three recoveries. Twenty-five had a double enterostomy (Mikulicz's procedure), with seven recoveries. There are an insufficient number of successful resections in this series (or in a collective review of the literature) to indicate whether primary anastomosis or Mikulicz's resection is the procedure of choice. Surprisingly enough, the successful resections for intussusception which could be gathered from the literature were treated in the majority of instances by primary anastomosis of the intestine. Our material to date tends to show that the Mikulicz procedure gives a little better chance of recovery.

Mikulicz's Resection: Technical Points.—If a Mikulicz type of resection is to be done, it should be performed so that absolutely no soiling of the peritoneal cavity takes place. In other words, the intussuscepted mass or the nonviable gut should be exteriorized and the abdominal wound completely closed around it before the diseased portion of the intestine is cut away. Catheters or glass Mixter tubes can then be sewed into the upper and lower loops to prevent contamination of the cutaneous wound and the abdominal wall. It is best to approximate the distal and proximal spurs with continuous sutures prior to closing of the abdominal cavity so that nothing can prolapse between these two loops when a crushing clamp is subsequently applied. Inasmuch as babies do not tolerate well the loss of succus entericus, the spurs should be cut down with a crushing clamp as soon as it is certain (in four or five days) that the two loops are firmly adherent to the abdominal wall.

"Preventive" Surgical Procedures.—Some surgeons have suggested procedures which are aimed at avoidance of recurrent intussusception, but it is doubtful if such undertakings are effective or desirable. They unduly prolong the operation for an already critically ill child. Furthermore, there is no assurance that the various measures which have been advised (tacking down the terminal ileum, anchoring the mesentery, etc.) will prevent recurrence. In two of our cases of recurrence an operation had been done previously (elsewhere) to prevent it. In our series, recurrence appeared in only 2 per cent of the individuals, and in each of these it was so quickly recognized by the parent, and the child brought to the hospital so early that it could be treated without mortality. In summary; the rather low incidence of recurrence, the inefficacy of preventive procedures, the possible increase in mortality at the original operation, and the lack of mortality in recurrent cases, make it evident that the various "preventive" surgical procedures should not be recommended.

POSTOPERATIVE TREATMENT AND COMPLICATIONS

Administration of Fluids.—If no parenteral fluids are administered before operation, they should certainly be given by intravenous and subcutaneous routes as soon as it is completed. Water, electrolytes, and carbohydrates should be given in this way at least twice a day for two or three days, and in some cases this period must be longer. It has been our practice to administer rectal taps every four hours for the first twenty-four hours. Three ounces are inserted each time, consisting of 5 per cent dextrose the first two times and warm tap-water for the subsequent four administrations.

Deflation of Stomach.—It is important to deflate the stomach to prevent vomiting and aspiration during or shortly after operation. Since the loss of several patients by this regrettable accident we have adopted routine aspiration of the stomach both before and immediately after the operative procedure.

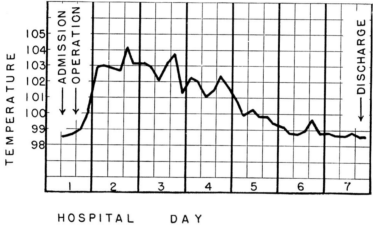

HOSPITAL DAY

Fig. 78.—Typical temperature chart of an infant with intussusception. Most patients have a fever of 103° or 104° F. for two or three days after operation.

Feeding.—For the first postoperative day, or as long as there is vomiting, only water in limited amounts should be given by mouth, for fear of aspiration pneumonia. After vomiting has ceased, equal quantities of milk and whey can be cautiously started. The full caloric or volume intake for the age and weight should not be offered until the fourth or fifth day. The intestinal tract has been extensively damaged and should not be subjected to its full normal activity until the reparative processes are well under way.

Postoperative Diarrhea.—Not infrequently a diarrhea develops during the first week of convalescence, because the traumatized intestine is more susceptible to infection and acute enteritis, particularly in the summer months of the year. It is therefore obvious that strict precautions must be taken to guard against exposure to other patients with dysentery or gastro-intestinal disorders. If such a complication develops, the oral intake of food should be reduced, sedatives administered, and fluids given by the parenteral routes.

Postoperative Peritonitis.—Shock, dehydration, and toxicity exact a high toll and fully four fifths of those who die have these factors listed as the immediate cause of death. Since such conditions cause most of the mortalities, the majority of deaths occur within forty-eight hours after operation. If the intestine has been opened during operation, peritonitis is the most important cause of death. Because of this fact, *chemotherapy* (sulfathiazole) should be instituted at once whenever any soiling of the peritoneum has occurred.

Postoperative Fever.—Almost universally some rise in temperature is found for the first three or four days after operation (Fig. 78). It is not uncommon to find a temperature of 103° or even 104° F. during the immediate postoperative course, but levels above 105° F. carry a grave and usually fatal prognosis. This postoperative pyrexia is presumably due to absorption of foreign proteins through the damaged intestinal wall or to assimilation of products of necrosis from the damaged intestine itself.

FACTORS IN PROGNOSIS

Early Treatment.—The most effective way to reduce the mortality of intussusception is to shorten the period between onset of symptoms and the initiation of treatment. This does not minimize the responsibility of the surgeon to improve the operative technic; nor does it imply that he is trying

TABLE 13

DURATION OF SYMPTOMS AND CORRESPONDING MORTALITY STATISTICS, 1928 THROUGH 1939

Symptom Duration	Operative Results		
	Number of Survivals	Number of Deaths	Mortality Percentage
0 to 12 hours.	66	0	0
12 to 24 hours.	44	0	0
24 to 36 hours.	20	6	23
36 to 48 hours.	12	6	33
48 to 72 hours.	15	4	21
72 to 96 hours.	8	5	38
More than 96 hours.	10	6	38
Totals.	175	27	13

to excuse a high mortality by stressing the necessity for earlier treatment. There are few illnesses in which the clinical history and physical findings are more suggestive of the correct diagnosis than intussusception of infancy. One may therefore reasonably expect the intelligent pediatrician and prac-

titioner to recognize this condition within the first twenty-four hours. The
direct relationship of the duration of symptoms to the corresponding

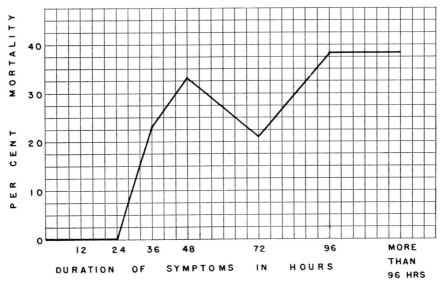

Fig. 79.—Graph showing relationship between duration of symptoms and corresponding mortality rates in 202 patients with intussusception treated from 1928 through 1939.
Operation was performed on 110 patients within the first twenty-four hours of illness
without fatality.

mortality figures is summed up in Table 13. In these 202 patients the overall mortality was 13 per cent, whereas in the 110 cases which were operated
upon within the first twenty-four hours of illness there was no mortality.

TABLE 14

IMPROVEMENT IN SURGICAL RESULTS IN PATIENTS WITH SIMILAR DURATIONS OF SYMPTOMS

Symptom Duration	Mortality Percentage	
	1908 to 1927 Series	1928 to 1939 Series
0 to 12 hours	7	0
12 to 24 hours	24	0
24 to 36 hours	49	23
36 to 48 hours	53	33
48 to 72 hours	53	21
72 to 96 hours	60	38
More than 4 days	54	38

These statistics are graphically represented in Fig. 79. In summary, symptom
durations up to twenty-four hours carried no mortality, symptom duration
of twenty-four to thirty-six hours carried a mortality of 23 per cent; whereas

illnesses of thirty-six to forty-eight hours had a mortality climbing to 33 per cent.

Improvement in Technic.—Recent advances in the treatment of intussusception may be attributed to greater effort on the part of both physicians and surgeons. The physicians' activity may be seen in the drop of the average symptoms duration from thirty-eight hours (1908 to 1927) to thirty hours (1928 through 1939). The surgeons' progress in operative technic

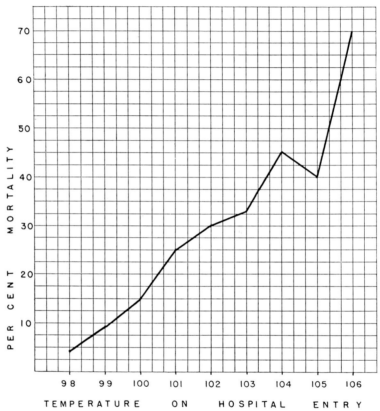

Fig. 80.—Graph of relationship between body temperature at time of hospitalization and corresponding mortality rate. Fever at the time of hospitalization implies a poor prognosis, presumably because it indicates severe dehydration or extensive intestinal damage.

and supportive care becomes evident when one compares cases of given symptom durations which were treated in the earlier period (1908 to 1927) with parallel cases treated from 1928 through 1939. In each symptom duration group (Table 14) there has been an appreciable reduction in mortality in the second period as compared to that of the first.

Patients in the private ward have always had a lower mortality rate than those on the charity service. In the period from 1908 through 1927 there were thirty recoveries and four deaths. In the period from 1928 through 1939 there were twenty-six recoveries and no deaths. These favorable figures can be partially attributed to the fact that the cases were all handled by senior service surgeons, but considerable importance is attached to the fact that intussusception is recognized earlier in private patients than in charity ones.

Preoperative Temperatures.—The temperature of these patients, prior to operation, has considerable prognostic value because it roughly reflects

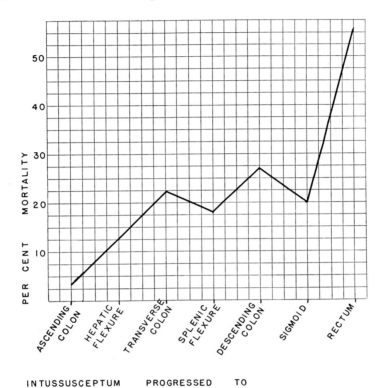

INTUSSUSCEPTUM PROGRESSED TO

Fig. 81.—Relationship between progress of intussusceptums and the corresponding mortality rates—irrespective of the origin of intussusceptions. The farther the mass has advanced along the colon, the higher is the expected mortality.

the existing degree of dehyration and toxicity. In general, the higher the temperature the greater is the likelihood of a subsequent death. As graphically shown in Fig. 80, a normal admission temperature is a good sign; a temperature of 100° or 101° F. carries a mortality expectancy of 20 to 25 per cent, and a temperature higher than 101° F. implies a rather poor outlook.

Distal Advancement of Leading Point.—If the origin of an intussusception is entirely disregarded and a tabulation is made of the most distal points to which intussusceptums have advanced, one finds that the farther along the leading point has progressed, the higher is the related mortality (Fig. 81). This increase in the probability of death as the leading point approaches the anus probably depends upon the increasing tension and damage to the mesentery as well as the increasing difficulty in operative treatment of the lesion.

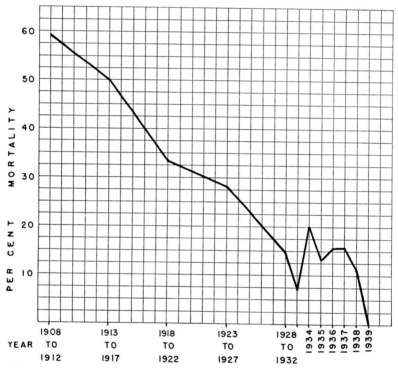

Fig. 82.—Mortality rate curve from 484 cases of intussusception treated at the Children's Hospital from 1908 through 1939. There has been a progressive decrease in the death rates during this period.

The death rates over a period of years in 484 cases are charted in Fig. 82. Beginning with a mortality of 59 per cent in the 1908 to 1912 period, a gradual decline has taken place, so that in 1939 twelve cases were operated upon without a fatality. This satisfactory improvement in results is due to a combination of earlier treatment and better surgical care.

CHRONIC INTUSSUSCEPTION

Subacute or *chronic intussusception* has been arbitrarily defined as that type in which the symptoms last from five days to two or more weeks. An intussusception which can persist this long without killing the individual must necessarily be of a form which does not completely obstruct the bowel. Indeed, such a patient may have occasional small bowel movements during the illness, and may not appear particularly sick. There may be irregular and intermittent vomiting, moderate abdominal pain, or passage of small amounts of blood in the stool. In short, partial obstruction produces symptoms which are not so pronounced and fulminating as those of acute intussusception, in which the bowel is completely occluded.

Not infrequently the chronic form of intussusception is seen in association with or following *acute enteritis;* accordingly any turn for the worse in a case of enteritis in a young child should arouse one's suspicions of the possibility of intussusception. When chronic intussusception is suspected, a barium-enema examination should be the deciding factor in establishing the diagnosis. The prognosis in these individuals is usually rather good, presumably because intestinal obstruction has been only partial and because the damage to the intestine and mesentery is minimal.

RECURRENT INTUSSUSCEPTION

Recurrence of the condition is found in a small percentage of patients with intussusception. The second attack may appear within a few days after the initial episode or it may be delayed for several years. In cases gleaned from the literature the longest interval between attacks was eight years and the shortest was thirty hours. The largest number of recurrences ever reported in one individual were in a child who required four operations. In our 484 patients there were ten individuals with a recurrence, an incidence of 2 per cent. Nine of these were treated by simple reduction of the second intussusception, but in one of them appendectomy was also performed. The tenth individual had simple reduction of an intussusception on three separate occasions.

Because of the low incidence of recurrence we believe that *it is not desirable to undertake procedures which are designed to prevent return of intussusception.* The chances of a second attack are so small that there is little justification for performing additional operative steps in a critically ill child. Another reason for not attempting them lies in the fact that recurrence does not necessarily take place in the same location as the original intussusception. Furthermore, it is questionable whether any of the steps which have been devised to date would be effective in preventing subsequent recurrence of the trouble. All of our recurrent cases were treated without mortality. We feel that this was primarily due to the acuity of the mothers, who invariably recognized the second attack as being similar to the first, and wasted no time in hospitalizing the children within periods when treatment could be given without appreciable danger.

BIBLIOGRAPHY

1. Arntzen, L., and Helsted, A.: Desinvagination unter Roentgendurchleuchtung bei akuter Darminvagination im Kindesalter. Acta chir. Scandinav., 65: 70, 1929.
2. Asbury, H.: Roentgenological Aspects of Intussusception. Am. J. Roentgenol., 18: 536, 1927.
3. Beaven, P. W.: The Occurrence of Chronic Intussusception in Young Children. Am. J. Dis. Child., 37: 373, 1929.
4. Clubbe, C. P. B.: The Diagnosis and Treatment of Intussusception. New York: Oxford University Press, 1921.
5. Hipsley, P. L.: Intussusception and Its Treatment by Hydrostatic Pressure. M. J. Australia, 2: 201, 1926.
6. Hutchinson, J.: A Successful Case of Abdominal Section for Intussusception. Tr. Roy. M. and Chir. Soc., 57: 31, 1874.
7. Kirsner, J. B., and Miller, J. F.: Roentgen Diagnosis of Intussusception. Radiology, 31: 658, 1938.
8. Ladd, W. E., and Gross, R. E.: Intussusception in Infancy and Childhood; A Report of Three Hundred and Seventy-two Cases. Arch. Surg., 29: 365, 1934.
9. Lehmann, C.: Ein Fall von Invaginatio ileocecalis im Röntgenbilde. Fortschr. a. d. Geb. d. Röntgenstrahlen, 21: 561, 1913.
10. McIver, M. A.: Intussusception of the Small Intestine with Special Reference to Meckel's Diverticulum as a Causative Factor. New England J. Med., 199: 453, 1928.
11. Mayo, C. W.: Spontaneous Expulsion of an Intussuscepted Bowel. Proc. Staff Meet., Mayo Clin., 7: 345, 1932.
12. Monrad, S.: Acute Invagination of the Intestine in Small Children. Acta paediat., 6: 31, 1926.
13. Montgomery, A. H., and Mussil, J. J.: The Treatment of Irreducible Intussusception in Children. Surg., Gynec. and Obst., 51: 415, 1930.
14. Perrin, W. S., and Lindsay, E. C.: Intussusception: A Monograph Based on Four Hundred Cases. Brit. J. Surg., 9: 46, 1921.
15. Peterson, E. W., and Carter, R. F.: Acute Intussusception in Infancy and Childhood. Ann. Surg., 96: 94, 1932.
16. Retan, G. M.: Nonoperative Treatment of Intussusception. Am. J. Dis. Child., 33: 765, 1927.
17. Robbins, F. R.: Acute Intussusception. Ann. Surg., 95: 830, 1932.
18. Schoenfeld, H. H.: Retrograde Intussusception. Virginia M. Monthly, 58: 242, 1931.
19. Southern, A. H., and Crawshaw, C. H.: Resection of Intestine for Acute Intussusception. Brit. M. J., 1: 266, 1921.
20. Stephens, V. R.: Ileocecal Intussusception in Infants, with Special Reference to Fluoroscopic Findings. Surg., Gynec. and Obst., 45: 698, 1927.
21. Stephens, V. R.: Acute Intussusception: Manipulation Under Fluoroscopic Control. Am. J. Dis. Child., 35: 61, 1928.
22. Sussman, M. L.: The Roentgenologic Aspect of Subacute and Chronic Intestinal Intussusception. Am. J. Roentgenol., 27: 373, 1932.
23. Thorndike, A.: Acute Recurrent Intussusception in Children. New England J. Med., 207: 649, 1923.
24. Wardill, W. E. M.: Polypi in the Bowel Causing Intussusception. Brit. J. Surg., 13: 158, 1925.

CHAPTER X

POLYPS OF INTESTINE AND COLON

Polyps of the alimentary tract are frequently encountered in childhood. They are found in any portion of the intestine or colon and give rise to symptoms which vary according to the position of the lesion. In the vast majority of cases, they are single, or else occur as a small group within a short segment of gut, but it is well known that polyps appearing at one site carry a certain implication that additional ones might concurrently exist in other parts of the intestinal tract. Polyps commonly present rather trifling symptoms and may be easily treated by minor surgical procedures, but in some instances they produce serious illness which requires the most major sort of surgery for adequate therapy.

PATHOLOGY

Size and Structure.—Polyps range from a few millimeters to several centimeters in diameter. Average ones are 1 cm. or less in maximum cross dimensions. They are soft and often friable. At first the base usually has a sessile attachment to the intestinal wall, but this later becomes pedunculated as the suspended and enlarging mass is pulled upon by the fecal current. The intestinal or colonic mucosa extends up over the stalk onto the polyp proper, and indeed many polyps appear to be little more than localized redundancies of the regional mucosa and submucosa. However, some of them exhibit definite evidence of neoplastic growth of a benign sort, and goblet, mucous-secreting cells are arranged in irregular, adenomatous formations. All polyps show some degree of edema, hemorrhage, and chronic inflammation. Surface ulceration and granulation-tissue formation are common.

Locations.—Polyps are most commonly located in the rectum, but they may occur at any point distal to the cardia of the stomach. In a series of ninety-two cases treated at the Children's Hospital, the lesions were distributed as follows:

In rectum only	78	cases
Sigmoid	3	"
Descending colon	2	"
Transverse colon	3	"
Cecum	1	case
Multiple polyposis of colon	3	cases
Ileum	1	case
Scattered through stomach, jejunum, and ileum	1	"

Multiple Polyps.—While polyps tend to be single or to be confined to a short segment of gut, they may be scattered diffusely throughout the alimentary tract. An example of this was encountered in an eight-year-old girl who at autopsy had four polyps in the stomach, fourteen in the jejunum, and four in the ileum. In unusual cases, polyps develop in enormous numbers, particularly in the colon. In a seven-year-old boy the colonic wall from the cecum to anus was found to have more than 400 of them of different sizes (Fig. 93). Some of these were sessile; others were pedunculated. Many had an adenomatous structure on microscopic examination.

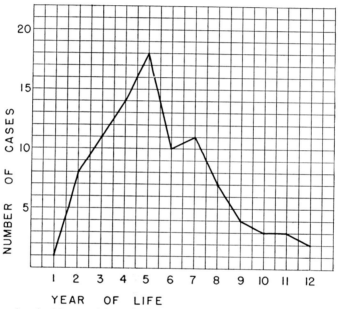

Fig. 83.—Age incidence of intestinal or colonic polyps in ninety-two children.

Complications.—Three important complications can result from intestinal or colonic polyps: (1) Surface erosion may produce hemorrhage, particularly if the pedunculated structures are large or multiple. (2) A polyp may act as the leading point of an intussusception, a sequence which was found in four of our cases. (3) Malignant degeneration occurs with considerable frequency. This danger is believed to be negligible in the small, isolated polyp such as is found in the rectum, but it is a serious hazard for those individuals with polyposis of the colon, in whom carcinomatous degeneration has been estimated to be as high as 50 per cent. If malignant changes appear, they seldom do so before adult life.

SYMPTOMS AND SIGNS

Bleeding.—*Melena* is the most frequent symptom. Polyps of the small intestine may produce occult blood in the stool which is demonstrable only by chemical tests, or there may be gross amounts of dark-red blood or tarry material intermixed with the excretions. Polyps of the descending colon, sigmoid, or rectum are particularly apt to bleed because they are constantly irritated and ulcerated by the more solid fecal concretions which lie in these parts of the colon. While polyps in these positions frequently bleed, it is unusual for more than a few cc. of blood to be passed at any one time. Polyposis of the colon causes almost continuous loss of small amounts of blood, which may induce a state of virtual exhaustion of red cells, hemoglobin, and blood proteins. In one of our children the red count had

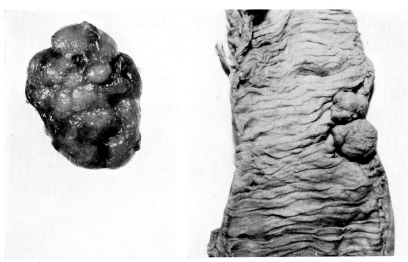

Fig. 84.—Intestinal polyps from a nine-year-old girl. *Left,* Three cm. long, adenomatous polyp from the jejunum which had been the leading point of an intussusception. *Right,* Two pedunculated polyps in upper ileum.

fallen to 2,500,000 and the serum protein to 2.7 gm. per cent. Furthermore, there was weakness, pallor, orthopnea, leg edema, and clubbing of the fingers.

A polyp of the rectum can usually be felt with the finger and is almost always attached to the posterior or posterolateral wall. If it cannot be palpated in this way, it can always be identified by proctoscopy.

Abdominal Pain.—Aside from bleeding and possible prolapse out through the anus, rectal polyps are usually silent, but lesions higher in the alimentary canal may produce *abdominal discomfort, cramps,* or even *severe pain.* Abdominal pain which is excruciating, colicky, and possibly associated with vomiting suggests that peristaltic activity has pulled a polyp into the intestine in such a way that an intussusception has been initiated.

Incidence.—*Age.*—Polyps are rarely discovered in the first year of life. They are most frequently seen from the ages of two to eight years, with a peak of incidence at four or five years. The age distribution of ninety-two cases is set forth in Fig. 83.

Sex.—Males are affected with somewhat greater frequency than females, the proportion being 54 to 38 in our series.

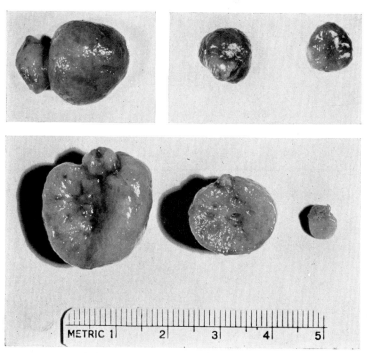

Fig. 85.—Photographs of colonic and rectal polyps removed from three patients.

Familial.—Individuals with polyposis are apt to have relatives with intestinal or colonic polyps, but this familial tendency is rarely found when a given patient has only one or two polyps.

ROENTGENOLOGIC EXAMINATION

The identification of one or several polyps in the rectum always raises the question of whether more of these lesions are present in other parts of the alimentary tract. It has been our policy to perform *barium-enema studies* routinely, but in only rare cases have additional polyps been detected higher in the colon. It would therefore appear to be acceptable practice to excise a presenting rectal lesion and perform roentgenologic investigation only if postoperative bleeding is subsequently encountered. When a child has melena and no rectal polyp can be felt, barium studies should of course be done. When there is polyposis of the rectum, a barium enema should always be given to determine the upper extent of the condition, and a gastro-intestinal series should be conducted to detect any polyps of the stomach or small intestine.

Polyps of the *colon* are found by fluoroscopic or film studies as filling defects during inflation of the colon with a barium mixture (Figs. 86, 91, and 95). In postevacuation films the polypoid mass may retain a thin coating of barium which outlines its borders. Polyps can be differentiated from *fecal masses* by the fact that they cannot be dislocated by manual palpation during the fluoroscopic examination, and by the fact that a filling defect

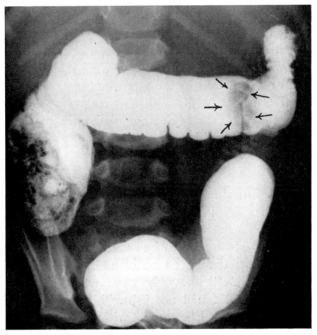

Fig. 86.—Roentgenogram following barium enema, showing single polyp (indicated by arrows) in transverse colon.

persists in a given region during different examinations. Double-contrast enemas—filling the colon with a barium mixture and later inflating it with air—are particularly effective in visualizing polyps.

DIFFERENTIAL DIAGNOSIS

Melena in childhood is a symptom of variable significance. In the vast majority of cases it signifies a minor ailment, but in some instances it may be the warning of a condition which threatens the individual's life.

Constipation is probably the most common cause of rectal bleeding in infants and young children. Dyschesia and bleeding may result from a small anal fissure if the stools are too hard, but these symptoms are completely alleviated by mild catharsis (mineral oil) for a few days.

A *Meckel's diverticulum* may give rise to bleeding which, when it appears, is usually copious in amount. It is rather typical for the hemorrhage to start suddenly and silently, persist for a day or two, and then terminate abruptly. The blood which is passed tends to be dark in color. Severe bleeding may occur on two or three occasions before it leads to laparotomy or exsanguination, but it is unusual for a Meckel's diverticulum to have frequent hemorrhages of small amounts of bright red blood—which are more suggestive of anal fissure or rectal polyp.

Intussusception usually has rectal bleeding as one of its cardinal symptoms. Sudden appearance of a bloody stool accompanied by severe abdominal pain, collapse, and possibly a palpable abdominal mass in a baby are usually sufficient to warrant making a diagnosis of intussusception.

Scurvy may cause rectal bleeding, but when it does so there is almost always evidence of the disease in the gums or long bones and a history of deficient vitamin C intake.

Blood dyscrasias are usually accompanied by hemorrhagic tendencies in other parts of the body and by some change in the platelet count, clotting time, or bleeding time.

TREATMENT

Treatments for intestinal or colonic polyps are divided into four types of operation, each of which is designed for a particular set of circumstances.

1. **Excision through Proctoscope.**—Excision of polyps through a proctoscope or sigmoidoscope is the most often used procedure (Fig. 87). By this means all polyps within the lowest 10 or 12 inches of the bowel can be easily removed. This should always be done under *general anesthesia,* to make certain that the child will not injure himself by moving while the instrument is in place. The *lithotomy position* is preferable to the knee-chest one since it gives the best view of the lesions which almost invariably arise from the posterior rectal wall. The bowel is *prepared* with a soap-suds enema the preceding evening, and by a second cleansing enema two or three hours before operation. If fecal material still obscures the view, the rectum can be further irrigated at the operating table, and the fluid then aspirated with a piece of tubing (connected to a suction apparatus) passed in through the proctoscope.

Polyps can often be grasped with an instrument and pulled down to a level where they can be directly handled through a short anoscope possessing a side slit. In this way the base can be transfixed before the pedunculated mass is cut off. This manipulation is often difficult because polyps tend to tear and bleed, or the rectal wall cannot be easily pulled down into a convenient position. Because of these troubles we have abandoned this ligature of the base in favor of snaring off the polyp with an elongated tonsil snare while simultaneously passing a *coagulating current* through the

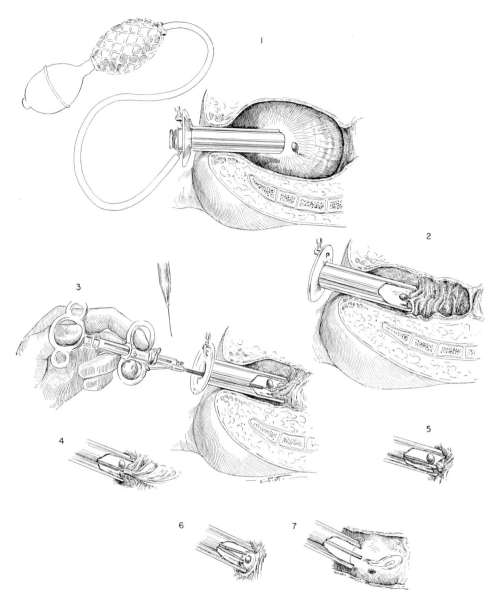

Fig. 87.—Method of removal of polyps from rectum or lower sigmoid. *1*, Patient in lithotomy position. Bowel inflated through proctoscope. Instrument placed so that its tip lies just distal to polyp. *2*, Air pressure released. Polyp prolapses into lumen of the proctoscope. *3*, *4*, Pedicle of polyp constricted with an elongated tonsil snare. Coagulating current passed through snare and pedicle of lesion. *5*, Alternate method of removing pedunculated polyp by grasping it with an alligator forceps through which a coagulating current is passed. The friable stalk can be severed by this squeezing and desiccation. *6*, Treatment of a sessile polyp by grasping it with an alligator forceps and then passing a coagulating current through it. *7*, Polyp and its base completely coagulated. Suction tube for removal of any smoke or fecal fluid which impairs vision.

9

instrument. A small polyp with a sessile base is best treated by grasping its central portion with an alligator forceps (through the proctoscope) and then passing a coagulating (endothermy) current through it. Coagulation is continued under direct vision until the entire polyp is charred white. Coagulation must be discontinued at this point to avoid perforation of the bowel wall. (We have never had a case of sloughing or perforation of the rectum or colon from this endothermy coagulation or snaring.)

2. **Abdominal Exploration with Ileotomy or Colotomy.**—Abdominal exploration with ileotomy or colotomy is employed for those polyps which lie

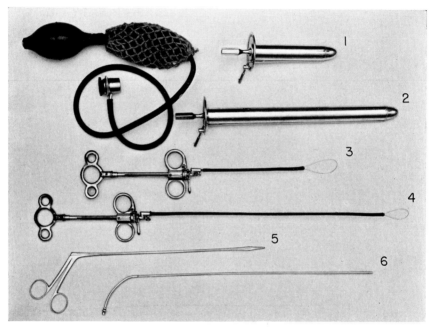

Fig. 88.—Instruments for excision of rectal polyps. *1*, Short proctoscope, 4 inches long, ¾ inch in diameter. *2*, Sigmoidoscope, 10 inches long. *3*, *4*, Tonsil snares with elongated stems. Thin rubber tubing is drawn over the stems for insulation. *5*, Long alligator forceps for grasping and coagulating sessile polyps or bleeding points. *6*, Metal suction tube for removing smoke or fecal fluid.

in a part of the tract above the sigmoid loop. When the abdomen is opened, the entire intestine should be carefully examined to determine accurately how many polyps exist. The segment of the intestine or colon which is to be treated is then drawn up into the wound and packed off carefully to avoid any subsequent soiling of the general peritoneal cavity. Rubber-covered clamps are placed across the proximal and distal ends of the exposed loop to prevent rushes of fecal material. Incision may be made opposite the polyp so that its pedicle can be tied, or an elliptical incision can be made around the base so that the entire mass (with its base) is removed. In either

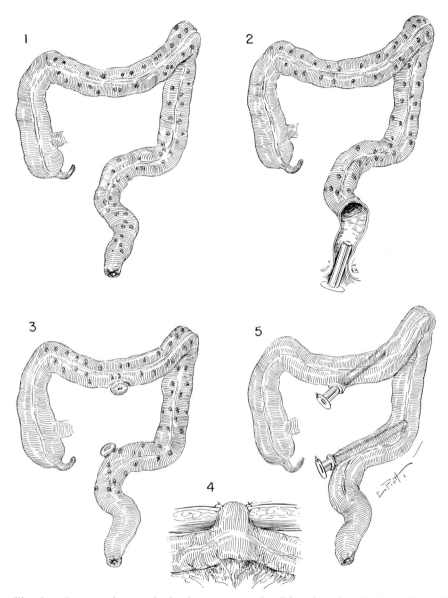

Fig. 89.—Conservative method of treatment of mild polyposis of colon when the lesions are scattered and are not numerous enough to warrant a colectomy. *1*, Outline of colon with scattered polyps. *2, First stage*—cleaning out all polyps from rectum and lower sigmoid through proctoscope. *3, Second stage*—establishment of colostomies (cecostomy, transverse colostomy, or sigmoidostomy: one or all three of these openings are made, depending upon positions of the polyps). *4*, Method of making colostomy. Unopened bowel wall is brought out through a small abdominal opening and is sutured to skin. This does not divert or obstruct the fecal stream. *5, Third stage* (ten days or more after second stage)—colostomies opened and polyps resected through proctoscopes.

case, the wall is closed with an inverting Connell continuous suture which is reinforced with a row of interrupted stitches.

3. **Temporary Colostomies.**—Establishment of one or several temporary colostomies provides avenues of attack on polyps of the colon (Fig. 89) which are too numerous for multiple colotomies and yet not numerous enough to warrant colectomy. Thus, a sigmoidoscope passed in through a *sigmoidostomy* allows the operator to remove polyps up to the splenic flexure by snare and endothermy coagulation. Similarly, a *transverse colostomy* permits treatment of lesions lying between the hepatic and splenic flexures; and a *cecostomy* gives access to those in the ascending colon. If

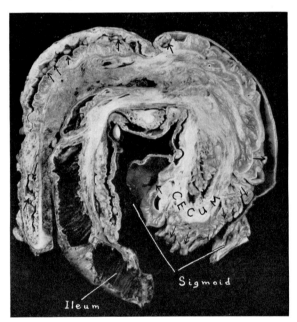

Fig. 90.—Opened specimen which was removed from a child with polyposis of colon and intussusception. Polypoid mass from cecum had led the intussusceptum around the entire colon to sigmoid. Arrows indicate some of the polyps.

necessary, all three of these temporary openings can be made, for through them and the anus scores of polyps can be removed from any part of the colon.

When this plan of treatment is undertaken, the colostomy (or colostomies) should be made in such a way that the fecal stream is not diverted out through the abdominal wall as is done in making a colostomy for obstructing colonic malignancies of the adult. It is necessary to make only a short incision—not over 1½ inches long—in the proper area of the abdomen, grasp the sigmoid (or transverse colon, or cecum), and pull the presenting surface of this up to the skin, to which it is stitched. An area of colonic wall about ½ inch in diameter is thus left exposed—at the periphery of which will be the sutures which anchor the bowel to the skin. If the abdominal wall opening is kept small enough, it will not be necessary to put any sutures in the peritoneum, muscle, or fascia. This entire procedure is aseptic and the fecal stream in the colon is not diverted or obstructed. After ten days or two weeks have elapsed, such a colostomy is opened by puncturing the exposed part of the bowel wall. A sigmoidoscope can then be introduced into the colon for removal of polyps. If these openings are suitably small, they contract spontaneously and seldom require secondary surgical closure.

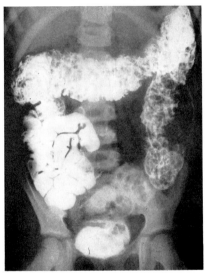

Fig. 91.—Roentgenogram from a seven-year-old boy with extensive polyposis of colon (compare Fig. 93 from same patient).

4. **Colectomy.**—Colectomy is the treatment of choice for cases of *advanced polyposis of the colon*. x-Ray irradiation has been tried in some of these, but on the whole it has given disappointing results. Resection of most of the colon can be performed in such a way that the rectum and anal sphincter are preserved. This is done by removal of all polyps from the terminal 6 or 8 inches of bowel, implantation of the terminal ileum into this prepared rectum, and then resection of the colon from cecum to lower sigmoid.

A variation of this procedure was employed in a seven-year-old boy (Figs. 91, 92, 93 and 94) whose colon, including rectum, contained over 400 polyps. This child had such severe and continuous bleeding that it seemed too hazardous to spend time cleaning out the rectum in the initial stages of treatment. Repeated transfusions raised the blood count to satisfactory levels, but the serum protein remained below the critical level and peripheral edema persisted. The following plan was therefore adopted with successful issue: *First stage.*—Transection of lower ileum, establishment of an ileostomy; resection of terminal ileum, cecum, and entire colon down to

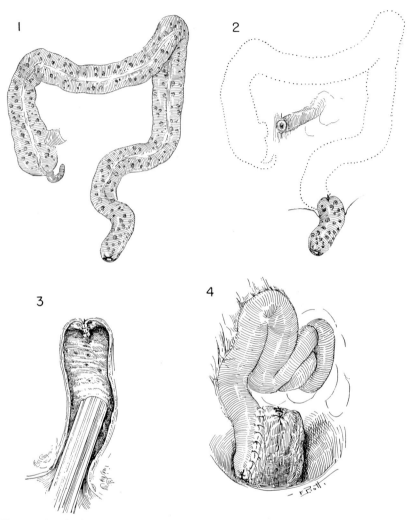

Fig. 92.—Method of treatment which was successfully employed for extensive polyposis of colon in a seven-year-old boy. *1,* Outline of colon which contained over 400 polyps, distributed from the cecum to the anus (see Fig. 93). *2, First stage*—division of terminal ileum. Establishment of ileostomy. Resection of dotted part of colon. Turning in lower sigmoid to leave a blind rectal pouch. *3, Second stage*—resection of polyps from rectal pouch by snare and coagulation method. *4, Third stage*—taking down of ileostomy and anastomosis of ileum to rectal pouch.

the lower sigmoid; turning in the lower sigmoid to make a blind rectal pouch about 6 inches long. (In this way the major portion of the bleeding was immediately stopped.) *Second stage.*—Per anal removal of all the polyps

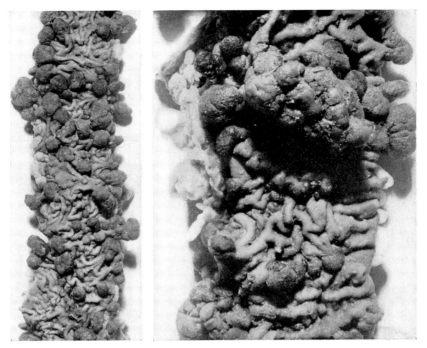

Fig. 93.—Portions of colon which was removed (Fig. 92) for extensive polyposis.

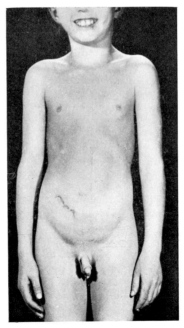

Fig. 94.—Photograph of patient treated as indicated in Fig. 92. Picture taken one year after colectomy and anastomosis of ileum to rectum.

from the rectal pouch by endothermy coagulation and snaring through a proctoscope. This required several sittings. *Third stage.*—Taking down the ileum from the ileostomy on the abdominal wall and anastomosing it to the prepared rectal pouch. The boy stood these procedures quite well and with slight limitation of fruits and green vegetables in the diet he has two or three semisolid bowel movements a day with good sphincteric control.

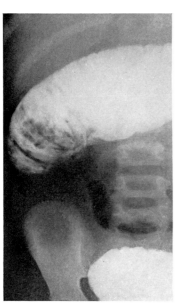 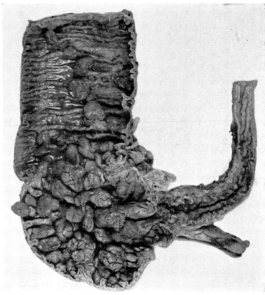

Fig. 95.—*Left,* Barium enema roentgenogram from a six-year-old boy with a filling defect in the cecum and ascending colon. *Right,* Photograph of the surgically removed specimen, showing mass of polyps in cecum. Patient successfully treated by right hemicolectomy.

BIBLIOGRAPHY

1. Coffey, R. J., and Bargen, J. A.: Intestinal Polyps: Pathogenesis and Relation to Malignancy. Surg., Gynec. and Obst., *69:* 136, 1939.
2. David, V. C.: Pathology and Treatment of Bleeding Polypoid Tumors of Large Bowel. Ann. Surg., *100:* 933, 1934.
3. Hedin, R. F.: Polypoid Disease of Colon; Anatomical Measurements of Colon Including Description of Colonoscope. Surgery, *6:* 909, 1939.
4. Lamson, O. F.: Treatment of Solitary Polyp of Colon. Northwest. Med., *38:* 119, 1939.
5. McKenney, D. C.: Multiple Polyposis: Congenital, Heredofamilial, Malignant. Am. J. Surg., *46:* 204, 1939.
6. Mayo, C. W., and Butsch, W. L.: Surgical Consideration of Solitary Polyps of Colon. Ann. Surg., *107:* 540, 1938.
7. Mayo, C. W., and Smith, C. H.: Transcolonic Removal of Polyps. Surgery, *5:* 942, 1939.
8. Shaw, E. A.: Polyposis of Small Intestine; Report of 5 Cases. New Eng. J. Med., *220:* 236, 1939.
9. Smith, N. D.: Rectal Polyps in Infancy. Surg. Clin. North America, *14:* 713, 1934.
10. Swinton, N. W., and Warren, S.: Polyps of Colon and Rectum and Their Relation to Malignancy. J. A. M. A., *113:* 1927, 1939.

CHAPTER XI

CONGENITAL MEGACOLON (HIRSCHSPRUNG'S DISEASE)

ETIOLOGY

Neurologic Imbalance.—Congenital idiopathic dilatation of the colon has long been associated with the name of Hirschsprung, who made an excellent description of the condition in 1886. As the name implies, the cause for the condition is not known, though there is accumulating evidence that the colonic portion of the parasympathetic innervation is deficient or else the sympathetic apparatus is overactive. It is difficult to prove which of these two explanations is the proper one, but there seems to be little doubt that a neurologic imbalance is the fundamental abnormality. Stimulation of the lumbar sympathetics is known to inhibit peristalsis of the colon and simultaneously to contract the internal anal sphincter muscle.

Reduced Bowel Sensitivity.—Aside from the alterations of peristalsis in the colon and the tone of the sphincter muscle, there is also a factor of reduced sensitivity of the bowel, because these individuals are not conscious of contractions of the colon which can be shown to exist by fluoroscopic examination or by colonimetric studies. Furthermore, distention of the colon by enemata does not produce discomfort unless the diaphragm and abdominal wall are stretched. The great diminution of peristaltic movements in these patients permits accumulation of enormous amounts of fecal material within the enlarged colon. This condition must be differentiated from dilatations of the colon which are solely the result of mechanical obstructions in the anus, rectum, or sigmoid. This latter type of case, called *pseudomegacolon* by some observers, is excluded from the following discussion.

PATHOLOGIC CONSIDERATIONS

The colon may be many times its normal caliber and it is not uncommon to find loops 6 or 7 inches in diameter in older children. Its wall has a leathery consistency and may be thickened to as much as $\frac{1}{8}$ or $\frac{1}{4}$ inch. The haustrations are largely or completely lost. Microscopic examination reveals *hypertrophy* of the longitudinal and particularly the circular smooth muscle coats. *Ulcerations* of the bowel mucosa are not uncommon. These erosions may be due to the continued pressure of fecal masses which do not move for long periods of time. It is not improbable, however, that the thickening of the gut wall reduces the size of the piercing blood vessels, so that ischemia is the forerunner of sloughing and mucosal ulceration.

These abnormalities may be found throughout the entire colon, but they are usually more marked in the left half of the organ. They may be localized to one part of the large gut, such as the transverse portion or particularly the sigmoid loop. The rectum is not universally involved, but shows some dilatation and thickening in most cases.

No morphologic changes have ever been demonstrated in the sympathetic or parasympathetic apparatus of the posterior abdominal wall, the mesocolon, or the colon proper.

The loops of the terminal ileum may be dilated but are not greatly thickened. This dilatation is presumably due to the obstruction which is caused by impaction of feces in the colon.

Occasionally *megalo-ureter* accompanies the condition of Hirschsprung's disease, and suggests that there has been an extension of the faulty innervation to involve the urinary tract.

CLINICAL FINDINGS

Hirschsprung's disease is a congenital lesion and symptoms are always present from birth or early infancy. When symptoms begin after the second year there is a strong possibility that some other condition is responsible for the dilated colon.

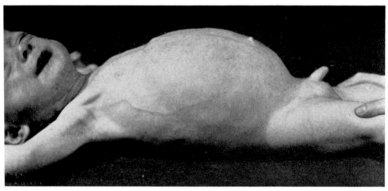

Fig. 96.—Photograph of three-month-old boy with Hirschsprung's disease, showing moderate abdominal protuberance. The abdominal distention was initially noticed in the first week of life.

Symptoms.—For many months the only abnormality noticed by the parents may be *enlargement of the abdomen* or *obstinate constipation*. There may be no movements for many days and, indeed, some of the patients often go as long as three weeks without defecation. While constipation is the rule, *diarrhea* may appear if fluid intestinal material is passed around the inert solid fecal masses which lie in the colon. In advanced cases *abdom-*

inal distention, fetid odor to the breath, *anorexia, lassitude,* and *malnour-ishment* are the rule. The diaphragm may be displaced upward and cause *atelectasis* of the lung bases. The distention may be so severe that respiratory and circulatory embarrassment culminate in death. *Vomiting* is seldom an outstanding feature. These individuals may have long periods with only moderate complaints, superimposed upon which there are episodes simulating acute intestinal obstruction. Hospitalization or medical advice may be first sought during one of these attacks.

Physical Examination.—By physical examination the abdomen is found protruding, and its skin is thin, tense, and shiny. Dilated veins may cross

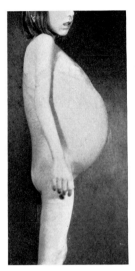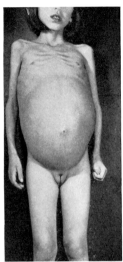

Fig. 97.—Photograph of seven-year-old girl with advanced degree of megacolon. Abdominal distention noted shortly after birth. This girl had extreme respiratory distress on entry to the hospital at which time the colon was even more dilated than indicated in the above picture.

over the abdominal wall. The umbilicus is often everted and pouting. *Auscultation* may reveal increased and high-pitched audible peristaltic activity, which at first gives the impression of acute intestinal obstruction. If the abdomen is very tense, *palpation* may be unsatisfactory, but more commonly an enlarged and thickened colon can be felt and outlined. On the basis of the physical findings the correct diagnosis can usually be suggested or made. Rectal examination reveals no obstruction in the anus or rectum. The dilated rectum contains impacted fecal material. Edema of the legs may be seen in severe cases. Orthopnea and dyspnea are present in extreme forms of the condition.

Varying degrees of the above clinical picture are encountered. In less severe cases, constipation and slight abdominal distention are all that is noticed and the child can get along without a physician's care. In more severe cases the condition will require some form of medical or surgical treatment. In advanced stages, the patient's malnourishment, toxemia, and respiratory embarrassment form a dire situation which demands urgent and effective therapy if a fatality is to be avoided.

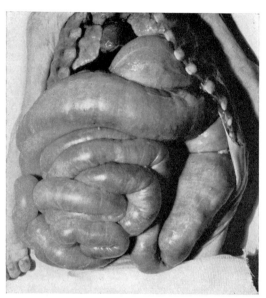

Fig. 98.—Postmortem photograph of a five-month-old boy showing moderate enlargement of the colon. (The small intestines are dilated because of obstructing fecal masses in the colon.)

ROENTGENOLOGIC EXAMINATION

The correct diagnosis is often suggested by a *plain film* of the abdomen which shows a markedly dilated colon (Fig. 101). The greatly distended organ may have a very mottled appearance if it contains inspissated feces.

Barium.—Examination with the use of a barium enema discloses no mechanical obstruction, but the colon is enlarged in diameter and in length. The great loops tend to overlie one another and seem to fill almost the entire abdomen. Haustrations are flattened out or are completely lost, and there is a diminution in peristaltic activity. A *postevacuation* film is important because this gives the best information concerning the capacity of the colon to empty itself and hence is an index of the severity of the lesion.

Examination with a barium enema must be done with some caution because the atonic gut may collect several quarts or indeed gallons of the barium mixture which the patient is then unable to expel. Some patients have great distress after such examinations and indeed a colostomy had to

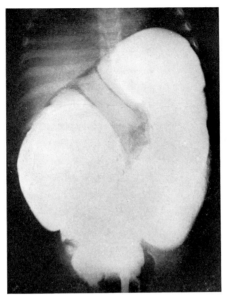

Fig. 99.—Roentgenographic visualization of a megacolon of moderate degree in a two-year-old boy. The haustrations are flattened out, except in the transverse colon.

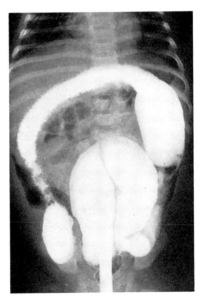

Fig. 100.—Barium-enema roentgenogram from a five-month-old boy with mild Hirschsprung's disease. The dilatation is limited to the descending colon, while the ascending and transverse portions of the colon have a normal caliber. (This child was subsequently effectively treated by a left lumbar sympathectomy.)

be made in one of our cases for prevention of what appeared to be impending death.

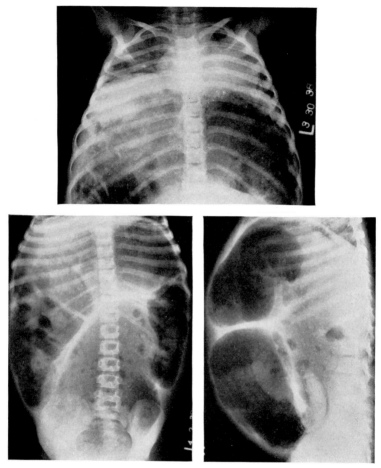

Fig. 101.—Roentgenograms from patient with marked megacolon shown in Fig. 97. The degree of respiratory embarrassment can be appreciated by noting the high position of the diaphragm on both sides. The anterior and lateral views of the abdomen show the enormously dilated loops of colon.

CONSERVATIVE TREATMENT

The type of treatment in a given case depends somewhat upon the severity of the condition. Many of these individuals are able to carry on an active life and to have an improved physical state if the *diet* is well controlled, *mineral oil* is constantly used, and *colonic lavages* are systematically employed. This regimen can be conducted at home if the parent is intelligent and cooperative, but occasional periods of hospitalization may be necessary if fecal impaction becomes troublesome, or if closer supervision is temporarily required to collapse the bowel.

Parasympathetic Stimulants.—The use of parasympathetic stimulants such as *physostigmine* has been rather disappointing, but *mecholyl,** *mecholyl bromide,†* and *doryl,‡* which are more potent activators of the parasympathetic system have given promising results in a few cases. These acetylcholine derivatives have an enhanced activity when combined with prostigmin. We have observed individuals with Hirschsprung's disease immediately after the administration of these drugs, and have found a greatly augmented activity of the colon. Within a few minutes the bowel begins to have contractions which are visible through the abdominal wall and which give rise to readily audible peristaltic sounds. Unfortunately, these contractions appear to be largely segmental ones and there is poor advancement of the peristaltic waves along the colon. Hence, little feces or gas are apt to be passed per anum. It is our impression that parasympathetic stimulants have a very limited use for the treatment of Hirschsprung's disease, but mild forms of the disease are slightly improved by the choline derivatives.

Dilatation of the Anus.—In occasional patients the atonic colon is found in association with a tight or spastic anal sphincter. There is no anal stricture, but the muscle has a tone which is greater than normal. This type of individual may benefit a great deal from anal dilatation. This is best done with hard-rubber or rigid, fingerlike dilators which are commercially available in a variety of sizes (Fig. 105). Starting with one about ½ inch in diameter, three or four increasing sizes are subsequently inserted, the largest being about 1¼ inches in diameter. The last large dilator should be left in place ten or fifteen minutes before it is withdrawn. Such dilations should be done each day for about a month, after which time they can be repeated two or three times a week, as the circumstances require. For the first few days the dilations may cause considerable discomfort and are better done by the physician, but after that time they can be easily continued by a nurse or parent. It is surprising to find that some children obtain remarkable relief and begin to have spontaneous bowel movements after these dilatations, even though no spasticity of the anal sphincter can be detected by digital examination. This experience in a few cases makes us feel that all patients with megacolon should be tried for several weeks on anal dilatations, and this regimen should be continued if effective.

SURGICAL PROCEDURES

While many individuals with this disease are relieved by supportive treatment, including dietary control, colonic lavage, and administration of drugs, there are a large number who must be treated by more radical meas-

---

* Acetyl beta methyl choline chloride.
† Acetyl beta methyl choline bromide.
‡ Carbamoyl choline chloride.

ures. Surgical procedures include three types of operation: (1) cecostomy; (2) resection of a dilated loop or a complete colectomy; (3) removal of a portion of the sympathetic apparatus.

1. **Cecostomy.**—In those patients with acute retention or severe distress, cecostomy may be a life-saving procedure. Opening the gut in this manner permits quicker deflation of the ascending colon and provides another route for administration of mineral oil, soapy solutions, and other fluids aimed at disintegration and removal of the impacted fecal masses. While cecostomy has its greatest value in acutely obstructed patients, it may also be used in other individuals when a thorough trial on a medical regimen has not been effective. In this latter type of patient, the cecostomy does not necessarily have to be a permanent one. We have treated several children by cecostomy (or appendicostomy) for periods of one to two years to allow the colon to regain some of its tone and have subsequently found that they have done rather well following closure of this stoma.

Cecostomy may be performed under local anesthesia, with either a McBurney or rectus-splitting form of incision. The cecum should be withdrawn and sutured to the abdominal wall before it is opened.

2. **Resection.**—*Local.*—Resection of a dilated sigmoid or transverse colon is an operation of some merit when the dilatation is largely confined to an isolated part of the colon. Selected individuals have considerable relief from such procedures for many years but there is always the possibility that the process may spread and subsequently involve other portions of the colon. Even so, the amelioration of symptoms for appreciable periods (fourteen years in one of our patients) makes local excision worth while when the disease is limited in extent. Segmental resection carries some risk of peritonitis, because of poor healing qualities at the line of anastomosis when a primary closure is attempted. A Mikulicz procedure should therefore be employed for local resections.

Complete Colectomy.—Complete colectomy may be justified in far-advanced cases when the gut is very thickened and dilated and all other forms of therapy have failed. If the colon has been properly cleansed and deflated the removal of the entire organ down to the lower sigmoid can be performed without undue shock. The great danger in colectomy lies in peritonitis, which is apt to result from disruption of the suture line when the terminal ileum is joined to the sigmoid or rectum.

3. **Sympathectomy.**—While the exact nature of the neurologic impairment in Hirschsprung's disease is not known, sympathectomy will often alleviate the symptoms, provided cases are properly selected for operation. If the condition is not greatly advanced and if the gut wall is not very thick, sympathectomy can be done with hope of mitigating the symptoms without producing any deleterious effects.

The abdominal sympathetic chains have an outflow through the first, second, third, fourth, and fifth lumbar ganglia, which lie on either side of the great abdominal vessels (Fig. 103). Repeated anatomic studies have demonstrated considerable variations in the number, size, and positions of these ganglia and their communications. Fibers pass medially from each ganglion to form a plexus over the aorta, the bifurcation of the aorta, and the promontory of the sacrum. The lower part of this network, called the *hypogastric* or *presacral plexus,* gives off branches which sweep downward along the posterior wall of the pelvis, to supply the rectum, pelvic viscera, and genitalia.

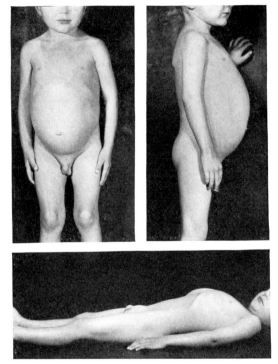

Fig. 102.—*Above,* Photograph of four-year-old boy with congenital megacolon and moderate distention of the abdomen. *Below,* Same patient following spinal anesthesia, showing great reduction in size of the abdomen.

Preliminary Study.—If sympathectomy is contemplated, it is well to study the patient first with a spinal anesthesia to determine what effects may be expected from eliminating the sympathetic control (Fig. 102). With anesthesia as high as the nipples, observations should be made to see if the colon has increased peristalsis, if flatus or feces are passed per anum, and if there is enhanced activity as shown by colonimetric readings. If the colon tends to empty itself or has an increased tone during spinal anesthesia, sympathectomy will probably be beneficial and advisable.

Methods.—The sympathetic supply to the colon may be interrupted in one of two ways. The lumbar chain, including second, third, fourth, and

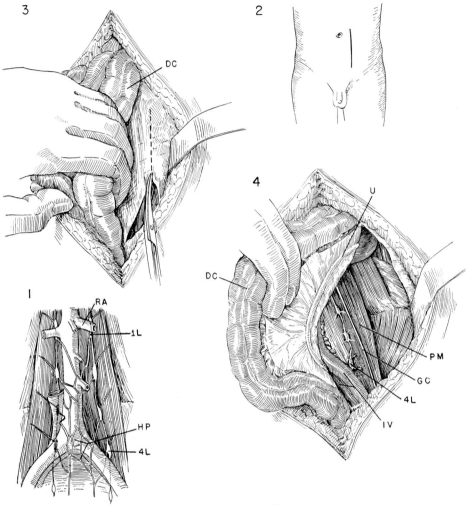

Fig. 103.—Sketches of lumbar sympathetic ganglia and operative removal of them by the transperitoneal route. *DC,* Descending colon. *GC,* Genitocrural nerve. *HP,* Hypogastric plexus of sympathetics. *IV,* Iliac vessels. *PM,* Psoas muscle. *RA,* Renal artery. *U,* Ureter. *1 L,* First lumbar ganglion. *4 L,* Fourth lumbar ganglion.

1, Position of the ganglia and their major connections. There is great variation in the number, size, position, and connections of these ganglia in different subjects. *2,* Position of operative incision in abdominal wall. *3,* The descending colon and sigmoid are retracted to patient's right so that the parietal peritoneum can be incised. *4,* Descending colon, sigmoid, and ureter reflected to patient's right to expose the posterior abdominal musculature, the aorta, and the sympathetic chain. The second, third, and fourth ganglia are the ones to be resected.

possibly fifth lumbar ganglia, can be excised (the chain on the left primarily affecting the left half of the colon). Thus, if the disease is limited to the descending colon a left lumbar sympathectomy is sufficient, but if the disease involves the whole colon, sympathectomy should be done on both sides. A second way in which the sympathetic supply to the colon can be interrupted is by a block removal of the hypogastric plexus and its branches. From a technical point of view this is a much easier operation to perform, but it should not be employed in the male because it interferes with the ejaculatory apparatus and produces sterility, while in the female it may interfere with sexual orgasm. Lumbar sympathectomy does not permanently alter the function of the bladder or of the reproductive system, provided the first ganglion is not disturbed. It does, however, produce vasodilatation of the leg on the operated side.

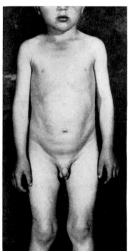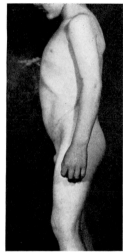

Fig. 104.—Same patient as shown in Fig. 102, following sympathectomy. Prior to treatment this boy often went three to four weeks without a bowel movement. After operation there was a spontaneous evacuation daily.

Technic of Lumbar Sympathectomy.—Lumbar sympathectomy can be done through an oblique, extraperitoneal incision similar to that employed for operations on the ureter. In children, who have little retroperitoneal and mesocolonic fat, a *transperitoneal approach* is quicker, adequate, and more desirable; it also allows direct inspection of the colon to determine the extent of pathologic changes. If the entire colon is then found involved a bilateral sympathectomy can be done at one stage, whereas with the extra-peritoneal approach a two-stage procedure would be necessary.

With the child in slight Trendelenburg position, a lower-abdominal, left *paramedian incision* is made (Fig. 103). The small intestines are walled off in the upper-abdominal cavity. The sigmoidal loop and lower part of the descending colon are then pulled toward the right and the peritoneum just lateral to these structures is incised. This incision allows mobilization of the lower descending colon and sigmoid which may be now reflected to the right with their mesocolon. The ureter usually adheres to and is reflected with the peritoneum. The genitocrural nerve stands out prominently on the psoas muscle and is a good landmark. Dissection is continued until the aorta and the common iliac artery are brought into view.

Groups of lymph nodes are encountered along the aorta. Between these nodes and the genitocrural nerve the sympathetic chain is exposed. The chain and its ganglia normally lie on the surface of the psoas muscle, but occasionally they are slightly buried within its substance. The first lumbar sympathetic ganglion rests just behind or below the vessels of the renal pedicle and the fourth ganglion is just above or behind the common iliac artery. The second, third, and fourth ganglia are now excised, removing as well the trunk which connects them. The colon is allowed to drop back into place and the peritoneum along its lateral border is sutured to prevent a retrocolonic hernia. If a *right* lumbar sympathectomy is performed, the cecum and ascending colon can be similarly freed by incising the peritoneum along their lateral border, reflecting them and the peritoneum toward the midline, and then exposing the sympathetic chain. The second, third, and fourth ganglia are excised.

RESULTS OF TREATMENT

To evaluate the results of therapy in Hirschsprung's disease is difficult. The mortality in any long series of cases is considerable, and it is axiomatic to say that no one has ever been permanently cured of this condition. While the final summary of results leaves much to be desired, one should not adopt a fatalistic attitude toward present-day methods of treatment. After any therapy a somewhat dilated colon may still be found by roentgenologic examination and the patient may have exacerbations of symptoms if not closely followed, yet a great deal can be accomplished toward diminishing the individual's troubles and improving his health. It must be emphasized that no one method of treatment will be effective in the care of these children. In mild cases, medical therapy will suffice, but much time and patience are required to control the diet, to supervise the disagreeable task of colonic lavage, and to establish regular habits of bowel evacuation—a routine which usually involves instructing the parent as well as the child. With more advanced forms of the disease surgical procedures are usually required but it will still be necessary to support these with continued medical care for protracted periods after operation.

Merely to list the outcome of various surgical undertakings results in figures of questionable significance because it does not take into account the original selection of patients on whom the various operations were done. However, a review of our material has partially crystallized our attitude toward these procedures and from this point of view it is of some value to list the findings to date.

1. **Cecostomy.**—Cecostomy (or appendicostomy) has been performed thirteen times with irregular consequences. In two patients it was a life-saving procedure when colonic dilatation had produced respiratory and circulatory embarrassment. One child died of peritonitis and in four others there was no improvement. In six there was moderate or considerable relief, for varying periods of time. In three of this latter group, the cecostomy was closed in one or two years, subsequent to which the patients have done fairly well at home under medical care.

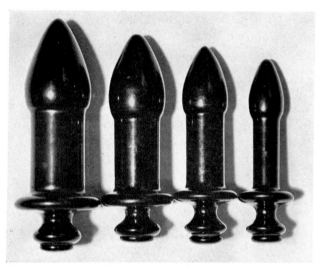

Fig. 105.—Set of four hard-rubber (Young's) anal dilators which are satisfactory for repeated stretching of a tight anal sphincter. (The largest dilator is about 1¼ inches in diameter.)

2. **Resection.**—*Local.*—Resection of a transverse colon or sigmoidal loop was performed in ten patients. One died of peritonitis. In one there was no improvement and in one there was slight improvement. One was improved, but died eight months later of endocarditis. One was greatly improved for fourteen years, after which there was recurrence and involvement of other parts of the colon. Five were greatly improved and in very satisfactory condition when last seen one, four, ten, eleven and twelve years, respectively, after operation.

Complete Colectomy.—Colectomies were done in three patients. In each instance all of the colon was removed except the rectum and lower sigmoid, which were anastomosed to the terminal ileum. Two of these died shortly after operation, from disruption of the intestinal suture lines. The third patient was extremely well for one year, after which time he developed ulcerations in the sigmoidal stump which perforated and produced a fatal peritonitis. While we were initially encouraged by the last boy, the final death of all three patients has now led us to abandon colectomy for treatment of this disease.

3. **Sympathectomy.**—Sympathectomies have been done in six of our cases. In two there was no significant improvement. In the other four there was a definite amelioration of symptoms which could not be classed as cures but which permitted a great reduction in the amount of medical care which was subsequently necessary. One of the latter children was found to have a somewhat spastic anus which the lumbar sympathectomy had failed to relieve; subsequent manual dilatation of the anus led to additional improvement. It is our impression that when restricted to early or only moderately advanced cases, sympathectomy is an excellent procedure.

Summary.—The treatment of Hirschsprung's disease might be summarized by pointing out that no one method or combination of methods is uniformly satisfactory in all patients, and indeed it is almost impossible to obtain a complete cure in any of these children. However, this note of pessimism must not obscure the fact that close medical supervision, combined with one or more of the surgical procedures when specifically indicated, can appreciably increase the emptying power of the bowel and can greatly improve the general health of the patient.

BIBLIOGRAPHY

1. Adson, A. W.: Hirschsprung's Disease; Indications for and Results Obtained by Sympathectomy. Surgery, *1:* 859, 1937.
2. Barrington-Ward, L.: The Abdominal Surgery of Children (Chap. 12). London: The Oxford Univ. Press, 1937.
3. de Takats, G., and Biggs, A. D.: Observations on Congenital Megacolon. J. Pediat., *13:* 819, 1938.
4. Judd, E. S., and Adson, A. W.: Lumbar Sympathetic Ganglionectomy and Ramisectomy for Congenital Idiopathic Dilatation of the Colon. Ann. Surg., *88:* 479, 1928.
5. Klingman, W. O.: Treatment of Neurogenic Megacolon with Selective Drugs. J. Pediat., *13:* 805, 1938.
6. Law, J. L.: The Treatment of Megacolon with Parasympathetic Drugs. J. A. M. A., *114:* 2537, 1940.
7. Morton, J. J., and Scott, W. J. M.: The Measurement of Sympathetic Vasoconstrictor Activity in the Lower Extremities. J. Clin. Investigation, *9:* 235, 1930.
8. Rankin, F. W., and Learmonth, J. R.: Section of the Sympathetic Nerves of the Distal Part of the Colon and the Rectum in the Treatment of Hirschsprung's Disease and Certain Types of Constipation. Ann. Surg., *92:* 710, 1930.
9. Stone, H. B.: Megarectum and Megasigmoid. Ann. Surg., *109:* 791, 1939.
10. Van Buskirk, E. M.: Roentgenological Studies of Megacolon Treated by Sympathectomy. Am. J. Roentgenol., *39:* 228, 1938.

CHAPTER XII

CHRONIC IDIOPATHIC ULCERATIVE COLITIS

Chronic ulcerative colitis is a poorly understood disease for which no really satisfactory method of treatment has yet been devised. While the condition is more common in early adult life, it is also found during childhood and may even appear in infancy. The *onset* is frequently acute but it may be rather insidious. The *course* is frequently severe, and leads to rapid emaciation, loss of strength, and possibly a fatal termination. However, not all cases are so serious; prolonged attacks may be followed by temporary recovery. In most instances the disease persists for a long period of years and seriously handicaps the health of the individual.

ETIOLOGY

Numerous theories have been advanced to explain the etiology of chronic ulcerative colitis. None seems to be entirely satisfactory, and no final opinion can be given concerning the cause of the disease. It is not impossible that the initial pathology or abnormal physiology is masked or overshadowed by secondary infection and inflammatory reaction.

Infection Theory.—Some investigators believe the disease to have an infectious origin. Numerous organisms have been considered to be causative agents. Bargen and his associates[1, 4] have described a gram-positive diplococcus which is thought to be the responsible organism. While the Bargen diplococcus can be obtained from a very high percentage of the lesions, it can also be found in an appreciable number of normal individuals and it is difficult to accept this organism as the primary factor in the disturbance.

Detailed bacteriologic studies have been made on many of our patients, principally by Dr. Leroy D. Fothergill. Cultures were taken from stools at frequent intervals and oftentimes they were made directly from ulcerations during proctoscopic examination. The results of these investigations have been very disappointing, because no single bacterium, or group of bacteria, of particular significance has been consistently isolated.

Neurogenic and Psychogenic Factors.—Lium[6, 7] has pointed out the possible neurogenic factor in chronic ulcerative colitis, and has put forth evidence to suggest that spasm of the colonic musculature compresses the perforating blood vessels so that local ischemia or hyperemia leads to necrosis and sloughing of the subjacent mucosa.

Contact with a group of these individuals clearly indicates that a large number of them have a complicated sociologic background or a psychogenic disorder. Behavior problems, familial maladjustments, or other complex psychologic disturbances can apparently manifest themselves by physiologic and later organic changes in some part of the alimentary tract, particularly the colon. Whether or not mental aberrations can initiate chronic ulcerative colitis is a question, but they certainly can aggravate the condition when it has once begun.

PATHOLOGY

The ulcerative process is subject to great variation in severity and distribution of the lesions. It usually originates and is more advanced in the rectosigmoid and descending colon, but a disease of some standing generally involves the entire colon. Occasionally the terminal ileum is also involved. The early appearance is that of a hyperemic and granular mucosa with small punctate *hemorrhages* and a loss of the normal glistening, moist surface. The mucosa has a diminished number of folds and bleeds after the slightest trauma; in the average case these are the only changes found by proctoscopy. *Ulcerations,* when they appear, are typically small and are placed quite close together, so that little unaffected mucous membrane exists between them. As the disease progresses, ulcerations become deeper and extend into the muscularis, which is destroyed or extensively scarred. All layers of the bowel can be penetrated; *perforation* with abscess formation or generalized peritonitis is the cause of death in many subjects. A large part of the colonic mucosa may slough away, leaving only islands of shaggy, swollen mucosa, so that initial inspection of the specimen suggests a polyposis of the colon. However, closer examination, verified by histologic study, shows that these nubbins are the only remnants of the mucosa.

Microscopic examination shows nothing which is characteristic of the disease process. The remaining mucosa is inflamed and possibly hypertrophic. Leukocytic infiltration is marked, particularly in the region of ulcerations. Inflammatory changes may be limited to the mucosa or they may extend through the entire colonic wall. Free perforation may be observed or diffuse scarring can be found through the muscularis and serosa.

CLINICAL FINDINGS

Symptoms.—In occasional patients the disease has a rather abrupt onset with what is thought to be an acute enteritis or enterocolitis. Commonly there is an insidious beginning and the first change is a gradual increase in *frequency of bowel movements,* which subsequently become more and more loose. They are accompanied by discharges of *mucus* and later of *blood. Tenesmus* is severe, and finally the majority of stools are largely blood and mucus alone. When ulcerations develop, hemorrhagic and purulent exudate is passed from the bowel. The defecations may be as often as fifteen or twenty times a day. *Abdominal cramps* and *discomfort* are common. A persistent low-grade *fever* is often observed, and higher temperatures appear if there is abscess formation or free perforation. *Pallor, weakness,* and *poor weight gain* are almost universal. In advanced cases there is extreme *weight loss,* emaciation, and retardation of physical development. The symptoms can continue for months or many years. Remissions and exacerbations are often observed; the symptoms seldom completely disappear during the periods of improvement.

Physical Examination.—On physical examination the patient exhibits moderate or advanced generalized debility. Pallor, weakness, and subnormal weight are evident. *Cachexia* and *wasting* are typical of advanced cases. There are few diseases which can produce the degree of emaciation which is characteristic of severe and longstanding ulcerative colitis. The abdomen is apt to be *tender,* particularly along the course of the colon. The firm tubelike bowel can sometimes be felt through the thin abdominal wall. Moderate or severe anemia is the rule.

Proctoscopic Examination.—Proctoscopic examination is preferably done under general anesthesia, for only in this way can one be certain that the end of the instrument will not damage the delicate wall of the colon and confuse the findings. Furthermore, tenesmus and discomfort of the individual make it impossible to insert a sigmoidoscope to its full length unless narcosis is induced. Grayish, mucopurulent, or hemorrhagicopurulent material may be found on the rectal or sigmoidal wall. When this is gently removed, the presenting membrane is congested and roughened; punctate hemorrhagic areas are scattered over it. No actual ulcerations may be observed, but if found they are apt to be quite small. The mucous membrane bleeds easily on the slightest trauma. These changes are diffuse and no normal mucosa is found between the lesions—a point of some importance in ruling out certain other ulcerative processes.

ROENTGENOLOGIC EXAMINATION

Chronic ulcerative colitis gives rather typical appearances by *barium-enema* examination. The haustrations are partly lost, and indeed there is often complete disappearance of segmentation. Because of spasticity or scarring of the wall, the lumen of the colon is greatly diminished. It is rather uniform in caliber; the colon is tubelike in contour and is shortened. The wide distribution of these changes throughout the colon is fairly diagnostic of the condition, and serves to differentiate it from amoebic colitis, which is more advanced in the right half of the colon, and is possibly limited to the cecum and ascending portions.

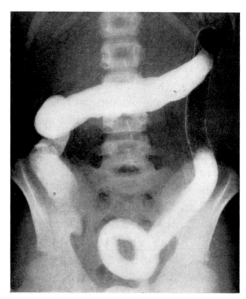

Fig. 106.—Barium-enema roentgenogram from an eleven-year-old girl with chronic ulcerative colitis, showing loss of haustrations, and a narrow, tubelike contour of the colon.

DIFFERENTIAL DIAGNOSIS

Chronic ulcerative colitis can be suspected in any child with a history of recurrent discharge of bloody mucoid material for a protracted time. Several conditions must be considered in the differential diagnosis.

Acute diarrhea, such as is caused by the dysentery bacilli and some members of the paratyphoid group, is usually typified by a sudden onset, short duration, and minimal general systemic reaction. The occurrence of diarrhea in other members of the family further suggests a self-limited, acute, and infectious type of colitis or enteritis.

Deficiency diseases, such as pellagra, beriberi, and sprue, must be considered when there is a history of dietary insufficiency. These conditions can be ruled out by adequate x-ray and proctoscopic studies.

Amoebic dysentery can generally be excluded by careful examination of several stool specimens by someone who is familiar with the cysts and the vegetative forms of Endamoeba histolytica. Such examinations must be made upon a warm stage and upon freshly collected material. If there is any question about the possibility of amoebic dysentery, a therapeutic trial with an emetine preparation is in order.

Tuberculous enteritis or *cecitis* can give rise to a chronic diarrhea with discharge of blood and pus. The *tuberculin test* is of great value in ruling out tuberculous enteritis in children. If the cutaneous test is negative with injection of 1 mg. of the substance, it is reasonably certain that tuberculous enteritis does not exist. If this reaction is positive, the patient must be carefully studied to determine whether lesions of other systems are responsible for the positive test. Tuberculous enteritis or cecitis is most apt to involve the Peyer's patches of the ileum and the lymphoid follicles of the cecum and ascending colon, and hence can usually be differentiated from idiopathic ulcerative colitis by suitable x-ray examination. If tuberculous enteritis can be reasonably suspected, properly prepared stool should be injected into guinea pigs for recovery and identification of the tubercle bacillus.

The diagnosis of idiopathic chronic ulcerative colitis is established only when the above-listed conditions have been excluded. Patients should have *serum agglutination tests* for Bacillus dysenteriae Shiga, B. dysenteriae Flexner, B. dysenteriae Hiss-Russell, B. dysenteriae Sonné, B. paratyphosus A and B, B. enteritidis, and B. abortus. Finally, barium-enema examination and proctoscopic study (under anesthesia) should always be done and the latter two procedures should be repeated if the findings are equivocal.

TREATMENT

There is a wide divergence of teaching concerning the most acceptable form of treatment of idiopathic ulcerative colitis. From the outset it must be recognized that the disease may have varying degrees of severity. In its mildest form a well regulated *medical regimen* can effect a complete and apparently permanent cure. More aggravated states can also be cared for medically; the symptoms and general health of the patient can be improved, even though some evidence of colonic disease persists. In severe cases *surgical relief,* by means of an ileostomy, can lead to great and possibly permanent improvement. Finally, in the most advanced forms, *neither* medical *nor* surgical regimens have much to offer and the mortality is astoundingly high.

Just where the line will be drawn between medical and surgical treatment is a matter of individual opinion. It is probably true that internists in general have leaned too far toward the conservative side, and have held patients under their care who might be improved by an ileostomy. Conversely, some surgeons have been too radical and have maintained that an ileostomy should be performed for the majority of these individuals. In the Children's Hospital series, approximately half of the patients have been under medical guidance, while the remaining half have had varying periods of medical care followed by an ileostomy.

Medical Treatment.—Adequate medical treatment requires *rest* and good general hygienic supervision, which in most instances can be obtained only by a prolonged *hospitalization.* Inasmuch as many of these children have important psychologic disturbances, every effort must be made to ferret out their troubles and to put them in rapport with the environment. Not infrequently this involves considerable readjustment on the part of a parent as well as the child.

Diet.—A low-residue diet will diminish mechanical irritation of the colon. Bland and simple foods with elimination of condiments and limitation of starches is desirable. Small feedings are better tolerated and are often more nourishing than large ones. Foods which are known to aggravate the symptoms should be scrupulously avoided. Attention must be paid to the adequate administration of *vitamins,* particularly the B complex.

Drugs.—Secondary anemia is combated by iron or in severe cases by transfusion. Paregoric or other opiates have no beneficial effect or else give only temporary relief. Soothing substances, such as bismuth subcarbonate, have very little to recommend them.

Colonic irrigations are worthless and painful; the possibility of perforating the bowel must be borne in mind. *Autogenous vaccines* made from cultures of the Bargen diplococcus isolated directly from the patients have had no therapeutic value in our hands.

Surgical Treatment: Ileostomy.—*Indications.*—Surgery may be necessary for the treatment of perforation, abscess, peritonitis, stricture, or superimposed malignancy. Aside from these complications which must be handled according to the requirements of the individual case, one must consider the possible benefits of procedures which are designed to alleviate the colitis itself. It is now agreed that *cecostomy* and lavage of the colon by this route has little or nothing to offer, and it has been generally abandoned. On theoretical grounds, supported by practical experience, placing the colon at rest by complete diversion of the fecal stream is of some value. An *ileostomy* will greatly ameliorate the symptoms in most cases, and indeed it may be a life-saving procedure for the patient who is rapidly declining with uncontrollable diarrhea. The establishment of an ileostomy unquestionably introduces several disagreeable features and some dangers, yet in properly selected cases the advantages outweigh the disadvantages.

Ileostomy should never be performed without an adequate trial on a well supervised medical regimen, during hospitalization, for at least two or three months and possibly longer. If permanent structural changes are beginning to appear in the colon, as roentgenologically indicated by shortening, loss of haustrations, and poor distensibility of the colon, surgical treatment should be thoroughly considered. Arrest of the disease before important structural changes have taken place gives the only hope of sparing the colon and allowing it to heal so that it can be ultimately reconnected with the intestinal tract. Unfortunately, permanent changes in the colon cannot always be avoided, even by early ileostomy.

Technic of Ileostomy.—Ileostomy can be established through a right lower quadrant McBurney or a rectus muscle-splitting incision. Temptations to explore and examine the colon must be assiduously resisted, because one never knows what part of the gut will rupture from the simplest manipulation. A loop of terminal ileum is grasped and the two limbs are sutured together (so that a crushing clamp can be applied if it subsequently becomes desirable to close the ileostomy). The loop is brought out through the abdominal wall, and the peritoneum, muscles, and fasciae are closed around it. If these are too tightly approximated, the ileostomy will be compressed and disagreeable symptoms of partial intestinal obstruction will result. Conversely, if the muscle and fasciae are left too loose, there may be a subsequent tendency for intestine to prolapse through the ileostomy. It is well to pierce the mesentery and separate the outer part of the two limbs by joining the skin between them. The intestine need not be opened for twenty-four hours or longer and in this way the wound will be sealed off before it is contaminated.

The ileum should never be transected and the distal loop closed and dropped back into the abdomen. It is well to have the distal loop opening on some portion of the abdominal wall, because one does not know when future developments in chemotherapy may bring forth a drug which can be conveniently run into the colon by this route. It has always been our practice to bring out the proximal and distal loops through the same wound, as above described. In this way it is relatively easy to reestablish the continuity of the intestinal-colonic tract if this should ever be warranted. If the operator contemplates a subsequent colectomy, the second stage will be made easier if (at the time of ileostomy) the ileum is completely divided and the distal branch is brought out above and medial to the proximal opening.

Postoperative Care of Ileostomy Patient.—When an ileostomy has been established, water and electrolyte loss through the orifice may be excessive and at first difficult to control, but with adequate administration of *parenteral fluids* a satisfactory balance can be reestablished in most cases. The withholding of solid food and fruit juices and the limitation of the diet to clear fluids, such as water, soups, beef broth, salt and sugar solutions for the first four or five days, will greatly diminish the tendency of an ileostomy to discharge excessive amounts of intestinal contents. *Paregoric* at three- or four-hour intervals during the early postoperative period is of some value in slowing down the intestinal peristalsis. While the ileostomy discharges are at first quite thin, green, and watery, there is a tendency for the ileum to take over some of the drying functions of the colon so that the material later assumes a semisolid form.

Protection of Abdominal Wall.—One of the most troublesome features of an ileostomy is concerned with the irritation or erosion of the abdominal wall by intestinal juices. The skin should be protected by some sticky, soothing drug, for which a combination of zinc oxide ointment, castor oil, and aristol, made up into a thick paste, serves admirably. It is well to point out that these cutaneous lesions are best treated by avoiding them. If the skin is adequately protected from the first, erosion seldom occurs. Thorough cleansing and painting of the skin every few days with tincture of benzoin and then reapplying the paste whenever the ileostomy bag is changed will keep the cutaneous surface in good condition in most instances. If ulceration has once developed, it is most quickly cured by placing the individual in a face-down position on a Bradford frame so that the ileostomy discharges can fall directly into a receptacle placed beneath the frame. The skin is thus kept completely dry and can be coated with medications to best advantage. Troubles with the abdominal wall can be greatly diminished if the ileostomy is made in such a way that a cuff protrudes beyond the abdominal skin (Cattell[3]) and fits into the rubber collecting-bag.

Subsequent Closure of Ileostomies.—The establishment of an ileostomy for chronic ulcerative colitis in the adult has been generally conceded to be an irrevocable step. A more optimistic view can be taken when one is dealing with patients in childhood, for in some cases the ileostomy can be closed after a variable number of years, and the fecal current returned through the colon without lighting up the local disease. One cannot predict which patients will be subjects for subsequent closure of an ileostomy. A short duration of symptoms before the establishment of an ileostomy does not imply that there will be a greater likelihood of subsequent closure of the opening. Indeed, some children with the longest standing lesions can have the ileostomy closed, whereas individuals who are surgically treated very early must have a permanent ileostomy. No prediction can be made regarding the length of time an ileostomy must be left open before it can be closed. In some cases there is sufficient improvement within a year to justify reestablishing the continuity of the alimentary tract; in others four or five years or more will be required before the ileostomy can be closed with any hope of success. In the majority of individuals the colon, while greatly improved, will never withstand having the fecal stream turned back into it.

Criteria for Determining Time of Closure.—The criteria for determining when an ileostomy can be closed are somewhat vague and as yet poorly defined. Study and reevaluation of the condition of the colon should be made at six-monthly or yearly intervals. Roentgenologic examination by barium enema may be of little importance in this regard, because increased amounts of fibrous tissue within the colonic wall will permanently keep its lumen small and tubelike. The clinical course of the individual is important. Adequate weight gain and establishment of a good general physical condition are essential but not sufficient. Rectal discharges of blood or pus indicate that the colon is still in a precarious state. Proctoscopic examination gives the best information concerning the repair in the colonic mucous membrane. Closure of the ileostomy should not be contemplated unless the rectal and sigmoidal mucosa appear normal by direct observation. Finally, as suggested by Stone,[9] the gentle introduction of a catheter into the anus and instillation of about a pint (depending upon the size of the individual) of physiologic saline which is then recollected will give considerable information. If the returned fluid is bloody by gross or microscopic study, active lesions can be assumed to exist in the lower colon.

RESULTS OF TREATMENT

It is impossible to compare the results from series of medically and surgically treated patients, because the types of cases are never analogous to one another. Within the medical group will be a certain number of individuals with exceptionally mild forms of colitis; the surgical patients will include advanced forms of the disease which have been refractile to all medical measures and which have been subjected to surgery in despair and even as a life-saving measure. Therefore, the number of fatalities will probably always be higher in the surgically treated group. A continuation of medical treatment in any given case does not necessarily insure against a fatality, because colonic perforation, marasmus, and superimposed infection take an appreciable toll of patients treated solely by conservative measures.

Therapeutic Possibilities of Ileostomy.—While there are certain advantages in the surgical treatment of this disease, the disadvantages of an ileostomy may make the treatment seem worse than the original complaint in the mind of patient or physician. Neglect of the ileostomy, development of cutaneous erosions around the intestinal opening, the unheralded discharges of fecal fluid or gas may all be extremely upsetting to the individual. However, with proper toilet and care of the dressing or ileostomy bag and with selection of a suitable diet, the disadvantages of an ileostomy can be minimized. While not belittling the disagreeable character of an ileostomy, the physician should not be blinded to the therapeutic possibilities of the procedure. It is surprising and gratifying to see many of these patients gain 40 to 50 pounds within a short space of time. In most instances the passages of mucus, pus, and blood from the rectum will gradually diminish in number, and while they may not completely disappear they are reduced to a tolerable level.

Some of the data from our surgically treated cases are presented in Table 15. It should be pointed out that an ileostomy has been closed in seven of these children. One died of peritonitis incident to the closure and another died of pneumonia. The remaining five were in good general health during the five years, five years, three years, fourteen months, and one year

TABLE 15

SUMMARY OF DATA FROM 22 CHILDREN WITH CHRONIC ULCERATIVE COLITIS TREATED BY ILEOSTOMY

Case	Sex	Duration of Symptoms	Age at Ileostomy	Result
				Fatal Cases
1	F.	1 year	4 years	For 2 years greatly improved. At 6 years ileostomy closed. Died 2 weeks later of peritonitis.
2	M.	8 months	8 years	Greatly improved. Three years later closure of ileostomy followed by colonic flare-up. Death 3 months later, respiratory infection.
3	M.	4 months	8 years	Some improvement. Nine months later colectomy, death from peritonitis.
4	M.	2 years	9 years	Died 1 month later, perforation of ulcers in ileum.
5	F.	7 months	9 years	Died 7 days later, perforation of colon.
6	M.	7 years	10 years	Excellent improvement for 2 years. Death from jejunal volvulus. Colonic mucosa almost normal at autopsy.
7	F.	4 years	11 years	Some improvement, then death 3 years later from adhesions and intestinal obstruction.
8	M.	7 years	13 years	Died, carcinoma of colon at 13 years.
9	M.	8 months	14 years	Died 5 days later.
				Surviving Cases
10	F.	2 months	4 months	Gradual improvement. Still has ileostomy and some symptoms at 6 years.
11	M.	4 months	11 months	Very satisfactory. At 3½ years ileostomy closed.
12	F.	5 years	6 years	Greatly improved, 15 months later ileostomy closed.* Entirely well in subsequent 5 years followed.
13	M.	4 months	7 years	Improved. No colon symptoms. Still has ileostomy at 12 years.
14	F.	2 years	8 years	Excellent result. At 10 years ileostomy closed. No recurrence in subsequent 5 years followed.
15	F.	3 months	8 years	Some improvement. Still has colon symptoms 1 year later.
16	M.	7 months	9 years	(Ileostomy too recent to evaluate result.)
17	M.	10 months	10 years	Improving in 8 months followed.
18	F.	3 years	10 years	Rapid improvement. At 18 years ileostomy closed.† Excellent health in subsequent 14 months followed.
19	F.	5 years	11 years	Very satisfactory. At 13 years ileostomy closed. Well for 1 year followed.
20	F.	9 months	11 years	Greatly improved. Asymptomatic 3 years later.
21	F.	11 months	11 years	(Ileostomy too recent to evaluate result.)
22	M.	4 years	14 years	Satisfactory improvement.

* Ileostomy and closure at another hospital.
† Closed at another hospital.

respectively since closure of the openings. There is, of course, no assurance that these patients will not have a subsequent exacerbation of colonic disease, but for the present at least they continue in a satisfactory state which has fully justified reestablishment of continuity in the ileocolonic tract.

BIBLIOGRAPHY

1. Bargen, J. A.: Chronic Ulcerative Colitis; Review of Investigations on Etiology. Arch. Int. Med., *45:* 559, 1930.
2. Cave, H. W.: Chronic Intractable Ulcerative Colitis—A Surgical Problem. J. A. M. A., *113:* 549, 1939.
3. Cattell, R. B.: New Type of Ileostomy for Chronic Ulcerative Colitis. Surg. Clin. North America, *19:* 629, 1939.
4. Jackman, R. J., Bargen, J. A., and Helmholz, H. F.: Life Histories of 95 Children with Chronic Ulcerative Colitis; Statistical Study Based on Comparison with Whole Group of 871 Patients. Am. J. Dis. Child., *59:* 459, 1940.
5. Ladd, W. E., and Fothergill, L. D.: Idiopathic Ulcerative Colitis in Children. Med. Clin. North America, *19:* 1673, 1936.
6. Lium, R.: Etiology of Ulcerative Colitis: II. Effect of Induced Muscular Spasm on Colonic Explants in Dogs, with Comment on Relation of Muscular Spasm to Ulcerative Colitis. Arch. Int. Med., *63:* 210, 1939.
7. Lium, R.: Observations on Etiology of Ulcerative Colitis. Am. J. M. Sc., *197:* 841, 1939.
8. McKittrick, L. S., and Miller, R. H.: Idiopathic Ulcerative Colitis. Ann. Surg., *102:* 656, 1935.
9. Stone, H. B.: Surgical Problems in the Treatment of Chronic Ulcerative Colitis. Arch. Surg., *41:* 525, 1940.

CHAPTER XIII

MALFORMATIONS OF THE ANUS AND RECTUM

Congenital anomalies of the anus and rectum are said to occur about once in every 5000 newly born babies. Some authors believe that such conditions appear as often as once in every 1500 infants, but this incidence is higher than is generally conceded. During the period from 1908 to 1939 inclusive, 155,997 patients entered the Boston Children's Hospital. In 214 of these there was an imperforate anus or an associated abnormality.

EMBRYOLOGY AND PATHOGENESIS

In the 7.5 mm. embryo (five weeks, Fig. 107) the tubular *allantoic duct* expands to form the bladder, which after receiving the *Wolffian ducts* continues caudally as the *urogenital sinus*. Posteriorly, this sinus has an extensive communication with the hindgut. Thus, there is a terminal cavity

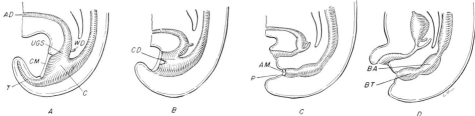

Fig. 107.—Normal development of the anus and rectum. *A*, 7.5 mm. stage. *B*, 9 mm. stage. *C*, 22 mm. stage. *D*, 42 mm. stage.

AD, Allantoic Duct	*CM*, Cloacal Membrane
AM, Anal Membrane	*P*, Proctodeum
BA, Bulbus Analis	*T*, Tail Gut
BT, Bulbus Terminalis	*UGS*, Urogenital Sinus
C, Cloaca	*WD*, Wolffian Duct
CD, Cloacal Duct	

common to both the urogenital and intestinal tracts, which is called the *cloaca*. The cloaca is a narrow, laterally compressed cavity which is closed off from the exterior of the body by the *cloacal membrane*. The intestinal tube extends beyond the cloaca into the tail, as the caudal intestine or *tail gut*. In either side of the cloaca, there is a longitudinal external groove with a corresponding internal ridge. Along this line of narrowing, the genito-urinary system will later become separated from the intestine.

In the 9.4 mm. stage there is further cleavage of the urogenital sinus from the intestine. This is accomplished by the downgrowth of a saddle of mesoderm between the urogenital sinus and the intestine, thereby reducing the opening between these two systems to a small passage called the *cloacal duct*. Normally, the process of separation continues so that this communication is closed off by the 16 mm. stage (seventh week).

In the 22 mm. stage (late in seventh week) a primary perineum is present. The perineum develops by the division of the cloacal membrane into the *urogenital membrane* anteriorly and the *anal membrane* posteriorly, and by a downgrowth and ingrowth of the mesenchymal elements between these two membranes. Late in the seventh week, the urogenital sinus has acquired an external opening, but the anal membrane does not rupture till later. A small dimpling of the anal pit forms the *proctodeum*, which inpocketing continues until the proctodeum and rectum join their lumina by rupture of the anal membrane. There is apparently a slight variation in the normal time of this rupture, but usually it takes place in embryos of about 30 mm. (eighth week).

In young embryos the rectal tube presents a spindle-shaped swelling which persists up to birth, although its form changes greatly. This upper bulbous enlargement (Fig. 107, *D*), termed the *bulbus analis,* has a position in the embryo which corresponds closely to that occupied by the rectal ampulla in the adult. Below the spindle-shaped portion just described, a second swelling develops which is much shorter and less well marked. It persists for only a brief period of embryonic life, and in specimens of 30 mm. it has largely disappeared. This lower enlargement, termed the *bulbus terminalis,* develops into the lower portion of the pars analis recti of the adult, namely the *zona intermedia.*

Pathogenesis.—Many of the rectal and anal malformations may well be interpreted as arrests or abnormalities of development arising in the seventh or eighth week of embryonic life. It is evident that an anomalous connection between the rectum and genito-urinary apparatus would be established if the cloacal duct failed to close. A rectoperineal fistula, however, would be formed if the anterior portion of the cloacal duct were obliterated, and if the remaining posterior portion were carried downward in the local growth of the region.

In the female, the rectal connections with the genital tract are doubtless formed in the following manner: The downward extension of the Müllerian ducts is at the expense of the posterior wall of the urogenital sinus, so that these ducts take over any already existing fistula to the rectum. The derivatives of the lower part of the Müllerian system, namely the vagina and uterus, can thereby attain an opening into the rectum.

Congenital anal stenosis (*Type 1*, Fig. 108) may occur at the anus or at a level 1 to 4 cm. above the anus. Such partial obstruction occurring at the anal site is the result of incomplete rupture of the anal membrane. A stenosis appearing within the terminal few centimeters of the rectum most likely arises because of incomplete development at the upper end of the bulbus analis or bulbus terminalis.

Membranous imperforate anus (*Type 2,* Fig. 108) results from a persistence of the anal membrane, an arrest at about the eighth week.

In those abnormalities in which the rectum ends blindly at a considerable distance above the imperforate anus (*Type 3,* Fig. 108) the embryologic origin is still obscure. Possibly the sequence is similar to that which Boyden[5] has carefully studied in the reduction of the hindgut of the ostrich. He has shown that as the tail gut disappears, excessive degeneration also involves the narrow, posterior, inferior part of the cloaca, which in man would correspond to the terminal portion of the rectum. Hence, if this resorptive process should extend to and involve the rectum, the upper portion of the rectum would end as a blind sac which is separated from the anus.

In those malformations in which the anus and anal pouch are normal, but the rectum ends blindly (*Type 4,* Fig. 108), an obliteration most likely occurs at the upper end of the bulbus analis, for this is the corresponding embryologic level. The common occurrence of such anomalies 3 to 4 cm. above the anus suggests a relationship to this embryonic constriction, which by its form leads one to believe that concrescence could easily take place at this point.

It should be emphasized that the *external* anal sphincter muscle develops from the regional mesenchyma, and is not dependent upon the presence of the terminal bowel. Hence, this sphincteric muscle is usually found in all the types of malformation under discussion.

TYPES OF ANAL AND RECTAL ABNORMALITIES

We have employed a classification of these cases which is valuable in determining the necessary form of treatment, and which is also useful for predicting the expected prognosis in a given patient. All of our cases have been placed, irrespective of any associated fistulas, into four groups, as follows, and as illustrated in Fig. 108. Classified as *Type 1* anomaly is the malformation having a patent anus and rectum, but with a stenosis either of the anus or of the rectum. As *Type 2* anomaly are grouped all conditions where there is an imperforate anus, the obstruction being membranous in character. In *Type 3* malformation, the anus is imperforate, and the rectal pouch ends blindly some distance above the anus. In the *Type 4* group, the anus and sphincter and lower portion of the rectum are all normal, but the upper portion of the rectum ends blindly and is separated by a variable distance from the lower pouch.

TABLE 16

DISTRIBUTION OF ANAL AND RECTAL ABNORMALITIES, IN MALES AND FEMALES

Type	Males	Females	Total
Type 1	13	11	24
Type 2	7	2	9
Type 3	75	87	162
Type 4	12	7	19
Totals	107	107	214

One hundred and seventeen of the patients (55 per cent of the series) had fistulas connecting the rectum with either the genito-urinary system or with the perineum; 45 per cent of the males and 64 per cent of the females had such fistulas. Four of these connections occurred in Type 1 cases, two

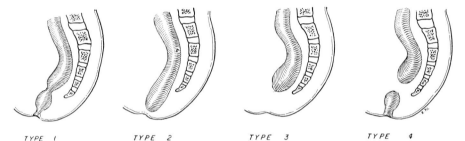

TYPE 1   TYPE 2   TYPE 3   TYPE 4

Fig. 108.—Types of anal and rectal abnormalities. *Type 1*—Stenosis at anus or at a point several centimeters above the anus. *Type 2*—Imperforate anus. Obstruction due to persistent membrane. *Type 3*—Imperforate anus. Rectal pouch ending blindly some distance above anus. *Type 4*—Anus and anal pouch normal. Rectal pouch ends blindly in hollow of sacrum.

in Type 2 malformations, and the remaining ones all had a Type 3 ano-rectal anomaly. In no case was there a fistula with a Type 4 malformation, but embryologically such a combination might be expected.

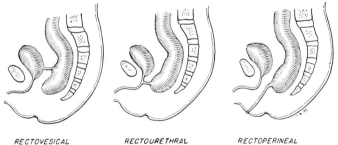

RECTOVESICAL   RECTOURETHRAL   RECTOPERINEAL

Fig. 109.—Types of fistulas encountered in forty-eight male patients.

In males, three kinds of fistulas are encountered (Fig. 109). The recto-vesical connections usually open into the trigone. The urethral fistulas open into either the prostatic or membranous portions (Fig. 111). The perineal openings usually appear just behind the perineoscrotal angle, but in one case there was a more anterior location with a bifid scrotum. We have had

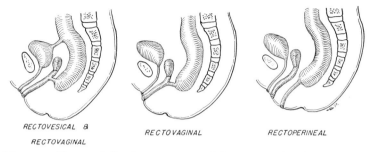

RECTOVESICAL &
RECTOVAGINAL

RECTOVAGINAL

RECTOPERINEAL

Fig. 110.—Types of fistulas encountered in seventy female patients.

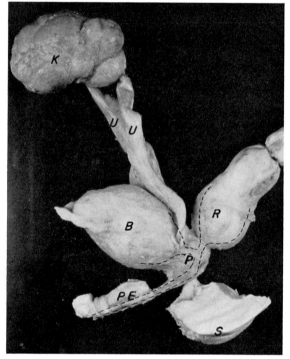

Fig. 111.—Autopsy specimen of imperforate anus. Type 3 anomaly of rectum and recto-urethral fistula from a male infant. The dotted lines indicate positions of lumina of rectum, bladder, and urethra. The rectum communicates with the prostatic portion of the urethra.

B, Bladder	*R*, Rectum
K, Fused Kidney	*S*, Perineal Skin and
P, Prostate	Subjacent Tissue
PE, Penis	*U*, Ureter

no case similar to those in the literature in which the rectal fistula opened on the undersurface of the penis.

In females (Fig. 110) the rectovesical fistula is a rare finding, and our only example of this occurred in conjunction with a rectovaginal one. The rectovaginal connections open anywhere along the posterior vaginal wall from the posterior fornix down to the labia, though they are particularly apt to appear in the lower third of the vagina. In one child with a septate vagina, there were two separate fistulas, with one to each side of the vagina. Many fistulas open into the fossa navicularis, just outside of the hymen. The perineal fistulas are seen from the fourchette back to the anal dimple.

TABLE 17

DISTRIBUTION OF FISTULAS IN MALES AND FEMALES

Types of Fistula	Males	Females	Total
Recto-urethral................	12	0	12
Rectovesical.................	16	1*	17
Rectoperineal................	20	10	30
Rectovaginal.................		59	59
Totals....................	48	70	118

* This female had both a rectovesical and a rectovaginal fistula.

There may be considerable variation in the *size* of these tracts. The external fistulas are often too small to permit evacuation of the rectum. Occasionally, only a small probe can be passed, while in other instances the opening is large enough to permit defecation if the stools are kept soft or liquid. Sixty-five of these 117 patients had such small fistulas that operative intervention was necessary in the first three to four days of life to relieve colonic obstruction.

SYMPTOMS

Complete Obstruction at Birth.—Since three fourths of the patients with anorectal malformations have acute obstructions from birth, they are seen in the first few days of life. These infants are brought to the hospital not only on account of symptoms of obstruction but also because the parent or the doctor notices that there is no anal opening, that stools have not been passed, or that meconium has come through an abnormal exit such as the penile urethra, vaginal outlet, or perineal fistula. The anal abnormality is often overlooked until the second or third day, when unsuccessful attempts are made to give the infant an enema or to take its temperature. The malformation is occasionally overlooked for months or even years when there is an associated fistula large enough to permit defecation.

Type 1.—These patients with stenosis of the anus or rectum naturally come for medical care later than those with complete obstruction. The *age* when they are first seen varies from a few days to two or three years, with an average of nine months. The chief complaint is usually related to difficulty in defecation. *Obstipation* is severe when enemata or cathartics are omitted. Not infrequently the stools are *"ribbonlike,"* because forcing of the soft stool through a constricted anus makes it emerge like paste squeezed from a tube. The parent often points out that the enema nozzle can be inserted into the rectum only with difficulty or at times cannot be inserted at all. *Abdominal distention* is commonly found in these cases, but vomiting is not a prominent feature.

Type 2.—These patients with an imperforate membrane are all seen within the first few days of life. The difficulty in each instance is apparent, for the obstetrician or parent discovers a complete anal block. There is no meconium staining on the diaper. For the first twenty-four to thirty-six hours of life the absence of bowel movements is frequently the only symptom noted, but at the end of that time *abdominal distention, vomiting,* and other evidence of obstruction develop.

Type 3.—In ninety-four of our 162 patients of this group, there was no associated fistula or else this tract was so small that it was ineffectual in emptying the rectum. Hence, these ninety-four cases had acute obstruction, and their symptoms were essentially the same as those of Type 2.

The remaining sixty-eight patients had fistulous openings large enough to support life for considerable lengths of time and were not seen as early in life as those in the last paragraph. The *age* when these first entered the clinic varied up to ten or eleven years, but the average age was fourteen months. Because of the relatively large size of the fistulas in these cases, there is rarely any complaint of nausea, vomiting, or distention. The patients are referred because of *pain on defecation,* difficulty in moving the bowels, or because the abnormal position of the rectal outlet has been discovered. The fistulous opening may be so large that incontinence develops.

Type 4.—The presence of a normal-appearing anus tends to make the parent and the attending physician overlook the possibility of this congenital malformation. Even with the administration of an enema the presence of a blind anal pouch is not always detected. Indeed, in only two of our nineteen cases was the information elicited that an obstruction had been noted inside of the anus. Repetitions of enemata and insertion of suppositories in the attempt to induce bowel movements tend to delay hospitalization. Thus, while Type 2 and Type 3 patients are often seen within eight or twelve hours after birth, these Type 4 patients are more apt to be brought in on the third, or fourth, or even fifth day of life. Therefore, the usual history includes marked *abdominal distention, refusal of food, vomiting, dehydration,* and *"toxicity"* of prominent degree. As a result, these infants are much poorer surgical risks than those of Type 1, 2, or 3.

PHYSICAL FINDINGS

Complete Obstruction.—A patient more than twenty-four or thirty-six hours old who possesses a complete occlusion has findings indicating lower bowel obstruction. These include the classical signs of *abdominal distention, intestinal patterning, borborygmus, tympanites, vomiting, dehydration,* and even *respiratory* or *circulatory collapse* in the later stages. If the infant is seen within the first twenty-four hours of life, the signs of intestinal obstruction are seldom found. In each instance the local examination of the anal region gives practically all the information necessary for classification into one of the four main types.

Recto-urethral Fistula.—A fistula connecting the rectum with the bladder or urethra is usually discovered immediately because of the passage of meconium or flatus through the urethra, but it may evade detection even with careful observation. This failure of early recognition is presumably due to plugging of the small passageway by inspissated meconium or to temporary closure of the tract by a flap of mucous membrane. Microscopic examination of the urine will show fecal débris or evidence of urinary tract infection in some cases in which a fistula has not been previously suspected. It has been our practice to repeat the urine examinations from time to time, because one negative urine sediment does not necessarily rule out a communication between the rectum and urinary systems.

More specific findings in the four types of rectal abnormalities are as follows:

Type 1.—When there is an incomplete rupture of the anal membrane, the opening is often no more than 2 to 3 mm. in diameter. In those cases with an obstruction higher in the anal canal, the anus appears normal but the stricture is felt a few centimeters above the anal orifice. When the stenosis is marked, the *perineum* is often seen to bulge downward as the child strains, and at the same time a *ribbonlike stool* is produced. The entire colon occasionally exhibits marked enlargement because of this anal or rectal obstruction.

Type 2.—The imperforate anal membrane is obvious. Because the obstruction is only membranous, a *dark discoloration* is imparted to the diaphragm by the meconium which lies against its inner side. The impaction of meconium against the membrane makes it bulge when the baby cries or strains.

Type 3.—These patients present a considerable variety of findings. The *perineum* occasionally has a small ridge in the region where the anus should be (Fig. 113), but a *dimple* at this site is a more common finding. This depression is of variable size and at times is large enough to admit a finger tip. *Puckering* of the skin is frequently observed when the external anal sphincter muscle contracts. If the blind rectal pouch is low in the pelvis, a finger placed on the anal region will detect an *impulse* when the baby strains or cries. A fistulous opening to the vagina, or the perineum, can give additional information concerning the position of the rectal pouch, because

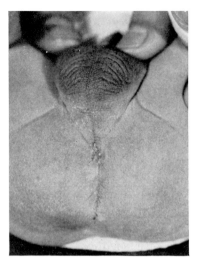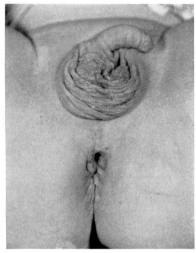

Fig. 112.—Male infant with imperforate anus (Type 3). *Left,* Appearance of perineum at one day of age, prior to operation. *Right,* Appearance of anus two months after proctoplasty (sphincter muscle has good tone).

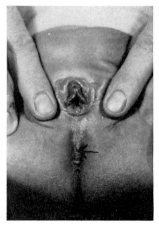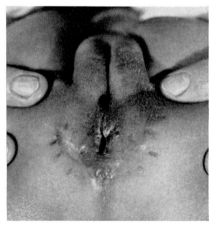

Fig. 113.—Female infant with imperforate anus (Type 3). *Left,* Photograph on first day of life. Arrow points to ridge of tissue where anal opening should be. *Right,* Appearance of perineum two weeks after proctoplasty employing a posterior curvilinear incision. (The anus has subsequently had good sphincteric action.)

a probe may be passed along this tract and then directed downward toward a palpating finger held on the anal skin.

Type 4.—These cases elude detection at first because the clinical picture of low intestinal obstruction with a normal-appearing anus arouses suspicion of a colonic atresia other than an anorectal abnormality. However, digital rectal examination always reveals a complete block within reach of the little finger. The anal sphincter is always present and possesses contractile power.

x-RAY EXAMINATION

Wangensteen-Rice Method.—In 1930 Wangensteen and Rice[29] published their ingenious method of determining the position of the blind rectal pouch in cases of imperforate anus by holding the infant with its head down and then making a roentgenogram of the abdomen and pelvis. The gas in the colon thus rises and outlines the distal extent of the rectal pouch, giving an indication of its position with relation to the anal membrane. Such in-

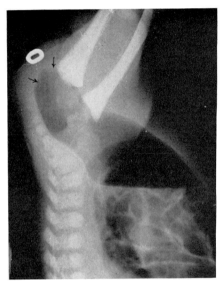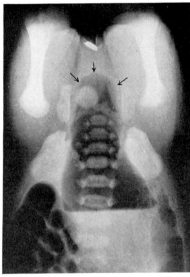

Fig. 114.—Roentgenograms of child with imperforate anus to show position of the rectal pouch (outlined with arrows) in relationship to anus (marked with an oval piece of lead). Child is inverted, so that gas will rise and indicate caudal extent of the rectal pouch.

formation is extremely valuable when deciding which approach (abdominal or perineal) is to be employed. We now use this method of examination routinely. Figs. 114 and 115 represent typical roentgenograms with the patients in the inverted position. Lateral films are better than anteroposterior ones for estimating the position of the rectal pouch.

Errors in Interpretation.—A word of caution must be said regarding this method of investigation. When this x-ray examination was first employed, we made two errors in diagnosis, for the leading point of intestinal gas had reached only to the terminal ileum in one instance, and to the mid-transverse colon in the other. We were therefore led to believe that atresias of the ileum and colon existed at these sites. Abdominal exploration of both

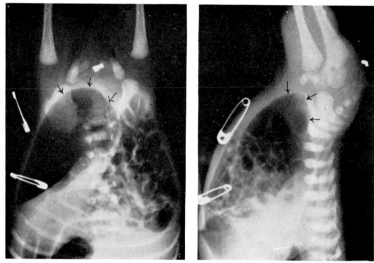

Fig. 115.—Roentgenograms to show position of a rectal pouch which is situated high in the pelvis. Child held head down. Gas outlines rectal pouch (marked with arrows). Lead marker placed on site of imperforate anus.

these babies revealed the fallacy of these interpretations. The errors in interpretation were made because gas had not yet been pushed along

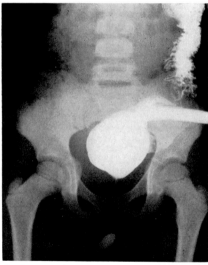

Fig. 116.—Roentgenologic examination of rectal pouch with barium placed in a colostomy. The metal coin indicates the anal region. An eight-year-old boy for whom a colostomy had been established (elsewhere) at one day of age. At subsequent operation, the high rectal pouch was brought down and opened in the anal area. Successful result.

through all of the sticky meconium at the ages of four and eight hours respectively. Thus, before fifteen to twenty hours of age, the absence of gas in the rectum cannot be taken as evidence of intestinal or colonic obstruction. However, by the end of the first day of life, an x-ray picture of the abdomen is an accurate method of determining the position of the blind rectal pouch.

Barium Colostomy Technic.—The x-ray is useful in another way, as is illustrated by Fig. 116. This case was typical of several others in the series. The patient was an eight-year-old boy who had been operated upon elsewhere at the age of one day, at which time the rectal pouch (Type 3) could not be found by perineal exploration, so a colostomy was resorted to. At eight years we first saw the child, and barium was placed in the colostomy to demonstrate the lower extent of the rectal pouch. Following this x-ray examination a successful perineal approach was made, at which time the pouch was brought down and sewed within the anal sphincter muscle. The colostomy was closed at a subsequent operation.

ASSOCIATED CONGENITAL ANOMALIES

Sixty patients (28 per cent of the series) had other congenital anomalies (Table 18) and some of these children had as many as seven or eight

TABLE 18

ASSOCIATED CONGENITAL ANOMALIES, WITH FREQUENCY OF THEIR OCCURRENCE

Abnormality	Frequency of Occurrence	Abnormality	Frequency of Occurrence
Congenital heart	10	Inguinal hernia	1
Harelip and cleft palate	4	Bicornuate uterus	2
Atresia of esophagus	5	Atresia of vagina	1
Hypertrophic pyloric stenosis	1	Septate vagina	4
Atresia of small intestine	4	Dermoid cyst of ovary	1
Meckel's diverticulum	3	Malformed vertebrae	4
Anomalous mesentery	2	Spina bifida	2
Stenosis of cecum	1	Pilonidal sinus	1
2 appendices	1	Meningocele	2
Atresia of colon	2	Supernumerary ribs	1
Transposition of colon	1	Supernumerary digit	2
Absence of gallbladder	1	Syndactylism	1
Absent kidney and ureter	2	Absent thumb	1
Polycystic kidneys	2	Bifid thumb	3
Horseshoe kidney	1	Absent radius	1
Ureteral valves	1	Absent metacarpal bones	1
Exstrophy of bladder	1	Dislocation of hips	3
Patent urachus	1	Extensive deformity of leg	1
Double penis	1	Absent metatarsal bones	4
Hypospadias	5	Clubfeet	2
Ectopic penis	5	Deformed ears	1
Undescended testes	3	Omphalocele	1
Bifid scrotum	2	Mongolism	2

other malformations. In seventeen cases, this *other* abnormality was directly responsible for death. Fifteen of these seventeen deaths were caused by a congenital heart anomaly, atresia of the small intestine, or atresia of the esophagus.

TREATMENT OF STENOSIS AND ATRESIA OF ANUS AND RECTUM

Type 1.—*Repeated dilatations* of the stricture usually suffice to overcome the obstruction and permit normal anal function. Such dilatations are performed with gum-elastic or metal dilators, the sizes of which are increased until the little finger can be employed. These dilatations are continued daily until the stools pass readily and until there is assurance that the trouble will not recur. This generally requires several weeks, but at the end of this period the parent is instructed to continue the procedure two or three times a week for four to six months. When the opening in the anal membrane is only a few millimeters in size, the obstruction is readily relieved by crucial incision of the remaining membrane and supplementing this with a few dilatations.

One patient had a marked stenosis about 3 cm. above the anal level. Because of extreme symptoms from this obstruction, it was deemed advisable to perform an *abdominal colostomy* first, and later to repair the local condition. The child unfortunately succumbed twenty-four hours after the first-stage operation. The suggestion has been made that this type of obstruction can be treated by making a *vertical incision* across the tissue and sewing this transversely to obliterate the constricting ring.

When a *fistula* is present, the entire rectum is freed from the surrounding structures, the fistulous tract is divided, and the rectum is brought down so that the rectal opening of the fistula can be exteriorized. This is the best way to insure against recurrence of the fistula.

We have had two deaths in the Type 1 cases, giving a mortality of 8 per cent. Of the twenty-four patients in this group, twenty-two are living from a few months to twenty-five years after operation, and all have a normally functioning anus.

Type 2.—This form of imperforate anus is easily treated by cruciate *incision* of the membrane followed by occasional *dilatations* with bougies or a small finger.

Our mortality in this group is 11 per cent. Of the nine cases, eight are living and have a normally functioning anus.

Type 3.—The form of treatment depends upon the position of the rectal pouch and the surgical possibility of reaching it by a perineal approach. When the pouch cannot be opened in the anal position, a colostomy must be resorted to. Of our 162 cases of Type 3 abnormality, 71 per cent have been amenable to treatment by a *perineal operation*. (If we include those cases who are now living with a colostomy, and on whom a perineal operation will be attempted later, we may consider that about 85 per cent of all Type 3 cases probably can be provided with a functioning anus.) The anal sphincter muscle is present in most of the cases, and an attempt should always be made to utilize it to control the rectal outlet.

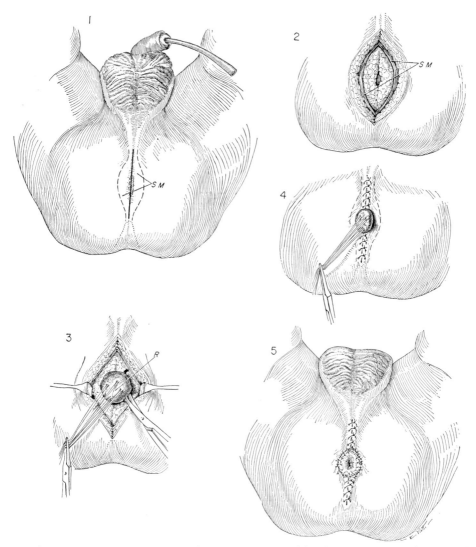

Fig. 117.—Plan of operation for imperforate anus with a Type 3 abnormality. *1*, Perineum viewed with legs drawn upward. Catheter in urethra so that urethra can be later palpated deep in wound. Dotted lines show position of underlying anal sphincter muscle (*SM*). Solid line indicates position of incision. *2*, Midline incision exposing deep perineal fat. Sphincter muscle (*SM*) separated into lateral halves. *3*, Blind rectal pouch (*R*) identified and pulled downward with traction sutures. Dissection continued so that rectum may be better mobilized. *4*, Rectal pouch drawn downward and skin closed anteriorly and posteriorly. Rectum thus brought between the lateral halves of the sphincter muscle. *5*, Rectal pouch opened, evacuated, and mucous membrane sewed to surrounding skin.

Extent of Perineal Exploration.—It is impossible to be dogmatic about how much one should attempt in perineal explorations. Certainly, a rectal pouch which is 1 or 2 cm. above the anal plate can be easily reached and brought down to the perianal skin. If the pouch is 3 cm. or more above the anal pit, the operator may experience great difficulty in mobilizing it in the tiny pelvis. In addition, there may be so much tension on the suture line that sloughing and a poor plastic result are produced. Therefore, we are now turning to the belief that a *primary colostomy* should be made when the general condition of the baby is poor or when the height of the rectal pouch augurs that difficulty will be experienced in reaching it. Undoubtedly, the mortality in any series will be less if this principle is adhered to and the proctoplasty is deferred until a second operation.

Technic of Perineal Operation.—For a perineal operation, the baby is placed in the lithotomy position (Fig. 117). An anteroposterior incision is made in the midline of the perineal floor, extending from the scrotum or vagina backward to the tip of the coccyx. This incision divides the external anal sphincter into two lateral halves. This splitting of the anal sphincter is necessary for an adequate exposure. Dissection is now made through the levator ani muscle and is carried up into the space normally occupied by the rectum. The fat here must be separated carefully; the dissection is carried close to the hollow of the sacrum to avoid injury to the genito-urinary tracts. A sound or catheter placed in the male urethra or in the vagina will aid in identifying these structures, so that dissection may be kept away from them. In some cases, a narrow and ill-defined fibrous cord leads upward and is attached to the blind rectum. When the pouch is identified, it is freed around its periphery so that it may be later pulled down to the perineum. Care is necessary at this stage to avoid opening the bowel, for if meconium leaks out the operative field is obscured.

Three or four traction sutures are placed through the tip of the pouch, each passing through all layers except the mucosa. Pulling on these strings brings the rectum down to the proper position between the lateral halves of the sphincter. The separated edges of the anal sphincter muscle and the perineal skin are sewed together anteriorly and posteriorly. The rectal sac is then opened and the rectal wall is sewed to the skin around the anal opening. Thus, the intestine has an opening *through* the external anal sphincter, and there is continuity of the epithelial surfaces of the mucous membrane and the skin. *It cannot be emphasized too strongly that the rectum must be adequately freed so that all tension is avoided when it is sewed to the perianal skin.* If tension is present, the sutures will almost certainly pull out and in a few days' time the rectum will retract upward, leaving a strictured zone which is almost impossible to cure by any subsequent operative procedure.

V-shaped or Curved Incision Posterior to Anus.—In two patients we have deviated from this operative approach by making a V-shaped or curved incision posterior to the anus (Fig. 113). This is so placed that the side arms pass lateral to and behind the anal sphincter. This incision has the advantage of giving a better exposure, but there is some danger of reducing the blood supply to the perianal skin. After this cutaneous flap has been raised, a stab wound is made through it at the anal area, and the rectum is threaded down through this opening before closing the posterior skin in-

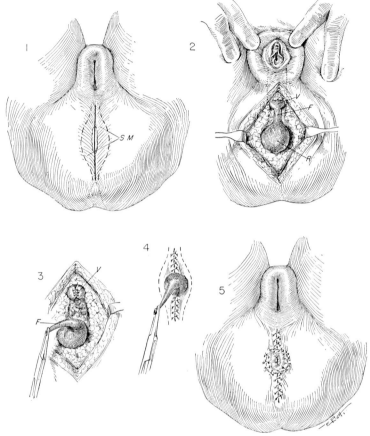

Fig. 118.—Type of operation performed for a Type 3 imperforate anus which has an associated rectovaginal fistula. *1,* Dotted lines indicate position of underlying anal sphincter muscle. Solid line shows position of incision. *2,* Dotted lines indicate lateral margins of vagina. The fistula *(F)* is exposed from blind rectum *(R)* to posterior vaginal wall *(V)*. *3,* Fistula *(F)* is severed and posterior vaginal wall *(V)* is turned inward with sutures. *4,* The mobilized rectum is brought downward so that the fistulous tract is exteriorized. Perineal skin closed anteriorly and posteriorly. *5,* Fistula cut off, rectum opened, and mucous membrane sewed to surrounding skin.

cision. In the two cases in which we have employed this incision and approach there has been no interference with the nerve supply to the anus and the functional results have been excellent. We intend to try this further in additional cases, but do not yet consider that we are fully justified in recommending it. Young[30] has suggested a transverse or curved incision in

12

the anterior part of the perineum. This would probably give an excellent exposure but great care would have to be exercised to avoid injuring the urethra or bladder if the patient is small.

Anal Dilatations.—About the tenth postoperative day, anal dilatations are begun and are continued until a functioning anus is obtained. The anal ring often becomes quite firm from postoperative reaction, and it seems that the anus will never be competent. But with persistence in dilatations, it is surprising to find that after three or four months the anal ring is pliable and possesses good muscle tone. The dilatations are conducted daily by the hospital staff for two or three weeks to make certain that no undue tension is put on the line of suture, but after that period the parent can be instructed to perform the task several times a week.

Dilatation of Associated Fistulas.—In eleven of our cases, there were associated fistulas to the lower vagina or perineum which, because of their large size, were dilated to permit defecation. These patients are being held over for operation on the anus and fistulas at an older age. Dilatation of a fistula has the great disadvantage of enlarging an abnormal opening, which is thus made more difficult to close at a later date. Dilatation of these fistulas should be done only if the child is in a precarious condition and cannot stand operative attack on the rectum.

Our total mortality in the group was 26 per cent. Of the 162 patients, 101 are living with a normally functioning anus, five are living with a permanent colostomy, and thirteen are living and awaiting further plastic procedures.

Type 4.—These cases are most difficult to treat because the rectal pouch is frequently so high up in the pelvis that it cannot be reached by a perineal approach. When the infant is in poor condition, a *colostomy* should be performed for relief of the intestinal obstruction, with the intention of performing a rectal repair at a subsequent sitting. Experience with this type of malformation leads us to the belief that it is better judgment always to defer the perineal operation until a second stage.

When the two blind pouches are separated from one another, their lumina can be joined by an *oblique anastomosis* to prevent postoperative constriction. Incision is made in the posterosuperior portion of the lower pouch and in the anteroinferior portion of the upper pouch. Suture along these adjacent edges gives a long, oblique union and an adequate lumen to the rectum.

Attempts were made to reach the rectal pouch *from below* in twelve cases. In eight of these (66 per cent) the continuity of the rectum could be established. However, in one of these a functioning anus was not obtained, and a permanent colostomy had to be established. Of the four unsuccessful perineal attempts, all had a colostomy performed at the same operation, and all the patients died. In seven patients who were in extremis on hospital entry, a colostomy was performed immediately without trying an anal repair; all but one of these died. In view of these discouraging statistics, it should be emphasized again that the best chances for recovery are assured by performing only a colostomy at the first operation.

Our total mortality in the group was 57 per cent. Of the nineteen patients, only six are living and have a normally functioning anus, and two are living with a permanent colostomy.

TABLE 19

METHODS OF TREATMENT IN FOUR TYPES OF ANAL AND RECTAL STENOSES AND ATRESIAS

Type of Abnormality and Treatment	Abnormality Cured*	Abnormality Uncured*
Type 1		
Repeated dilatations..............................	17 (1)	0
Stenosed area excised and rectum sewed down to skin through anal sphincter.............................	6	0
Sigmoidostomy...................................	0	1 (1)
Totals..	23 (1)	1 (1)
Type 2		
Incision of membrane, followed by dilatations......................	9 (1)	0
Type 3		
Rectum sewed down to skin through anal sphincter....................	111 (13)	0
Unsuccessful perineal attempt, followed by colostomy..................	0	13 (11)
Colostomy at first operation, perineal operation later...................	5 (2)	3
Colostomy, without perineal attempt............................	0	11 (8)
Dilatation of associated fistulas (perineal operation to be done at eight or nine years of age)...	0	10
No operation—died on entry.................................	0	9 (9)
Totals..	116 (15)	46 (28)
Type 4		
Perineal operation only...	4	0
Unsuccessful perineal attempt, followed by colostomy at same operation..	0	4 (4)
Colostomy at first operation, perineal operation later..................	2	1
Combined abdominal and perineal approaches at one operation..........	1 (1)	0
Colostomy, without perineal attempt..............................	0	7 (6)
Totals..	7 (1)	12 (10)
Totals for all 4 groups...	155 (18)	59 (39)

* Numerals in parentheses represent the number of patients who died.

TREATMENT OF RECTAL FISTULAS

The higher incidence of recto-urethral and rectovesical fistulas in the males implies that the results following treatment of fistulas were less satisfactory in boys than in girls. Because of different anatomic and operative considerations, the statistics vary considerably in the two sexes, and one must study them separately to gain accurate knowledge of the problems encountered and the results obtained. Tables 20 and 21 summarize the number of cured and uncured patients with the various forms of treatment.

TABLE 20

METHODS OF TREATMENT OF FISTULAS IN FEMALES

Type of Fistula and Treatment	Abnormality Cured	Abnormality Uncured*
1. Rectovesical:		
Attempt to close fistula at same time imperforate anus was treated.	0	1
2. Rectovaginal:		
Attempt to close fistula at same time imperforate anus was treated..	21	13 (2)
Repair of fistula at second operation.	1	1 (1)
Dilatation of fistula, nothing else done.	0	4
Dilatation of anus (Type 1); nothing else done.	2	1 (1)
No operation; died on entry.	0	5 (5)
No operation; to be done at eight to nine years of age.	0	11
3. Rectoperineal:		
Attempt to close fistula at same time imperforate anus was treated.	10	0
Totals.	34	36 (9)

* Numerals in parentheses indicate deaths.

Fistulas in Females.—*Rectovesical fistula* was unsuccessfully treated in one case by attempting to close it at the same time a Type 3 imperforate anus was operated upon by perineal approach. Unfortunately, the patient has been lost track of and no secondary repair has been attempted.

TABLE 21

METHODS OF TREATMENT OF FISTULAS IN MALES

Type of Fistula and Treatment	Abnormality Cured	Abnormality Uncured*
1. Rectovesical:		
Attempt to close fistula at same time imperforate anus was repaired.	4	13 (7)
2. Recto-urethral:		
Attempt to close fistula at same time imperforate anus was repaired.	1	7 (5)
Repair of fistula at a second operation.	1	3 (2)
3. Rectoperineal:		
Attempt to close fistula at same time imperforate anus was repaired.	14	0
Dilatation of fistula, nothing else done.		4
No operation; died on entry.		1 (1)
Totals.	20	28 (15)

* Numerals in parentheses represent deaths.

When one encounters a rectovesical fistula, it is probably better to make no attempt to correct it until the child is older. This plan is suggested, because it is almost a technical impossibility to close such a tract in a newborn infant. Furthermore, if the anal obstruction is completely relieved, the fistulous tract to the bladder will sometimes become spontaneously obliterated and thus obviate the necessity for secondary operation. It is true that this course may lead to urinary infection which may be severe and even fatal, yet it is surprising to find how often a rectovesical communication can be tolerated with little or no urinary disturbance. Thus, while it is not ideal to leave the fistula, it is the treatment of choice in a young baby.

Rectovaginal fistula can be repaired in about half of the cases at the same time the imperforate anus is operated upon (Fig. 118). This is particularly true if the fistula is at the lower end of the vagina. In the remaining cases a high fistula must be left until the local parts are large enough to permit satisfactory dissection. This is then begun by identifying the tract, and thoroughly freeing it and the rectum from the vagina and surrounding structures. The opening into the vagina which had been caused by the fistula is now closed. A suitable perineal body is built up. The fistulous opening in the rectum is now dilated so that it can be stitched to the skin at the site of the sphincter, to form the anal opening. Thus, there is no chance for the tract to reestablish itself.

Rectoperineal fistula is easily amenable to treatment by a mere excision of the entire tract and a suturing down of the rectal pouch to the skin in such a way that the site of the old opening is brought outside of the anal sphincter. In four cases we have dilated these low fistulas to permit evacuation of the rectum, but in view of the ease of attaining operative cure of the imperforate anus and the fistula, it would have been better to make the relatively simple repair in the first few days of life.

Fistulas in Males.—*Rectovesical fistula* in the male presents extreme technical difficulties because of the small size of the local structures and because adequate exposure is hard to obtain through the relatively small perineal wound. Of fifteen attempts to close such a fistula at the time the imperforate anus was repaired, there were only four in which the tract did not become reestablished. Of the thirteen unsuccessful cases, six patients are living and further attempts will be made to close the defect at an older age, when the larger structures will permit adequate operative exposure. Preliminary suprapubic cystostomy and possibly colostomy would aid the healing when the sinus is closed.

Recto-urethral openings in the male involve almost the same problems as do the rectovesical variety, and the same may be repeated concerning their treatment.

Rectoperineal fistulas, however, offer little difficulty at early operation, and a satisfactory repair can be uniformly obtained when this is attempted in the first few days of life. In four instances we have repeatedly dilated such fistulas in order to delay performance of the anoplasty, but there is little merit in such a choice, since permanent and good results can be expected from early recourse to surgery. The method of operative treatment is the same as that in females.

RESULTS OF TREATMENT

The essential in treatment of these rectal and anal abnormalities is to establish a continuity of epithelium between the rectum and skin and thus prevent scar formation and constriction. To provide adequate anal control, the external sphincter muscle must always be utilized. In the stenoses (Type 1) repeated dilatations are usually all that is necessary, but when the anal canal is unyielding, it must be excised and the rectal mucosa brought down to cover the defect. In the membranous imperforate anus (Type 2) simple cruciate incision and dilatations suffice. The rectal atresias (Types 3 and 4) are treated by a perineal operation (when the pouch is low enough) and the rectum is brought down to the skin through the anal sphincter muscle. When the pouch is high and prohibits a successful perineal operation, a colostomy should be resorted to. In Type 3 atresias, about 85 per cent of the cases are amenable to treatment by the perineal approach. In Type 4 atresias, approximately 66 per cent of the cases are amenable to treatment by the perineal operation provided that a colostomy has been previously made.

There were fifty-seven deaths in the Children's Hospital series, giving a mortality of 26 per cent. At least seventeen of these deaths were directly due to other associated congenital abnormalities and their complications. By groups the mortality rates were: Type 1, 8 per cent; Type 2, 11 per cent; Type 3, 26 per cent; Type 4, 57 per cent.

The lower fistulas (rectoperineal and rectovaginal) are relatively easy to close when the rectal obstruction is corrected in the first few days of life. The higher fistulas (recto-urethral and rectovesical), however, are very difficult to reach through a perineal incision in a newborn infant; hence it is found best to delay treatment of such communications until the patient attains an age of six to nine years.

BIBLIOGRAPHY

1. Barney, J. D.: The Urological Complications of Imperforate Anus. Trans. Am. Assoc. G. U. Surg., *21:* 393, 1928.
2. Berman, J. K.: Congenital Anomalies of the Rectum and Anus. Surg., Gynec. and Obst., *66:* 11, 1938.
3. Bevan, A. D.: Imperforate Anus. Surg. Clinics Chicago, *4:* 21, 1920.
4. Bodenhamer, W. H.: Congenital Malformations of the Rectum and Anus. New York: Wood, 1860.
5. Boyden, E. A.: The Early Development of the Cloaca in Ostrich Embryos with Special Reference to the Reduction of the Caudal Intestine. Anat. Record, *24:* 211, 1922.

6. Brenner, E. C.: Congenital Defects of the Anus and Rectum. Surg., Gynec. and Obst., *20:* 585, 1915.

7. Cripps, H.: Diseases of the Rectum and Anus. New York: Macmillan, 1914, p. 26.

8. David, V. C.: Embryology and Malformations of the Rectum. In Nelson's Loose Leaf Living Surgery, *5:* 161.

9. David, V. C.: Congenital Stricture of the Rectum in Children. Surg. Clin. North America, *3:* 1115, 1923.

10. David, V. C.: The Treatment of Congenital Openings of the Rectum Into the Vagina—Atresia Ani Vaginalis. Surgery, *1:* 163, 1937.

11. Felix, W.: The Development of the Urinogenital Organs. In Keibel and Mall's Manual of Human Embryology. Philadelphia: Lippincott, 1912, *2:* 752.

12. Fichet, S. M.: Imperforate Anus. Boston M. and S. J., *195:* 25, 1926.

13. Hunter, R. H.: Observation on the Development of the Human Female Genital Tract. Carnegie Inst. of Washington; Publ., *414:* 91, 1930.

14. Johnson, F. P.: The Development of the Rectum in the Human Embryo. Am. J. Anat., *16:* 1, 1914.

15. Keibel, F.: Zur Entwicklungsgeschichte des menschlichen Urogenitalapparatus. Arch. f. Anat. u. Entwcklngsges., 1896, p. 55.

16. Keibel and Mall: Manual of Human Embryology. Philadelphia: Lippincott, 1912, *2:* 306.

17. Keith, Sir A.: Malformations of the Hind End of the Body. Brit. M. J., *2:* 1736, 1908.

18. Keith, Sir A.: Malformations of the Human Body from a New Point of View. Brit. M. J., *1:* 489, 1932.

19. Ladd, W. E. and Gross, R. E.: Congenital Malformations of Anus and Rectum. Am. J. Surg., *23:* 167, 1934.

20. Lewis, F. T.: The Development of the Digestive Tract. In Keibel and Mall's Manual of Human Embryology. Philadelphia: Lippincott, 1912, *2:* 306.

21. Parin, B.: Atresia Ani Urethralis. Arch. f. klin. Chir., *166:* 386, 1931.

22. Pohlman, A. G.: The Development of the Cloaca in Human Embryos. Am. J. Anat., *12:* 1, 1911.

23. Politzer, G.: Ueber die Entwicklung des Dammes beim Menschen. Ztschr. f. Anat. u. Entwcklngsges., *97:* 622, 1932.

24. Retterer, M. E.: Mode de cloisonnement du cloaque chez le cobaye. Bibliog. Anat., *1:* 184, 1893.

25. Stieda, A.: Ueber Atresia ani congenita und die damit verbundenen Missbildungen. Arch. f. klin. Chir., *70:* 555, 1903.

26. Thunig, L. A.: Atresia Ani Urethralis. Arch. Surg., *38:* 501, 1939.

27. Tourneux, F.: Sur le mode de cloisonnement du cloaque. Bibliog. Anat., *2:* 99, 1894.

28. Tuttle, J. P.: Diseases of the Anus, Rectum and Pelvic Colon. New York: Appleton, 1906, p. 47.

29. Wangensteen, O. H., and Rice, C. O.: Imperforate Anus—a Method of Determining the Surgical Approach. Ann. Surg., *92:* 77, 1930.

30. Young, H. H.: Imperforate Anus: Bowel Opening into Urethra; Hypospadias. A Presentation of New Plastic Methods. J. A. M. A., *107:* 1448, 1936.

CHAPTER XIV

PRIMARY PERITONITIS

Grouped together as cases of "secondary" peritonitis are those which originate from a focus in some abdominal viscus, such as an inflamed appendix, a perforated Meckel's diverticulum, or an ulcerated colon. Quite distinct from these is the condition of "primary," "idiopathic," or "metastatic" peritonitis, which has no focus of infection within the peritoneal cavity and which presents quite a different problem of diagnosis, treatment, and prognosis. The responsible organism in these cases is almost invariably a pneumococcus or a hemolytic streptococcus; the latter is about twice as common as the former.

Primary peritonitis has been described in all age groups and has been observed in elderly individuals, but it is essentially a disease of infancy and early childhood. Two thirds of the cases occur within the first four years of life. Peritonitis of this type carried an extremely high mortality rate until a few years ago, but the more recent use of chemotherapy, antipneumococcus serum, improved supportive treatment, and a more logical surgical approach are continually increasing the number of recoveries.

PATHOLOGY AND ETIOLOGY

Exudate.—The inflammatory process diffusely affects the parietal and visceral peritoneum and small accumulations of fluid appear between the intestinal loops. This exudate is thin, slightly cloudy, and contains small flecks of fibrin if the streptococcus is present. If a pneumococcus is present, the fluid tends to be a little thicker early in the course of the disease. Later, the pneumococcal exudate becomes definitely fibrinopurulent or even plastic and the visceral and parietal peritoneum becomes coated with a thick layer of fibrin similar to that found in cases of pneumococcal empyema. The mesenteric lymph glands are pale, swollen, and usually prominent.

Not infrequently, a surgeon opens the right lower quadrant of one of these abdomens, and finding the appendix red and injected, will suppose that the peritonitis originated there. The appendix in such cases is no more involved than are other viscera, and appendectomy is a useless, and indeed a harmful, procedure. Collection of the exudate into isolated pockets of pus occurs much less frequently in cases of primary peritonitis than it does in those of the secondary type. Walled-off *abscesses* are occasionally formed, but it is more characteristic for the peritoneal infection to kill the individual quickly, or to disappear completely and leave no traces.

Causative Organisms.—In a series of 120 patients at the Children's Hospital, the peritoneal fluid contained a hemolytic streptococcus in eighty-five and a pneumococcus in thirty-five. The types of pneumococci involved have not been noted in the majority of previous publications, but the available studies show a preponderance of Type I. In seventeen of our patients for whom typing was performed, there were five of Type I, four of Type VI, two of Type V, and one each of Types IV, VIII, X, XI, XVIII, and XXII. No conclusions could be drawn relating the type of pneumococcus to the severity of the peritonitis.

Paths of Invasion.—The avenues by which organisms enter the coelomic cavity cannot be accurately determined. Some authors have conjectured that bacteria invade the female *genital tract* and ascend by way of the uterus and its tubes into the pelvic peritoneum. This theory, of course, utterly fails to explain the mode of infection in males. It is our belief that invasion by way of the uterus occurs but rarely, because autopsy examination of our fatal female cases has never shown evidence of ascending genital tract infection. The *gastro-intestinal tract* may serve as a source of infection in rare cases in which pathologic examination has shown a severe inflammation of all of the enteric coats. The *transdiaphragmatic lymphatics* have also been incriminated, but they certainly cannot be a common portal of infection because a preceding pneumonia or empyema is rarely a part of the picture.

The *blood stream* is probably the path by which bacteria reach the peritoneum in most cases. This belief is supported by the frequent occurrence of an upper respiratory infection during or just preceding the peritonitis and by the number of bacteremias which can be demonstrated by cultural means. Blood cultures were made on thirty-one of our patients. Twelve of these had a pneumococcal infection of the peritoneum and the same organism was recovered from the blood stream of ten; nineteen had a Streptococcus hemolyticus infection of the peritoneum and this organism was found in the blood of five. In short, about half the individuals had a known blood stream infection, and repeated or earlier cultures would probably have uncovered more cases with a transient bacteremia.

The somewhat higher incidence of primary peritonitis among charity patients than among private ones suggests that lowered standards of living and a diminished resistance might play a role in susceptibility to this type of infection.

SYMPTOMS AND SIGNS

Primary peritonitis appears with about equal frequency in males and females.

Symptoms.—Infants or young children are most frequently affected, for the majority of patients are less than four years of age. The illness commonly, but not always, begins with a head cold or other *respiratory tract* *infection.* The onset of abdominal symptoms is sometimes masked by the respiratory infection or an accompanying diarrhea. When the abdominal involvement has become established, the symptoms are severe and rapidly progressive. Older children may complain of diffuse *abdominal pain;* babies exhibit this by crying, restlessness, or irritability. *Vomiting* is frequent and may produce marked *dehydration.* A *fever* higher than that found in other types of peritonitis and excessive perspiration are common. *Diarrhea* is found in about half of the cases, particularly during the first day of intestinal irritation, but it is apt to be followed by constipation.

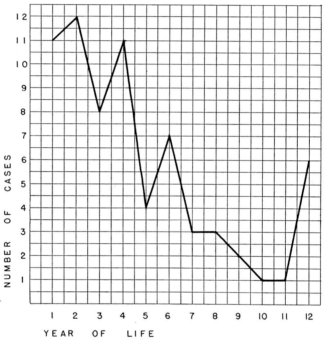

Fig. 119.—Graph showing age incidence of primary peritonitis in sixty-nine patients. The disease is most common in infancy and early childhood. Two-thirds of the patients are less than four years of age.

Physical Findings.—On physical examination, the individual appears extremely ill. The *facies* is drawn and worn, and the eyes are sunken and listless. An upper respiratory infection may be present. The *temperature* is elevated to 104° or 105° F. and the *pulse* is correspondingly rapid. The abdomen is diffusely *tender.* Should an inguinal hernia be present, there may be thickening and tenderness along the sac which extends downward in the inguinal canal. In older individuals the abdomen may have a board-like rigidity, but in babies it is more apt to be soft and *"doughy."* Some degree of *distention* is the rule, and a protuberant and slightly tender abdomen may be the only local findings if the patient is an infant. Shifting dullness of abdominal fluid can be made out but rarely. Peristaltic activity may be found to be increased by auscultation during early stages of the infection, but it is greatly diminished in later periods. Dry mucous membranes, sunken eyes, inelastic skin, and dry, coated tongue are evidences of dehydration. Rectal examination reveals diffuse tenderness, but usually there is no pelvic mass.

The *white blood count* is almost invariably elevated, and varies between 20,000 and 50,000; the polymorphonuclear leukocytes are 80 to 90 per cent or more. The *red blood count* may be slightly or moderately depressed, particularly in the streptococcal infections of several days' standing. Urinalysis commonly shows an acetonuria, but is otherwise not remarkable.

DIFFERENTIAL DIAGNOSIS

There is no way definitely to differentiate clinically between *pneumococcal* or *streptococcal forms* of peritonitis. If throat smears or cultures show a predominance of one of these organisms, the same bacteria may be responsible for the peritoneal infection, but one can be misled by such an assumption. A positive blood culture gives good presumptive evidence of the type of organism which is affecting the abdomen. While it is usually impossible prior to operation to differentiate between streptococcal and pneumococcal forms of peritonitis, these can usually be distinguished from secondary peritonitis. In the present series a correct preoperative diagnosis of primary peritonitis was made in 68 per cent of the cases.

Primary peritonitis is most likely to be confused with *generalized peritonitis* which is secondary to a ruptured appendix. In the latter condition the symptoms are maximal on the right side of the abdomen at the beginning of the illness, whereas in primary peritonitis the pain and tenderness are generalized from the outset. An age of less than three years, initiation of the illness by a chill, and a very stormy course from the start, are all suggestive of a primary type of infection. Fever and leukocytosis are usually higher with the primary form. It is uncommon for patients having peritonitis of appendiceal origin to have a temperature over 103° F., while those having a primary peritonitis commonly show a temperature of 104° or even 105° F., and rarely one below 103° F.

The other condition which is particularly difficult to differentiate from primary peritonitis is *pneumonia* in its early stages. This is especially so in small infants, and, in fact, it is not too uncommon for the two conditions to coexist. In early pneumonia all the symptoms found in peritonitis are likely to be present—vomiting, chill, high temperature, and high leukocyte count. The chest signs in pneumonia may be slight and hard to demonstrate, and the abdomen is often distended and resistant. An unduly elevated respiratory rate and lack of abdominal tenderness are the two most important factors lending support to a diagnosis of pneumonia. An x-ray examination will usually clarify this confusing picture.

TREATMENT

Forms of treatment advocated for primary peritonitis vary from abdominal exploration and appendectomy on the one hand to recent suggestions of no operation and chemotherapy on the other. We do not agree with either of these extremes and believe that a middle course is usually productive of the best results. Certainly, there can be no question about the harm inflicted by extensive packing, retraction, and manipulation within the abdominal cavity in the attempt to find a source of peritoneal infection. Appendectomy under such circumstances is certainly to be condemned. Such operative measures are followed by a forbidding mortality which in some published series has run as high as 100 per cent.

Operation versus Chemotherapy.—The present tendency to advise against operation and to rely entirely on chemotherapy and supportive measures may prove in the long run to give the most favorable results, but we have not subscribed to it for three reasons: (1) It is desirable to have a specimen of the peritoneal exudate to direct more intelligently the administration of chemotherapy and serum treatment. Thus, if a streptococcus is present, sulfanilamide is preferred, but if a pneumococcus is found sulfapyridine (or sulfathiazole) and possibly an antipneumococcus serum will be more efficacious. A sample of peritoneal exudate for this study can be obtained by abdominal tap. Risk of injury to the bowel is completely avoided by making a tiny abdominal opening and obtaining the material under direct vision. (2) The peritonitis may not be a primary one, as supposed, and considerable harm may be done by allowing a ruptured appendix to seed the peritoneal cavity continually with highly infected material. (3) The insertion of a drain into the abdominal cavity provides an escape for exudate, which diminishes the patient's toxicity.

Abdominal Exploration and Drainage.—For these reasons we advise operation—of a very limited sort—for such patients. Under morphine sedation and local novocain infiltration of the abdominal wall a small, rectus-splitting incision ¾ inch long is made in the right lower quadrant (Fig. 120). With two narrow finger retractors to separate the wound edges, the peritoneum can be adequately exposed and slit open for about ½ inch. Without disturbing intestinal loops, the operator is now able to obtain a sample of peritoneal fluid on a swab, or to suck it up in a syringe. If this is odorless and has the other characteristics of pneumococcal or streptococcal pus, a primary form of peritonitis should be suspected at once, and nothing further done until an assistant can smear, stain, and microscopically examine some of the pus.

If pneumococci or streptococci are thus identified, a single Penrose (cigarette) drain is gently inserted down into the pelvis (without additional

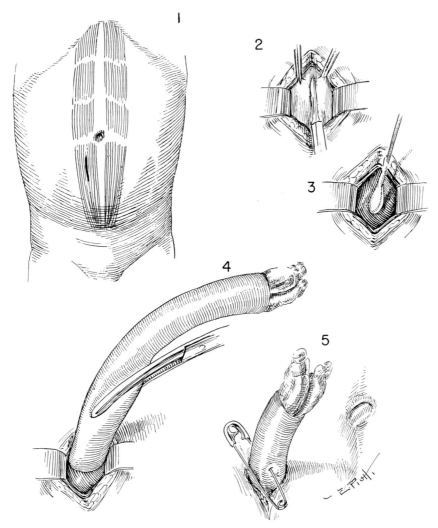

Fig. 120.—Surgical treatment of primary peritonitis. *1*, Under local anesthesia, a right rectus muscle-splitting incision not over 2 or 3 cm. long. If this is made below the inferior tendinous inscription (which is opposite the umbilicus), very little bleeding is encountered. *2*, Muscles retracted. Peritoneum being opened. *3*, Intestines presenting; these are not disturbed. Exudate then taken for culture and immediate smear. *4*, If pure pneumococcus or streptococcus is seen on smear, nothing more is done, except to insert a drain down into the pelvis. *5*, Soft cigarette drain just fills the wound. No sutures are necessary.

anesthesia) and a dry sterile dressing is applied. If this minor procedure is properly done it is not shocking. With the short incision, as recommended, the abdominal opening will be just large enough to accommodate a drain without placing a single suture in the wound. The information gained from this simple exploration permits immediate institution of intelligent specific therapy for primary peritonitis. If the small opening reveals a foul-smelling pus, a ruptured appendix can be suspected, ether anesthesia can be given, the incision enlarged, appendectomy performed and drainage instituted.

Should Supportive Treatment Be Given First?—On the assumption that peritoneal drainage is of value—and we believe that it is definitely so—the question arises of whether it is better to perform this immediately or to defer it for some days or weeks while general supportive ("Ochsner") treatment is administered. Prior to 1929 it was our custom to undertake immediate operation and the overall mortality was 65 per cent. From 1929 until 1936 we experimented with more conservative treatment, which consisted of Fowler's position, sedation, gastric suction, withholding of food, administration of parenteral fluids, etc., with postponement of operation

TABLE 22

MORTALITY RATES WITH DIFFERENT FORMS OF THERAPY IN 120 CASES OF PRIMARY PERITONITIS

Type of Peritonitis	Immediate Abdominal Drainage (Prior to 1929)	Supportive Treatment— Abdominal Drainage Some Days or Weeks Later (1930–1936)	Early Abdominal Drainage plus Chemo- therapy or Serum Therapy (1937–1940)
Pneumococcal peritonitis.............	66%	83%	12.5%
Streptococcal peritonitis.............	65%	70%	22.2%
All cases of primary peritonitis.........	65%	73%	17.6%

for some days. In a few cases abdominal drainage was not done until two or three weeks later. With this change in treatment several patients for whom little hope was held at the time of hospitalization happily recovered. However, upon extension of this series it was found that the overall mortality was higher than it had been previously with early operation. Therefore, since 1936, we have returned to early operation in all cases, following this whenever possible with sulfanilamide, sulfapyridine, sulfathiazole, or antipneumococcus serum, as seems best for the particular case. The various mortality figures in these three periods of therapeutic practice—(1) immediate operation; (2) delayed operation; and (3) early operation plus specific therapy—are summed up in Table 22.

We do not wish to imply that these children should be rushed into the operating room as soon as they are hospitalized. Severe toxicity and dehydration should be first controlled by administration of subcutaneous and intravenous fluids, saline or glucose. If anemia is marked or shock is evident, a transfusion is in order. Gastric lavage will diminish retching, vomiting, and the dangers of aspiration. A few hours spent in this way are extremely beneficial, and "early operation" is meant to include this pre-operative treatment when it is indicated.

Aftercare.—The aftercare of the patient is of utmost importance. A high Fowler's position should be constantly maintained. *Morphine* every four hours by the clock for a day or two will give much-needed rest. *Constant gastric siphonage* should be instituted and continued as long as there is any intestinal or bile-stained fluid returned by the tube. Water may be drunk as desired, for it helps to moisten the mouth and keeps the suction apparatus clean. Milk and solid foods must be withheld. A flaxseed poultice or hot-water bottle on the abdomen every two or three hours is helpful. A tent with high concentration of *oxygen* (90 to 95 per cent) is a valuable adjunct in the treatment of abdominal distention. The *water balance* is maintained by intravenous injections of 10 per cent dextrose solution and hypoder-moclyses of physiologic solutions of sodium chloride. *Blood transfusions* are liberally employed for anemia or hypoproteinemia.

The constant gastric suction may be necessary for four or five days or more. After it is discontinued, semisolid food should be started *with caution.* Physicians sometimes interpret a falling temperature, a flat abdomen, and disappearance of vomiting as sure signs of recovery, and hence prescribe the return to a normal diet. All too often this decision is followed by reap-pearance of distention and fever which might have been avoided by restrict-ing the intake of food for several more days. The wound should be dressed frequently enough to keep it dry. The abdominal drain should be loosened from its bed on the fifth day and pulled out a little each succeeding day so that it is completely removed by the eighth or ninth day. It is of interest that only three patients in our series required an enterostomy for intestinal obstruction following primary peritonitis.

Chemotherapy.—*Streptococcal Peritonitis.*—In primary peritonitis of the streptococcal type, specific treatment with *sulfanilamide* should be started as soon as the patient is returned from the operating room. At first the drug may be given by hypodermoclysis of an 0.8 per cent solution in physiologic sodium chloride, and later it is continued by oral administration of crushed tablets when the patient is able to tolerate fluids by mouth. During the first day of treatment doses of about 2 grains per pound of body weight in twenty-four hours will usually be sufficient to establish an optimum level of about 10 mg. per 100 cc. of blood. After twenty-four hours, the dose should be reduced to about 1 grain per pound for each twenty-four hours that it is continued. Since the drug is excreted rapidly, a calculated twenty-four-hour dose should be divided into four portions which are given at six-hour intervals.

The fluid balance in these extremely sick patients is apt to change rapidly and accordingly the blood concentration of sulfanilamide is apt to rise above or fall below the optimum concentration. It is therefore essential to determine the blood sulfanilamide level frequently as a guide for subsequent dosage. Regardless of any disturbing cyanosis or delirium, sulfanilamide should be continued in maximum dosage until there is distinct clinical improvement. If it is discontinued before the fever has fallen below 100° F., there may be a recrudescence of the infection. It is not possible to state dogmatically how long drug therapy must be maintained, but in our cases the average was five to six days, while in one individual it was as long as ten days. Some degree of anemia develops in almost all of these patients since red cell destruction results from both streptococcal infection and drug reaction. Repeated small transfusions should be given to maintain the red cell count between 4,000,000 and 5,000,000.

Pneumococcal Peritonitis.—In those patients with pneumococcal infection it has been our policy to employ chemotherapy, and also serum therapy whenever this is available. Because of the superior bacteriostatic activity of *sulfapyridine* and *sulfathiazole* against the pneumococcus, these drugs are preferred to sulfanilamide. Sulfathiazole is less toxic to the patient and yet apparently has about the same potency as sulfapyridine against the pneumococcus. Sodium sulfapyridine and sodium sulfathiazole* are highly soluble and can be easily administered by the intravenous route as a 1 to 5 per cent solution in physiologic saline.† A massive initial dose of 1 grain per pound of body weight is given. In the following twenty-four hours 1 grain per pound of body weight is given, and this dose is divided into at least four parts, to be administered at six-hour intervals. The concentration of sulfapyridine or sulfathiazole in the blood is apt to build up quickly; hence, it is important to determine this figure after the first twenty-four-hour period, and to reduce the subsequent administrations to about ½ grain per pound for each twenty-four hours. Blood levels of 4 to 6 mg. per 100 cc. are optimal for sulfapyridine or sulfathiazole.

Serum Therapy in Pneumococcal Infection.—When lanceolate, grampositive diplococci are seen in a smear of the peritoneal exudate, a Neufeld typing should be done immediately on the fresh material; or if this is not possible, the test should be made on organisms grown from a culture. If a serum can be procured for the specific type which is identified, arrangements should be made for employing it at once. Fortunately, many pneumococci invading the peritoneum are of Type I, for which serum is widely available from state bacteriologic laboratories and commercial drug houses.

---

* Kindly supplied to us on trial by E. R. Squibb and Sons.

† These drugs apparently lose their effectiveness if heated in glucose solutions.

Type I serum is usually prepared from the horse, but some of the other types have now been obtained from rabbits.* The use of rabbit serum has considerable advantage in that one rarely finds a patient who is already sensitive to it and hence the serum can be administered without delay. Furthermore, rabbit serum will not sensitize the individual to equine pro-teins—a fact of some importance if some subsequent illness should require the use of a horse serum.

Serum Sensitivity.—Before specific antipneumococcus sera are injected, precautions must be taken to determine the presence of any existing sensi-tivity. A careful inquiry should be made regarding previous injections of serum or manifestations of allergy. An intradermal or an ophthalmic test should be made with $\frac{1}{10}$ cc. of a 1:10 dilution of the serum which is to be employed. If this is negative in one-half hour, therapeutic doses can be started, but epinephrin solution should always be available for immediate use.

Administration and Dosage.—Serum is given exclusively by the intra-venous route. Initially, 1 cc. (approximately 1000 units) of the serum in 10 cc. of saline is given slowly to ascertain that the intravenous injection of this protein will not have any undesirable effects. If there is no untoward reaction to this in an hour, 50,000 to 100,000 units (according to the patient's toxicity and size) are then administered. This is repeated at twelve-hour intervals until there is significant abatement of the fever.† The total doses of serum in our cases averaged 350,000 units, ranging from a min-imum of 66,000 units (in a thirty-one-month-old girl) to a maximum of 900,000 units (in a seventeen-month-old girl). The total amount in most cases was administered during twenty-four to forty-eight hours, but in some instances it was distributed over a four-day period. The amount of antibody required appears to vary greatly from patient to patient, so that the clinical course of the individual is the best guide for directing the specific therapy, which should not be discontinued until definite improvement has been manifested.

To minimize reactions, *slowness of injection* is deemed of great im-portance. This is facilitated by diluting the serum in from 5 to 10 volumes of physiologic solution of sodium chloride. Small quantities can be delivered from a standard syringe. If the antecubital veins are inaccessible or throm-

---

* Rabbit antipneumococcus sera for Types I to XXXIII inclusive are now commer-cially prepared by the Lederle Laboratories, Inc. Types VI and XXVI, and Types XV and XXX are considered to be identical.

† In adults the *Francis skin test* (with capsular carbohydrates from the type of pneu-mococcus under consideration) indicates in fifteen or twenty minutes if the patient has a sufficiently high antibody titer. If the test is positive, the individual has circulating free antibodies and it is unnecessary to administer more serum. Unfortunately, this test is not reliable in the first two or three years of life.

bosed, a 24-gauge needle can be used and the serum injected into small veins of the extremities or scalp. Large amounts of serum are better given through a standard intravenous infusion set by injecting the material into the rubber tubing of a constant intravenous drip.

Antisera Plus Chemotherapy.—It is probably unnecessary to give both antisera and chemotherapy to all cases of pneumococcal peritonitis in order to obtain satisfactory results. Both of these have been given to most of our patients, since it was thought advisable to employ all of the weapons which were at our disposal. More recently, a few patients have been treated by chemotherapy alone and have recovered satisfactorily. This raises the possibility that the expense of sera (which is considerable in some communities) may be avoided by using only chemotherapy. If a given patient is not too ill, sulfapyridine or sulfathiazole can be tried with the idea of adding antisera twelve or twenty-four hours later if the clinical course is not satisfactory.

RESULTS OF TREATMENT

Mortality rates in primary peritonitis have been universally high until the last few years. Some estimate of published statistics can be gained from Table 23.

TABLE 23

MORTALITY RATES IN PNEUMOCOCCAL AND STREPTOCOCCAL PERITONITIS

Author	Year Reported	Pneumococcal Peritonitis	Streptococcal Peritonitis
Lipshutz and Lowenburg	1926	100%	100%
Ladd	1930	66%	65%
Donovan	1934	75%	78%
Cole	1937	54%	
Leopold and Kaufman	1937		91%
Ladd and Gross*	1940	12%	22%

* Series by early drainage, supportive treatment, and specific chemotherapy or serum therapy.

The reduction of mortalities in our series to 12 per cent and 22 per cent, respectively, for pneumococcal and streptococcal peritonitis reflects the efficacy of the program of treatment, which may be summed up as follows: (1) Early incision and drainage of the peritoneal cavity under local anesthesia with minimal manipulation. (2) Rapid identification of the organism from the peritoneal cavity. (3) Immediate postoperative institution of sulfanilamide therapy by hypodermoclysis for streptococcal infections. (4) Immediate postoperative intravenous administration of sodium sulfapyridine (or sodium sulfathiazole) and specific antiserum (if one is available) for pneumococcal infections. (5) Use of constant gastric siphonage and high-concentration oxygen tent to relieve abdominal distention and vomiting. (6) Maintenance of adequate fluid and caloric intake by parenteral routes. (7) Repeated small blood transfusions to combat anemia and hypoproteinemia.

BIBLIOGRAPHY

1. Barnett, H. L., Hartmann, A. F., Perley, A. M., and Ruhoff, M. B.: The Treatment of Pneumococcic Infections in Infants and Children with Sulfapyridine. J. A. M. A., *112:* 518, 1939.

2. Carey, B. W., Jr.: The Use of Para-Aminobenzenesulfonamide and Its Derivations in the Treatment of Infection Due to the Beta Streptococcus Hemolyticus, the Meningococcus, and the Gonococcus. J. Pediat., *11:* 202, 1937.

3. Cole, W. H.: Pneumococcus Peritonitis. Surgery, *1:* 386, 1937.

4. Donovan, E. J.: Surgical Aspects of Primary Pneumococcus Peritonitis. Am. J. Dis. Child., *48:* 1170, 1934.

5. Glazier, M. M., Goldberg, B. I., and Weinstein, A. A.: Primary Pneumococcic Peritonitis: Recovery of the Acute Serous Type Following Type I Serum Treatment Without Surgical Intervention. Ann. Int. Med., *10:* 1042, 1937.

6. Ladd, W. E., Botsford, T. W., and Curnen, E. C.: Primary Peritonitis in Infants and Children. A More Effective Treatment. J. A. M. A., *113:* 1455, 1939.

7. Ladd, W. E.: The Acute Surgical Abdomen in Children. Pennsylvania M. J., *34:* 153, 1930.

8. Leonardo, R. A.: Primary Pneumococcus Peritonitis. Ann. Surg., *83:* 411, 1926.

9. Leopold, J. S., and Kaufman, R. E.: Acute "Primary" Streptococcus Peritonitis. J. Pediat., *10:* 45, 1937.

10. Lipshutz, B., and Lowenburg, H.: Pneumococcic and Streptococcic Peritonitis. Report of Twenty-three Cases in Infancy and Children. J. A. M. A., *86:* 99, 1926.

11. McCartney, J. E., and Fraser, J.: Pneumococcal Peritonitis. Brit. J. Surg., *9:* 479, 1922.

CHAPTER XV

APPENDICITIS

Incidence.—Inflammation of the vermiform appendage is the most common lesion requiring intra-abdominal surgery in childhood. Appendicitis is still a highly important problem because of the great frequency of the condition, and because it continues to be responsible for many preventable deaths. Although the mortality rates in first-class hospitals have been grad-

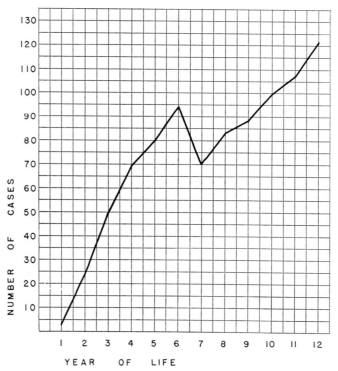

Fig. 121.—Graph showing age incidence of acute appendicitis in 940 children. The condition is rare in the first year and is uncommon in the second year of life (in contrast to idiopathic peritonitis, Fig. 119).

ually improving, this does not reflect the state of affairs in the population at large. According to Sperling and Myrick,[12] appendicitis accounts for 20,000 deaths (patients of all ages) annually in the United States, the highest mortality rate in any civilized nation of the world. The general death rate in Massachusetts per 10,000 children under ten years of age was 669 in 1920, 324 in 1930, and 180 in 1936; and the death rate for children with appendicitis was 8.2 in 1920, 15.9 in 1930, and 10.6 in 1936. Only pneumonia and accidents exceed appendicitis as a cause of death in this age group. Of each eighteen or twenty children who now die, one succumbs to appendicitis.

Differences in Appendicitis in Children and in Adults.—While appendicitis is the same disease in the adult and the child, the reactions may be quite different in these two types of individuals. The physician who tries to fit the same therapy to both groups will often invite, and frequently meet, disaster. In children an accurate and early diagnosis is more difficult, and generalized peritonitis occurs in a high percentage of cases. To obtain reasonably good results with appendicitis in children it is necessary to recognize that the criteria for establishment of a diagnosis are different, that the untreated disease runs a more rapid and deadlier course, and that somewhat different therapeutic principles must be used for combating the condition.

PATHOLOGY

Inflammation of the appendix begins in the mucosa or submucosa with leukocytic infiltrations, vascular engorgement, edema, and hemorrhage. This progresses to ulceration of the mucosa and accumulation of purulent exudate within the appendiceal lumen. It is characteristic for the process

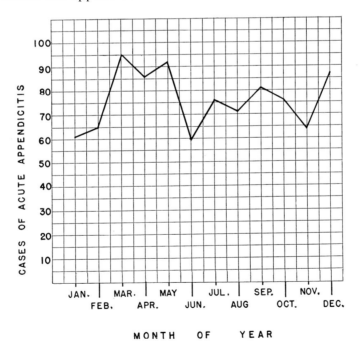

Fig. 122.—Incidence of acute appendicitis by months of the year. The greater frequency of the disease during March, April, and May is possibly related to the prevalence of respiratory infections during these spring months.

then to spread outward to involve the muscularis and serosa. Distention of the appendix or thrombosis of its vessels diminishes the blood supply to the organ so that gangrene and rupture may follow. In the course of the disease fibrin is poured out on the serosal surface so that light adherence to near-by structures tends to take place, particularly to the omentum if it is

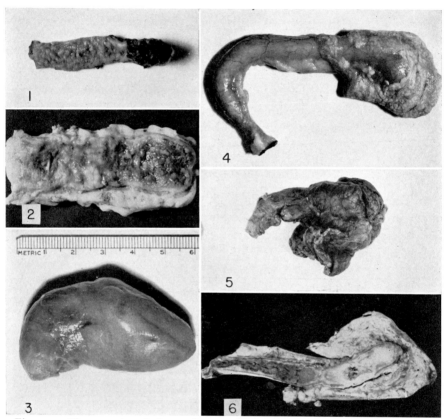

Fig. 123.—Photographs of six specimens which were removed because of acute appendicitis. The base of the appendix is at the left in each picture. *1*, Opened appendix, necrosis of mucosa only at the tip of the organ. *2*, Opened appendix, with diffuse necrosis of entire mucosal lining. *3*, Acutely inflamed appendix, with marked swelling and edema. *4*, Appendix with inflammation limited to its bulbous tip. *5*, Acutely inflamed appendix surrounded by a protecting sheath of adherent omentum which was excised with it. *6*, Longitudinal section of a gangrenous appendix and a protective mass of omentum which encased the distal half of it.

long enough to reach to the iliac fossa. This defense mechanism for localizing infection is efficient in older children and adults, but it is poor in infants and younger children in whom the omentum is short, thin, and almost devoid of fat.

Fluid is poured into the peritoneal cavity when the appendiceal veins are thrombosed, or when the appendiceal lumen is blocked by exudate, fecalith, or swollen mucosa. For a few hours this is clear, but soon fibrin and leukocytes accumulate and make it a thin, cloudy, odorless but sterile *exudate*. Bacteria may then invade such a medium by rupture of the appendix, or by traversing a highly inflamed but still intact appendiceal wall.

In the natural course of the disease, checking of the inflammation will depend upon the immunity of the individual and upon the availability of mobile structures for *walling off* the process. The complete encirclement and enclosure of the appendix in a protective omental sheath takes place in some fortunate cases. A less effective mode of defense appears when loops of intestines, mesentery, cecal wall, or parietal peritoneum become adherent to one another to form a pocket which encases the appendix and any pus which may surround it. If these walling-off reactions fail to limit the infection, *rupture* of the appendix contaminates the general peritoneal cavity. Once this has occurred, the spread is very rapid because of the fluid medium which is present by this time. While a generalized peritonitis is a supreme menace to the life of the individual, a final defense is still possible by a gathering of the exudate into one or more regions of the abdomen to form *localized abscesses*.

Much has been said about the *danger of purgatives* in patients with acute appendicitis. There is adequate statistical evidence to show that castor oil or other active laxatives will greatly increase the intestinal and appendiceal peristalsis so that perforation and dissemination of infection are more likely to occur.

The *bacteriology* in cases with abscess or peritonitis is variable. In many such peritoneal cultures there are doubtless important organisms which are lost sight of when there is a luxuriant overgrowth of colon bacillus. In a series of 336 peritoneal cultures which showed subsequent growth, the following identifications were made:

Colon bacillus	202
Enterococcus	4
Streptococcus haemolyticus	5
Streptococcus nonhaemolyticus	1
Staphylococcus aureus	3
Pneumococcus	4
Mixed (intestinal)	95
Other organisms	22

ETIOLOGY

Not much is known about the etiology of acute appendicitis. The greater frequency of the disease at certain periods of the year when respiratory infections are common suggests that certain organisms have a predilection for localized invasion of the vermiform appendix, but there is little statistical evidence to support such a hypothesis. However, a history of respiratory infection preceding the onset of acute appendicitis is not un-common. The fact that early stages of appendicitis do not show uniform involvement of all layers of the organ is rather against the theory of a hematogenous origin of the lesion.

The frequency with which inflammation originates in the inner coats of the appendix tends to support the thesis that *obstruction to its lumen* is important in causing appendicitis. Wangensteen and his colleagues ex-teriorized and artificially obstructed appendices in humans (adults) and then demonstrated sufficient formation of mucus to raise the intra-ap-pendiceal pressure to figures approaching the systolic blood pressure. This rising tension of the entrapped secretory products was sufficient to bring about ischemia and necrosis of the appendiceal walls. It is therefore reason-able to believe that a *fecalith* or *inspissated material* which obstructs the appendiceal lumen plays an important part in the onset of inflammatory disease of the organ. The frequency with which fecaliths are found in gangrenous or ruptured appendices lends strong support to this view. That this is not a universal factor is proved by those cases in which no fecalith, foreign body, hyperplastic lymphoid tissue, or other form of obstruction can be demonstrated.

There is a strong impression that an appendix which has been once acutely inflamed and allowed to subside spontaneously is quite apt to have another infection at a subsequent time. This is presumably true because *scar tissue* forms in a place in which it blocks the drainage of the organ.

SYMPTOMS AND SIGNS

Difficulty in recognition of acute appendicitis in young children has been often emphasized, but the more skill one has in managing patients of this age the rarer will be the errors in diagnosis. Certainly it is possible in most cases to identify the condition before peritoneal involvement has taken place. To do this in the less clear-cut instances requires careful examination by an experienced physician or surgeon. If the diagnosis is in question and it is impossible to reexamine the child at home at one- or two-hour intervals, it is wise to advise hospitalization for a day or two to permit adequate observation. Certainly the triad of *abdominal pain, vomiting,* and *slight fever* must be considered as appendicitis until proved otherwise.

Age and Sex Incidence.—The youngest individual in the Children's Hos-pital series with acute appendicitis was six months old, but younger patients have been reported. Appendicitis is quite rare in the first year of life, is infrequently found in the second year, but from then on it becomes com-mon. More cases are seen in the period from six to twelve years than in the period from one to six years. The disease is slightly more frequent in males than in females—54 per cent against 46 per cent in our series. This ratio is somewhat higher than the predominance of males over females in the general population.

Symptoms.—*Pain.*—The usual history is one of acute abdominal pain, followed by nausea and vomiting. The pain is apt to begin around the umbilicus or in the epigastrium, but often children are vague and inaccurate about describing their complaints and the physician fails to elicit a story of early periumbilical discomfort. After a variable number of hours, the pain is most intense in the *right lower quadrant.* When a child is seen in this stage the severity of his current troubles may make him forget and even deny that he previously had any periumbilical symptoms. Pain of appendiceal origin is occasionally maximal in the *right upper quadrant* because of an incompletely rotated colon. If the inflammation advances to a spreading involvement of the peritoneum, pain will become diffuse and severe. Appendiceal pain is apt to be constant, but it may be colicky because of obstruction of the *appendiceal lumen* (by fecalith, swollen mucosa, or a kinking of the organ).

Vomiting.—This is an almost universal finding in acute appendicitis with children, and only rarely is it absent. Vomiting may occur only once or twice, or it may be repeated and persistent. Fever of 100° to 101° F. is the rule, but the temperature may be normal, particularly if the child has been exposed to cold while being brought to the physician or hospital.

A *temperature* above 102° F. is rare unless peritonitis has set in, in which case it may reach 103° F. or more. The bowel movements may be normal, but *constipation* is common. An inflamed appendix which lies against the lower sigmoid, or a spreading peritonitis which irritates the intestinal tract, will both produce a *diarrhea.* Urinary symptoms are usually absent, but frequency or pain on voiding suggests that an inflamed appendix lies against the right ureter or the urinary bladder.

A history of recent *upper respiratory infection* is obtained in about one-fifth of the cases. This may be only incidental, but one often gains the impression that the preceding respiratory disease was the forerunner of the abdominal infection. Intestinal disorders, principally *acute enteritis,* are found in some cases and any important changes for the worse in a patient with gastro-enteritis should arouse the physician's suspicions of a superimposed appendicitis. Appendicitis may occur at any time during the *acute exanthemata* of childhood, particularly measles. Hence, the onset of abdominal symptoms during one of these infections should make one mindful of this possibility.

Technic of Physical Examination.—To mention here the technic of physical examination in children may appear superfluous, but if the physician is mindful of a few details he will be able to gain the maximum amount of information from this portion of his study. An examination which is hurried, rough, and in the wrong order will only agitate the child and produce a crying, alarmed, and uncooperative patient. The common routine of starting with the head, gagging the child with a throat stick, upsetting him with a cold stethoscope, and then suddenly palpating the abdomen with a heavy hand is almost certain to give an unreliable impression of the presence or absence of abdominal inflammation. The findings under such circumstances are apt to be misleading and the resulting diagnosis is often incorrect. It is essential to gain the child's confidence before proceeding with the examination, in spite of the fact that this may take as long or longer than the actual examination itself. A great deal of patience is often required to accomplish this, but the time is well spent.

Everything which can be learned by *inspection* should be noted first: The general appearance of the child, the luster or sunkenness of the eyes, the dryness or perspiration of the skin, the position of the legs, the manifestations of pain and the rate of respiration will frequently give considerable information regarding the seat of pathology, the extent of the lesion, and the degree of toxicity.

Very gentle superficial *palpation* must precede deep palpation and will usually give more valuable information than the latter, which may throw the whole abdominal musculature into spasm. If one part of the abdomen appears to be tender, this should be avoided until all other parts are examined. A warm hand which is applied slowly and gently and kept on a tender area without moving will often give more information and upset the child less than will a palpating hand which is hastily moved from one region to another. If pneumonia or pleuritis is the basis of the patient's complaints, abdominal spasm will gradually disappear if the observer's hand takes over the function of splinting the lower chest wall. Spasm which remains in spite of continued manual pressure on the abdomen is an indication of peritoneal irritation. Palpation should always include bimanual examination of the kidney regions to rule out renal disease.

Abdominal *auscultation* may reveal augmented peristalsis if there is a spreading peritonitis, or a diminished peristalsis if there is a local infection or a longstanding peritonitis.

A complete general physical examination should follow the abdominal inspection and palpation. *Digital rectal examination* should be left until the last.

Tenderness.—The appendix of the child is larger in relation to the size of the abdominal cavity than is that of the adult, and the mesoappendix is correspondingly longer and less fixed. Therefore, the *point of maximal tenderness* may vary more in location than it does in the adult. It may appear near the midline, well down in the pelvis, or even out in the right flank. If tenderness is accompanied by involuntary muscle spasm, this is evidence of inflammatory involvement of the parietal peritoneum. A low-lying pelvic appendix may give exquisite tenderness by rectal examination which is not felt by abdominal palpation. If the disease has been present for five or six days or more, a walled-off abscess may possibly be felt by rectal or abdominal palpation. If generalized peritonitis complicates the picture, tenderness is widespread and marked. Elicitation of rebound tenderness is difficult except in older and more cooperative children.

Likewise a *positive psoas* or *obturator sign* may be hard to detect. Irritation of the psoas muscle by an abscess or inflamed appendix is more apt to be recognized by noting what position the child assumes when left undisturbed, for there will be a tendency to lie with the right thigh partially flexed.

LABORATORY DATA

Routine laboratory procedures should include a white blood cell count, a differential count, and a urine examination. *Leukocytosis* to levels of 12,-000 to 20,000 is common; counts above the latter figure are apt to imply that a local or generalized peritonitis exists. The polymorphonuclear ratio is commonly increased to 85 or 95 per cent. While leukocytosis of some degree is practically always found in acute appendicitis, gangrene or even spreading peritonitis without leukocytosis is found in rare instances.

Urine examination usually shows acetone or other ketone bodies. The sediment should be examined to rule out infection of the urinary tract, but it must be remembered that irritation of the ureter by adjacent appendicitis can make a few white or red blood cells appear in the urine.

Roentgenologic examination has been used in some clinics to determine the question of free gas in the peritoneal cavity in order to differentiate ruptured from nonruptured appendicitis. This procedure is unwarranted and has little practical importance. x-Ray studies of the chest have great value in cases of suspected appendicitis when there is any question of detecting and ruling out a central pneumonia.

DIFFERENTIAL DIAGNOSIS

The commonest diseases which offer difficulties in differential diagnosis are bronchopneumonia, pyelitis, idiopathic peritonitis, acute (nontuberculous) mesenteric adenitis, and acute enteritis. It is important to recognize pneumonia and urinary tract infections, because an erroneous diagnosis of appendicitis in such cases may lead to operations which are harmful. If a child should have idiopathic peritonitis the incorrect diagnosis of appendicitis is not particularly harmful because laparotomy and drainage (without exploration of the abdomen) is the procedure of choice. In the presence of mesenteric adenitis, operation for a supposed appendicitis is not particularly harmful, but it is not very satisfying to the surgeon to open the abdomen unnecessarily.

Bronchopneumonia.—This may be suspected by a higher fever, a higher leukocytosis, and an increased respiratory rate. In early stages of the disease or if the pneumonia is central in location, auscultation and percussion of the chest may give normal findings. Abdominal spasm may accompany pneumonia, but will gradually disappear if a supporting hand is laid on the abdomen and maintained there steadily for a few minutes. When this differential diagnosis is in question, a roentgenogram of the chest should always be obtained.

Pyelitis.—Pyelitis or other infection of the urinary tract can usually be differentiated by a higher fever, white cells in the urinary sediment, and tenderness which is maximal over one of the kidneys.

Idiopathic Primary Peritonitis.—When this results from streptococcal or pneumococcal infection of the peritoneum it almost always produces a high fever (104° to 105° F.), generalized tenderness, and a doughy abdomen in infants or a spastic one in older children. As a rule this condition is more common in the first year or two of life, but when it does occur in older, cooperative individuals, the history may indicate that the pain was generalized at its onset and did not begin around the umbilicus or in the right lower quadrant as would be the case with appendicitis. Leukocytosis is usually higher in primary than in secondary peritonitis. In pneumonia, pyelitis, or idiopathic peritonitis the illness may be ushered in by nausea, vomiting, and abdominal pain, but the temperature is apt to be 103° F. or more; whereas in appendicitis the temperature is rarely over 101° F. and is usually not above 103° F. even when complicated by peritonitis.

Acute Mesenteric Adenitis (*Nontuberculous*).—This is the most common condition which must be differentiated from acute appendicitis. It almost invariably accompanies a respiratory infection, so that examination of the pharynx, nose, and chest is important. The abdominal pain may be generalized or may be localized to any region where the swollen lymph nodes are located. Since the involved nodes are larger and more numerous in the mesentery of the terminal ileum, the abdominal pain and tenderness are more marked in the right lower quadrant. Nausea is often present, but vomiting occurs in a rather small percentage of individuals. Fever is low grade or absent. Tenderness is only slight and is usually not as marked or as localized as that found in acute appendicitis. The white blood count is rarely above 10,000.

When mesenteric adenitis is suspected, observation of the child for several hours is usually sufficient to indicate that the process is stationary or subsiding, and hence is not typical of acute appendicitis. Thus, a mild course which is indicated by (1) minimal tenderness on repeated examinations of the abdomen, (2) normal or only slightly elevated temperature, and (3) white counts which are not appreciably elevated, will finally convince a conscientious physician that there is no pathology within the abdomen requiring surgery. Several hours' delay in making such observations will usually do no harm, even if appendicitis is present, and a number of useless laparotomies can be thereby avoided. However, if any reasonable suspicion persists about the possibility of appendicitis, laparotomy should be undertaken.

Constipation.—Constipation can cause abdominal pain, nausea, and even vomiting, which may be confused with appendicitis. A normal temperature and white blood count are the rule, but there may be slight tenderness in the right lower quadrant when the cecum is distended. If the bowels have not been moving well, or if fecal concretions can be felt within the rectum or along the sigmoid, it is permissible to prescribe a warm soap-suds enema and observe the child again within an hour or two. If constipation is the cause of the complaints this treatment will almost certainly relieve the symptoms, whereas little or no risk is involved if acute appendicitis really exists.

Gastro-enteritis.—This may be confused with appendicitis. A history of a similar condition in other members of the family, or a diarrhea without significant abdominal tenderness, tend to rule out appendicitis. Gastro-enteritis and vomiting may give mild or diffuse abdominal tenderness by retching and straining of the abdominal wall, but there is little or no localization of the tenderness such as is the case with appendicitis. If diarrhea is a manifestation of an inflamed pelvic appendix or a spreading peritonitis, these should be readily suspected by marked tenderness on rectal or abdominal examination.

Anomalies of the Right Ureter.—A kidney which is blocked by a stricture at the ureteropelvic junction, by an aberrant blood vessel crossing the ureter, or by a ureteral stone, may give fever, nausea, vomiting, and abdominal pain, but the pain and tenderness are maximal in one of the flanks. The urine may or may not contain white cells, according to the presence or absence of superimposed infection. If the abdominal complaints have been recurrent or if there is a reasonable possibility of urinary tract pathology, it is desirable to perform intravenous pyelography. A considerable number of patients come to the attention of urologists for complaints which persist after appendectomy, and adequate studies then make it evident that the ureter has actually been the seat of the important pathology.

Chronic Cicatrizing Enteritis.—This is a chronic inflammatory condition which has been described under many names, including "regional ileitis," and "nontuberculous granuloma of intestine." It may involve the colon or small intestine, particularly the latter, and is most common in the terminal ileum. Ulcerations, the etiology of which is not understood, appear in the mucosa and inflammatory cell infiltration and fibrosis may involve all layers of the intestinal wall so that it is narrowed, stiffened and tubelike. A pannus of mesenteric fat grows up around the sides of the intestine and tubercle-like lesions develop on the serosal surface. In late stages the lumen is markedly diminished.

While much more common in adult life, this pathology can occur in childhood. It manifests itself by symptoms of great chronicity, chiefly characterized by recurring bouts of abdominal pain, possibly vomiting, and occasionally diarrhea. x-Ray examination is often negative, but there may be evidence of partial obstruction. Barium studies (gastro-intestinal series or enema) may visualize the narrowed intestine. The inflammatory reaction has been known to disappear spontaneously; recurrence has often been observed after surgical resection. Surgery is indicated only for treatment of complications such as perforation or obstruction. The single case we have encountered in childhood was a nine-year-old boy with a history of intermittent complaints since the age of nine months; there was involvement of a few inches of the jejunum and 9 or 10 inches of the terminal ileum. The chronicity of symptoms in these patients serves to differentiate clearly between cicatrizing enteritis and any form of appendicitis.

TREATMENT

When the diagnosis of acute appendicitis has been made, there should be no question about the form of treatment, for *immediate appendectomy* carries very little risk and is followed by a short convalescence.

Dangers of Expectant Treatment.—When the inflammatory process has spread beyond the appendix and a generalized peritonitis has developed, there is some divergence of opinion concerning when to operate, how to operate, whether to drain, and what the aftercare should be. There has been a recent tendency to return to treatment by the "Ochsner" method, that is, delaying of operation for some days or weeks in the hope that a localized abscess will be formed which can then be drained. This expectant treatment in childhood will often result in death of the patient from overwhelming infection before any abscess develops. In a child, an appendix which is ruptured and is seeding the abdominal cavity with infected material is a constant menace, and if it can be quickly and gently removed the individual has an improved chance for combating the peritonitis which already exists.

Immediate Appendectomy Is Indicated.—We are strongly of the opinion that most cases of generalized peritonitis run a smoother course, have a better chance of recovery, and have a shorter hospitalization, if the appendix is removed and adequate *supportive measures* are employed in the postoperative period. This course of treatment is necessarily one which requires constant supervision by a competent staff. It implies that appendectomy must be performed with a minimum of trauma, with little or no disturbance of other intraperitoneal structures, and with as short an operating time as is consistent with safety. In general, we conform to the policy of appendectomy and drainage for all cases with peritonitis. However, in those patients who are unusually toxic, several hours can be profitably spent before operation in combating dehydration and ketosis by administration of subcutaneous saline and intravenous glucose.

In some clinics a definite *symptom duration,* such as thirty-six hours, is used to decide the question of immediate operation or delayed operation (some weeks later). We do not agree with this arbitrary method of dictating forms of treatment, because some patients may still be in good general condition forty-eight to sixty hours after the onset of appendicitis symptoms, whereas others will have a ruptured appendix and spreading peritoneal infection in less than twelve. Each case should therefore be considered individually and should be treated according to the conditions which are thought to be present.

In a series of 940 cases of acute appendicitis, it was possible to remove the appendix from 896 at the initial operation (95 per cent). In 43 instances the operator considered it better not to search out and remove the appendix and of these 29 were later readmitted for appendectomy. The following types of operation were done:

Appendectomy	433
Appendectomy with drainage	463
Drainage without appendectomy	43
Not operated upon	1
	940

Drainage of Appendiceal Abscess.—If an appendiceal abscess has been formed during the time prior to hospitalization, this is an indication that the individual's powers of resistance are good and that intestinal loops, omentum, or other viscera have fortunately become adherent to one another to limit the spread of infection. After any existing dehydration or ketosis has been properly combated, careful drainage is in order.

Incision should be made directly over the presenting mass. If the abdominal cavity should be traversed before the abscess mass is come upon, it may be better treatment to close the wound and make a more lateral one which will enter the abscess from the side by a *retroperitoneal approach* and thus avoid soiling of the general peritoneal cavity. If an abscess is in a position which necessitates opening it across the abdominal cavity, this does relatively little harm if a sucker is available for immediate removal of purulent material as soon as it appears. If the appendix presents itself and

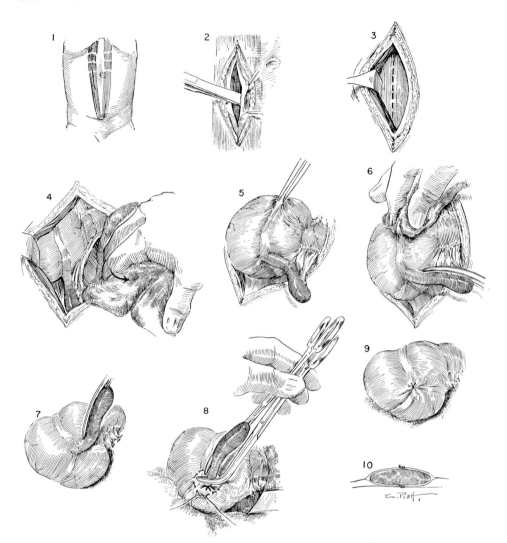

Fig. 124.—Method of operation for acute unruptured appendicitis.

1, Position of operative wound, with its upper end just above level of the umbilicus.

2, Anterior rectus sheath opened midway between its medial and lateral borders. Freeing medial edge of rectus muscle by blunt dissection with handle of forceps.

3, Rectus muscle retracted laterally. Posterior rectus sheath and peritoneal wall will be opened along the dotted line.

4, Lateral retraction of wound. Intestine covered with a single gauze sponge and then swept to the left side of the abdomen with one or two fingers introduced into the wound.

5, Presenting cecum grasped with smooth forceps and pulled up into the wound.

6, Cecum held up by right hand of assistant during remainder of operative procedure. A half-length clamp is placed along the mesenteric border of appendix, its tip running well down to the appendiceal base.

7, Appendix can be handled with the single half-length clamp. It is never allowed to touch wound edges or surrounding structures. Its mesentery is divided and the vessels ligated.

can be readily excised, it is best to do so. If it is surrounded by vascular *granulation tissue* or by dense *adhesions* it is wiser merely to insert a drain, and defer appendectomy until four to six months later when it can be performed with safety.

Appendectomy.—*Anesthesia.*—Anesthesia is preferably *ether* or *nitrous oxide-oxygen* with ether. These may be advantageously combined with a basal dose of avertin (90 mg. per kilogram of body weight, without morphine) if there is a concurrent respiratory infection. *Spinal* anesthesia has no place in childhood cases and *local* anesthesia is only satisfactory when it is proposed to make a small opening solely for inserting a drain into an abscess.

Exposure of Appendix.—The position and type of operative incision are of some importance.

McBurney Incision.—While the McBurney incision—or some modification of it—is quite suitable for most adults, it often gives poor exposure in young subjects and its advantages are greatly outweighed by its disadvantages. In a child the surface area of the right lower quadrant between the linea semilunaris and anterior-superior spine is relatively small. Therefore, the division of the external oblique muscle, the internal oblique muscle, and the transversalis along the direction of their various fibers finally produces an opening which is generally too small to work through safely unless the appendix happens to lie immediately beneath this area. In an appreciable number of children the appendix is tucked up under the liver when the cecum is incompletely rotated. In such cases a gridiron opening in the right lower quadrant is hard to enlarge upward without considerable destruction of the abdominal wall, whereas a paramedian incision can be easily extended.

A McBurney incision is good for drainage of a palpable abscess or for the removal of an appendix which can be accurately localized because of tenderness limited to this region, but its habitual use in childhood will often lead the surgeon into operative difficulties. This small opening, with the forceful and brutal retraction which might be required to get exposure, often leads to a stormy convalescence which could be avoided by a wider exposure through a paramedian incision which permits gentleness in treat-

---

8, Appendix held with the half-length clamp. Right-angle clamp placed on its base. Handles of these two instruments can then be conveniently held together. Appendiceal base ligated. Purse-string suture has been placed. Gauze placed under the cecum to prevent subsequent soiling of peritoneal cavity.

9, Appendix cut off (between ligature and right-angle clamp). Purse-string suture drawn up.

10, Horizontal section of closed rectus sheath. The muscle belly becomes interposed between the continuous peritoneo-posterior rectus-sheath suture and the interrupted anterior rectus-sheath sutures. This gives a stronger wound than if the muscle had been split.

14

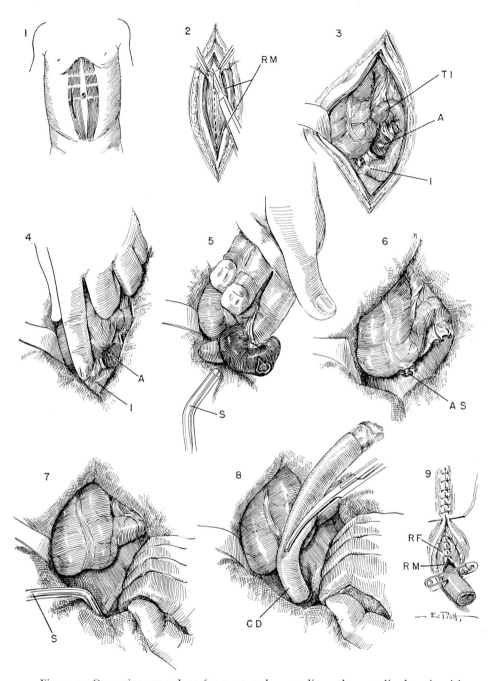

Fig. 125.—Operative procedure for ruptured appendix and generalized peritonitis.

A, Appendix	*RF,* Rectus Fascia
AS, Appendiceal Stump	*RM,* Rectus Muscle
CD, Cigarette Drain	*S,* Sucker
I, Intestines, adherent to cecum	*TI,* Terminal Ileum

ment of the tissues. Our infrequent use of the McBurney incision (less than 5 per cent of the cases) and our low mortality record are of interest in view of the opinion so often expressed in surgical literature that reduced death rates are to be ascribed to the routine use of this incision.

RIGHT RECTUS INCISION.—In 95 per cent of our cases a right rectus incision was used, usually retracting the muscle but splitting it when drainage was contemplated. Retraction of the muscle medially, if properly performed, gives an excellent exposure of the appendix; but if it is ruthlessly done a part of the nerve supply to the rectus may be severed. Medial retraction of the rectus is advantageous for some cases, but it is preferable to pull the muscle belly laterally. The abdominal incision should be made with its upper end opposite to or just above the umbilicus, so that the somewhat higher cecum of the child can be rolled up into the wound to allow easier treatment of the appendiceal stump.

Excision.—The actual removal of the appendix presents no special problems in most cases, but the dislodging of a high retrocecal, deeply embedded, inflamed appendix may be a most difficult surgical task. Not infrequently it is easier to sever the appendix at its base before dividing the meso-appendix. Great care must be exercised to avoid rupturing an acutely inflamed, edematous, and friable organ. If an appendix is surrounded by a wad of *adherent omentum* (Fig. 123, Nos. 5 and 6) this fatty protecting sheath should not be dissected off because it probably encloses a gangrenous organ, the exposure of which would contaminate the operative field. Such adherent omentum should always be left attached to the appendix and should be excised with it.

It is best in the majority of cases to *invert the cecum* with a purse-string silk suture, since this probably reduces the chances of establishing a fecal

---

1, Position of incision.

2, Rectus-muscle split (because subsequent drainage is contemplated). Posterior rectus sheath and peritoneum will be opened along dotted line.

3, Lateral retraction of wound. The inflamed appendix is buried in fibrinous adhesions. Loop of intestine lightly adherent to tip of cecum.

4, Wound edges and peritoneal cavity walled off with gauze. Blunt dissection of fibrinous adhesions with finger tip. No more adhesions than necessary are disturbed.

5, Swollen, ruptured appendix dissected bluntly from its bed and flipped forward with a finger. Sucker ready to catch any exudate, blood, or extravasated fecalith.

6, Appendix removed. Stump often cannot be safely inverted because of edema of cecal wall.

7, Cecum rolled up posteriorly to bury the appendiceal stump against the posterior peritoneal wall. Medial side of wound and presenting intestines held toward patient's left so that a sucker can be passed into pelvis for removal of any remaining exudate.

8, Intestines held toward left. Cigarette drain passed down into pelvis and allowed to rest against the lateral wall of the pelvis.

9, Wound closure. Drain led out inferior part of wound. Safety pin through drain to prevent it from slipping inward.

fistula. In those cases in which the caput of the cecum is diffusely inflamed, thickened, and edematous, it is folly to attempt inversion of the stump, for the suture will pull out, undue bleeding will result, and considerable damage may be inflicted on the cecal wall.

Drainage.—The peritoneal fluid which may accompany an acutely inflamed but unruptured appendix does not necessarily contain bacteria. If it is odorless or if an immediate smear shows no organisms, all of the obtainable fluid should be sucked away and the abdomen closed without drainage. If, however, there is any question about the presence of bacteria in this fluid, the operator will be wise to insert a single cigarette drain or soft rubber wick down into the pelvis which may be withdrawn in twenty-four or forty-eight hours if the peritoneal cultures subsequently show no growth.

The question of drainage for *generalized peritonitis* is a moot one. In recent years a few authors have inclined toward the closure of such abdomens without drainage, but with this view we are distinctly in disagreement. While a drain is admittedly ineffective in evacuating the general abdominal cavity after a few days' time, there appears to be little doubt that individuals with generalized peritonitis of appendiceal origin convalesce better if the abdomen is drained. Such an avenue of escape allows pus to be discharged which would otherwise have to be absorbed by the general circulation. Furthermore, subsequently formed collections of pus in the iliac fossa or pelvis can break into this drainage tract and discharge themselves.

Stiff rubber tubing as a drain should be decried because of the danger of pressure erosion of near-by intestines. A thin, pliable rubber (*Miller*) wick with a center core of loose gauze (a *Penrose* drain) will not erode or damage surrounding structures. Drains should not be indiscriminately placed among coils of intestines, but they should be laid along the lateral wall of the abdomen and thereby led down into the pelvis. To avert the formation of fecal fistula, a drain should be placed so that it does not rest against the appendiceal stump.

POSTOPERATIVE CARE

Following simple appendectomy for acute, unruptured appendicitis, little in the way of special treatment is necessary during the postoperative course. Vomiting may be troublesome for twenty-four or thirty-six hours, during which time the oral intake is best limited. In the average case, fluids can be taken as desired after the first day and soft solids after the second day. Because of the rapidity of wound healing in the young patient, the individual may be safely allowed out of bed in eight or nine days.

Gastric and Duodenal Aspiration.—Following operation for an appendiceal abscess or generalized peritonitis the postoperative period requires the utmost vigilance. The intestinal tract should be put at rest by withholding all solid food until there is clinical evidence that the infection has subsided and is under control. Abdominal distention is combated or prevented by the use of an *inlying gastric aspiration tube*. If no suction apparatus is available, the free end of the Levine tube can hang over the side of the bed to form a gravity system for decompressing the upper alimentary tract.

A suction apparatus of the *Wangensteen* type is most desirable for aspiration. A satisfactory modification of this is the three-bottle system shown in Fig. 127. One bottle is used to collect the aspirated fluid, so that the doctor or nurse can tell at a glance how much has been withdrawn from the patient. A second water-filled bottle on the bedside table forms a suitable reservoir for the gravity system. A column of water extends from this into the third vessel on the floor.

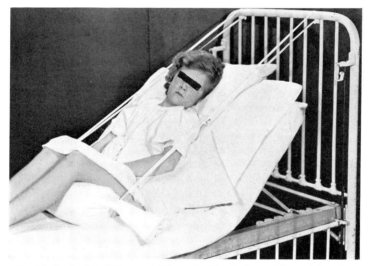

Fig. 126.—Method of holding a child up in Fowler's position with a knee roll.

For young children a No. 12 or 14 French urethral catheter is sufficient for the inlying gastric tube, but in older patients the longer Levine tube will be necessary. Since it is much easier to avoid distention than to treat it after it has appeared, we have routinely inserted an in-lying gastric tube in all cases with peritoneal infection. When this is in place and the patient regains consciousness he is allowed to drink water or clear fluids as desired. These fluids keep the oral and esophageal mucous membranes moistened, irrigate the stomach, and cleanse the suction tubing as they wash back through it. Any patient who has constant gastric suction for more than a day or two should have the blood chlorides checked so that lost salt may be replaced by parenteral solutions if necessary.

The double lumen *Miller-Abbott tube* has some limitations in the childhood group because of the size of the tube in relation to that of a child's nostril. The smaller tubes of this type can be used with a modicum of success in older children, but they become repeatedly plugged by intestinal contents and are difficult to keep working properly. On the whole, therefore, Miller-Abbott tubes have a very limited usefulness for children.

Oxygen Tent.—A valuable adjunct in combating abdominal distention is a tent (Fig. 128) which contains 90 to 95 per cent of oxygen. Fine and his co-workers[5] have demonstrated that trapped, inert intestinal nitrogen

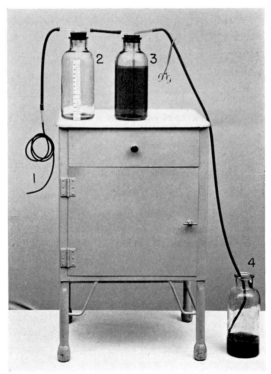

Fig. 127.—A satisfactory type of gastric suction apparatus. *1*, The gastric tube. *2*, Bottle for the aspirated material. *3*, Water reservoir for gravity system. *4*, Bottle for collecting water.

(from swallowed room air) may be removed rather effectively if the patient is placed in an atmosphere where the concentration of oxygen is high and that of nitrogen is low. It is helpful in all cases in which distention is present or appears to be imminent. To gain effective results the tent must be employed for twelve to twenty-four hours, but we have yet to observe any deleterious effects on the lungs when continued as long as four or five days. While this form of treatment may be expensive, troublesome, and often disappointing for the adult patient, it is much more satisfactory for the child. The amount of oxygen required depends upon the individual's consumption, leakage from the apparatus, number of times the tent is opened, etc., but with good equipment the oxygen does not cost more than $4 to $6 for a twenty-four-hour period. While the patient is in such a tent, constant gastric suction should be simultaneously employed to remove any fluid which accumulates in the upper intestinal tract.

Other Postoperative Measures.—*Fowler's Position.*—An erect position of the patient in bed is believed to aid in keeping any peritoneal exudate from the upper part of the abdomen. Some observers deny this, but we are strongly in favor of maintaining Fowler's position (Fig. 126) when peritoneal infection is known to exist. Under this regimen, subdiaphragmatic

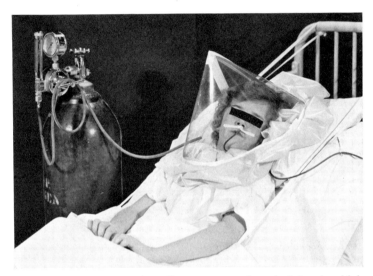

Fig. 128.—A satisfactory type of small oxygen tent for administering high concentration (90 per cent) oxygen. The transparent celluloid cone is closed inferiorly with a cloth which can be drawn tightly around the neck. Gastric suction is concurrently employed. Because of the continuous flow of oxygen, a cooling apparatus is seldom necessary. If it is desirable to cool the oxygen it can be led through a wide-mouthed stoppered bottle containing ice.

abscesses are extremely rare and localization of infection to the pelvis appears to be better than when the individual is allowed to lie in a horizontal position. Certainly the upright position permits a better discharge of exudate from the abdominal cavity when drains are employed. Furthermore, the sitting position allows the individual to breathe more easily and probably helps to reduce the incidence of pulmonary complications.

Heat to Abdomen.—Heat applied to the abdomen at two- or three-hour intervals has a soothing effect, possibly aids in reducing abdominal infection and distention, and certainly helps in resolving any inflammation which might develop in the surgical wound.

Morphine.—This has an important place in the postoperative care. In the uncomplicated cases it may be given every three or four hours, as indicated, to control pain and restlessness. When a peritoneal abscess or peritonitis exists it should be given by the clock at four-hour intervals for the first day or two to keep the patient in a somewhat stuporous condition. Treatments at this time are much facilitated if the child is relaxed and quiet, instead of thrashing about, attempting to pull out the nasal tube, or hindering the administration of parenteral fluids. Aside from this consideration, adequate sedation permits rest which is so beneficial. After the first twenty-four to forty-eight hours, discomfort can be controlled with smaller and less frequent injections of morphine.

Administration of Parenteral Fluids.—In recent years when so much stress has been laid upon the administration of parenteral fluids, this aspect of the treatment need hardly be emphasized. Fluids by *intravenous* or *subcutaneous* route two or three times per twenty-four-hour period are usually sufficient to maintain a positive fluid balance, electrolyte level, and caloric intake. If intravenous therapy is difficult to administer, a constant *venoclysis* may be employed. When this is used, the needle should not be left in any one vein for more than a twenty-four-hour period because thrombosis, thrombophlebitis, or troublesome infection in the cutaneous wound is likely to develop which may even lead to a bacteremia.

The *amount* of solution administered will depend upon the exigencies of the case. With a patient who is critically ill, who has fever and extensive infection, who has a constant gastric suction, and at the same time is having fluids administered by parenteral routes, it is essential to keep a written balance sheet of the fluids which are given and which are excreted or sucked away. Such a tabulation enables one to evaluate quickly the fluid status of the patient at any time. Rough estimates of the degree of hydration can be gained by the frequency and the amount of urinary voidings.

If suction is maintained or if parenteral fluids are administered for more than two days, the level of *blood chlorides* and *serum protein* must be checked at appropriate intervals. If the chloride level is low, more saline solution should be ordered. If the serum protein begins to fall below 6 gm. per 100 cc. of plasma, a transfusion or serum infusion (depending upon the red blood count) is indicated. In cases of overwhelming infection repeated small *blood transfusions* are beneficial, even though the red blood cell level is satisfactory.

Removal of Drains.—If drains have been used, they should be loosened slightly from their bed about the fifth day and should be withdrawn about an inch each succeeding day so that they are completely removed seven or eight days after operation. After this period a drain is of little use and should not be left in place longer. There is no advantage in the painful process of daily removing and reinserting abdominal drains, and such a practice is likely to spread rather than localize infection.

Chemotherapy.—Chemotherapy will probably have a larger role in the treatment of these cases in the future than it has at present. It is impossible to believe that it will replace properly performed operative procedures, but it should be an important adjuvant to surgical therapy. *Sulfanilamide* given in a small group of our postoperative cases of generalized peritonitis changed the results so little that we were not encouraged to undertake studies of a long, controlled series to see if any appreciable reduction in the mortality would accrue. *Sulfathiazole,* however, has been quite promising. Our series with the use of this drug is not long enough to warrant any final conclusions, but there is a definite impression that it reduces the toxicity of these patients and has been an important factor in the treatment of many recovered cases. It is doubtful if the introduction of these drugs directly into the peritoneal cavity has much superiority over the adequate administration of them by parenteral routes.

SUMMARY OF TREATMENT

Our treatment of peritonitis of appendiceal origin can be summarized as follows: (1) Immediate operation (except in rare cases) with delay only for the administration of parenteral fluids, if needed. (2) Primary appendectomy in 95 per cent of the cases. (3) A rectus-retracting or muscle-splitting incision. (4) Introduction of a drain for peritonitis or local abscess. (5) Postoperative use of gastric suction. (6) Liberal administration of parenteral fluid. (7) Adequate sedation with morphine. (8) High-concentration oxygen tent for combating distention. (9) Fowler's position. (10) Application of heat to the abdomen. (11) Blood transfusion for low serum-protein levels, anemia, or overwhelming infections.

COMPLICATIONS

Paralytic Ileus.—Ileus may result from a spreading peritoneal infection, from undue trauma to the intestines during operation, or from low levels of blood chloride and protein. Recognition of the early stages of adynamic ileus is important because it is easier to ward it off than it is to treat it after it is established. Constant gastric suction, high-concentration oxygen tent, hot abdominal poultices, and rectal tubes are effective in most cases. While prostigmin, pituitrin, and other such drugs are at times advantageous, their use is contraindicated in the presence of infection or any mechanical form of obstruction. Enterostomy for paralytic ileus has little or nothing to offer, because it usually deflates only the local loop.

Intestinal Obstruction.—*Mechanical* intestinal obstruction may occur at two periods after operation for a ruptured appendix. *Early* obstruction may

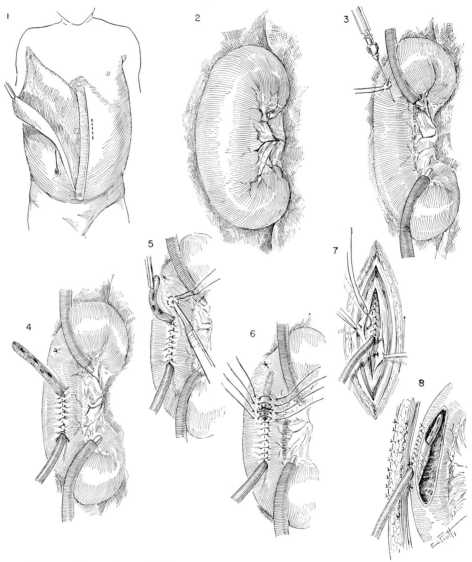

Fig. 129.—Operative method (Witzel enterostomy) for relief of intestinal obstruction from plastic fibrinous adhesions during convalescence from peritonitis.

1, Appendiceal drainage wound walled off with a towel which is stuck along the midline of the abdomen with a strip of adhesive tape. Operative incision for enterostomy to be made along the dotted line.

2, Presenting loop of distended intestine brought out through wound and walling off gauzes carefully placed.

3, Rubber-covered intestinal clamps placed across either end of exteriorized loop. Deflation of bowel between clamps with a needle attached to sucker or large syringe. Purse-string suture in place around puncture site.

4, Puncture wound closed. Catheter, with multiple holes in tip, laid on bowel and partially covered with interrupted embedding sutures.

appear a week or two later, when intestines become adherent to one another by plastic fibrinous exudate. *Late* obstruction occurs after several months or years, when a firm fibrous band compresses or strangulates an intestinal loop.

Early and late obstructions require entirely different forms of therapy. In the *early form of obstruction* no attempt should be made to explore the abdomen widely, for doing so involves a high risk of spreading an infection which nature is doing its best to wall off. Conservative treatment by constant *gastric suction* will tide many patients with early obstruction over the critical period, but if this fails, an *enterostomy* of the Witzel type may be a life-saving procedure. This can be carried out under local anesthesia, by entering the left side of the abdomen, grasping a presenting dilated loop of intestine, and inserting a soft urethral catheter into it, which is led out through the abdominal wall as depicted in Fig. 129. If this catheter is irrigated gently at frequent intervals, the intestine can be deflated and a safety valve provided during the subsequent weeks when most of the plastic fibrinous adhesions are absorbed and the intestinal obstruction is spontaneously relieved. When normal flatus and bowel movements are passed per rectum, the catheter may be withdrawn and the tract in the abdominal wall will promptly close. *In the late type of obstruction* the abdomen must be extensively explored, the obstructed loop identified, and the constricting bands severed.

Localized Abscess.—A localized abscess is occasionally found after subsidence of a generalized peritonitis. When pain, tenderness, and swelling show that an abscess is forming in the lower abdomen or in the pelvis, a gentle daily examination will indicate whether it is resolving itself or whether it is accumulating more exudate which must be evacuated. Considerable judgment is required to determine the optimum time for instituting drainage. If fever is maintained or is climbing, if there is increasing local pain, or if there is increasing intestinal obstruction (from a loop which is involved in the inflammatory mass) *incision* and *drainage* should be resorted to. In general, there is no need for haste in opening one of these abscesses; what often appears to be an abscess will spontaneously subside.

5, Purse-string suture placed, bowel punctured, catheter ready to be pushed into intestine.

6, Purse-string suture tightened. Completion of catheter embedding with additional stitches.

7, Catheter leading out from intestine, which is now anchored in several places to the inner surface of the peritoneum. Catheter should come out through peritoneum in central part of wound.

8, Parasagittal section of abdominal wall and drained intestine. The catheter pierces the abdominal wall in an oblique manner, so that the tract will quickly and spontaneously close when the catheter is subsequently withdrawn.

It is then evident that the swelling consisted mainly of edematous, matted intestinal loops or swollen peritoneal leaves without an actual accumulation of pus.

If an abscess appears in the *pelvis,* no attempt should be made to open it through the rectum until definite fluctuation is detected by digital examination, and until the mass is large enough to impinge upon the adjacent pelvic nerves and paralyze the anal sphincter muscle. A low-lying collection of pus often spontaneously ruptures into the vagina or rectum or it can be satisfactorily evacuated through the rectum and the resulting wound heals with remarkable rapidity. It is well to remember that a rounded, soft mass presenting against the rectum may prove to be a loop of intestine which is stuck in the pelvis. The surgeon should be confident of the nature of the mass before plunging a knife into it.

MORTALITY FACTORS

Type of Appendicitis.—Acute, unruptured appendicitis has a well standardized method of treatment and is attended by a death rate which is negligible. Appendicitis with peritonitis, however, is a major surgical problem, and continues to carry a high risk. Acute appendicitis of all forms at the Children's Hospital from 1928 through 1939 had an overall mortality of 3.1 per cent. When further analyzed according to the extent of the infectious process, the figures given in Table 24 are obtained.

TABLE 24

RELATIONSHIP BETWEEN TYPE OF ACUTE APPENDICITIS AND MORTALITY RATE: 1928 THROUGH 1939

Type of Appendicitis	Cases	Deaths	Mortality Percentage
Acute, unruptured, without fluid......................	386	1	0.2 ⎫ 0.37
Acute, unruptured, with peritoneal fluid..............	149	1*	0.6 ⎬
Acute, ruptured with local or diffuse peritonitis..........	405	28	6.9 ⎭
Totals.......................................	940	30	3.1

* Death from hemophilia.

Duration of Symptoms.—It is at once evident that before rupture has taken place acute appendicitis carries an excellent prognosis, but that invasion of the peritoneal cavity itself implies a serious menace to the patient's life. Since *rupture* of the acutely inflamed organ is the dangerous turning point in appendicitis, it is of some interest to know when this takes place in most cases. In 893 cases in whom the duration of symptoms were known, the condition of the appendix shown in Table 25 was found at operation.

These figures show that even within twelve or twenty-four hours some appendices have already ruptured, and that after twenty-four hours the incidence of rupture rises sharply. It is apparent that great responsibility rests upon the pediatrician or general practitioner to make a diagnosis within the first twenty-four hours if the disease is to be treated while rupture is uncommon and good results are to be expected. This challenge is further evident from Table 26, which points out an acceptably low mortality when

TABLE 25

RELATIONSHIP BETWEEN TYPE OF APPENDICITIS AND DURATION OF SYMPTOMS

Type of Appendicitis	Duration of Symptoms					
	Less than 12 hours	12–24 hours	24–36 hours	36–48 hours	48–72 hours	More than 72 hours
Number of cases without rupture....	76	173	107	31	50	54
Number of cases with rupture.......	16	22	44	49	101	170
Percentage of cases with rupture.....	17%	11%	29%	61%	66%	75%

hospitalization and operation took place in the first twenty-four hours. It is appalling to note that approximately one quarter of the individuals were not hospitalized until seventy-two hours or more had elapsed.

Age of Patient.—The individual's age, *per se,* is not believed to be a factor in mortality rates, for in very young children the results following

TABLE 26

RELATIONSHIP BETWEEN DURATION OF SYMPTOMS AND THE CORRESPONDING MORTALITY RATES IN ACUTE APPENDICITIS

Duration of Symptoms before Operation	Cases	Deaths	Mortality Percentage
Less than 12 hours...............................	92	1	1.0 ⎫ ⎫
12–24 hours......................................	195	0	0.0 ⎬0.4 ⎪
24–36 "	151	2	1.3 ⎭ ⎬0.6
36–48 "	80	3	3.7 ⎪
48–72 "	151	5	3.3 ⎭
More than 72 hours...............................	224	18	8.0

treatment of acute unruptured appendicitis are as good as those in older subjects. However, the more rapid progression of inflammation to a generalized peritonitis in the young, and the greater difficulty in arriving at a correct diagnosis in these individuals, gives rise to a mortality of 11 per cent for all children under four years of age as compared with 1.6 per cent for all those above this age (see Table 27).

TABLE 27

RELATIONSHIP BETWEEN TYPE OF ACUTE APPENDICITIS, AGE OF PATIENT, AND MORTALITY RATE (1928 THROUGH 1939)

Patient's Age	Acute, Unruptured, with or without Fluid	Acute, Ruptured, with Local or Diffuse Peritonitis	Totals
Less than 1 year:			
Cases		2	2
Deaths		1	1
Mortality		50.0%	50.0%
1—2 years:			
Cases	2	22	24
Deaths	0	5	5
Mortality	0.0%	22.7%	20.8%
2–4 years:			
Cases	26	94	120
Deaths	0	11	11
Mortality	0.0%	11.7%	9.1%
4–6 years:			
Cases	74	96	170
Deaths	1	5	6
Mortality	1.3%	5.2%	3.5%
6–12 years:			
Cases	390	184	574
Deaths	1	6	7
Mortality	0.2%	3.2%	1.2%
12–16 years:			
Cases	43	7	50
Deaths	0	0	0
Mortality	0.0%	0.0%	0.0%
Totals:			
Cases	535	405	940
Deaths	2	28	30
Mortality	0.3%	6.9%	3.1%

PINWORMS AND APPENDICITIS

Pinworms or their ova were recognized in 3 per cent of our surgically removed, acutely inflamed appendices, but only rarely was there histologic evidence of burrowing of worms into the submucosal tissues which might have initiated the inflammatory process.

Symptoms.—Pinworms are often found in appendices which show no inflammation despite the fact that the patients have clinical findings which are highly suggestive of acute appendicitis. Such symptoms include *nausea, vomiting, abdominal pain,* mild right lower-quadrant *tenderness,* a degree or two of *fever,* and a mild or moderate *leukocytosis.* Mechanical obstruction of the appendix by a bolus of the parasites undoubtedly accounts for this syndrome which is often indistinguishable from that of acute appendicitis.

The frequency with which pinworm infestation of the appendix gives rise to symptoms will undoubtedly vary with the prevalence of the disease in the particular community and the stratum of society from which patients are drawn. A recent survey at the Children's Hospital revealed that approximately 18 per cent of the general ward population harbored these parasites; indeed, this figure should probably be set much higher. In the last few years we have encountered one patient with abdominal symptoms from pinworms to about each ten children who had acute appendicitis.

Treatment.—In a given case, if symptoms are equivocal and the abdominal tenderness is minimal, a *vermifuge* may be tried, but if there is any lighting up of abdominal signs, *appendectomy* should be undertaken. As a general rule, it is not wise to administer a vermifuge to patients with appendiceal symptoms. It will seldom empty an appendix of worms, and furthermore the patient may actually have appendicitis. The safest treatment of appendiceal symptoms due to pinworms is appendectomy.

APPENDECTOMY FOR RECURRENT ABDOMINAL PAIN

Any physician who undertakes the care of children is familiar with the frequency and worrisome character of recurrent and unexplained abdominal pain. These bouts of discomfort may appear alone, may be accompanied by nausea, or may be followed by vomiting. Fever is usually absent or minimal. Individual attacks as a rule are not severe, but the nagging and repetitious quality of the symptoms is finally sufficient to arouse the parents' apprehensions. These cases also provide considerable anxiety for the practitioner, as well as the surgeon, who wants to avoid unnecessary operation and yet give the patient any benefit which surgical treatment might offer.

Preoperative Study of Patient.—A case of this sort requires careful consideration and study before any surgery is contemplated. The possibility of *constipation* as a cause of complaints should be completely eliminated. If there is any question of incomplete elimination, daily administration of mineral oil over a period of two or three weeks should be tried. *Pinworms* as a source of complaints must be investigated. A history of perianal itching, finding of worms around the anus, or the identification of ova in the stools calls for a course of vermifuge treatment.

Provided constipation and parasitic intestinal infection have been excluded, three investigations should be made: (1) The *stool* should be examined by benzidine or guaiac tests, for occult bleeding may turn attention to an unsuspected polyp or Meckel's diverticulum. (2) A *roentgenologic examination* of the colon by barium enema should rule out colonic polyp or incomplete rotation of the colon. These fluoroscopic and film studies of the abdomen should incidentally reveal any calcification which might be present in tuberculous mesenteric lymph nodes. Examination of the upper intestinal tract by roentgenologic means is so seldom productive of positive findings in the childhood ages that such an examination may be omitted in most cases (unless there are specific indications for doing it). (3) *Intravenous pyelography* should be performed in all these cases even though the urine is normal. An unsuspected hydronephrosis, ureteral stricture, or aberrant renal vessel may be uncovered. All too often is an abdomen explored and the patient subsequently brought back with persistent symptoms which are found to arise from the urinary tract.

Surgical Treatment.—Provided these studies are all negative and the child's symptoms are severe enough, *laparotomy* is justifiable and indeed advisable—if the operator is willing to perform a thorough exploration. The small intestine from the ligament of Treitz to the ileocecal valve should be carefully inspected to make sure there is no polyp, Meckel's diverticulum, obstructing band, or other abnormality. The gallbladder should be palpated for stones. Any undue mobility of the cecum should be corrected. Finally, after the entire examination has been completed, *appendectomy* can be undertaken. A satisfactory exploration implies that a rectus incision is employed; a McBurney opening gives an entirely inadequate exposure for this undertaking.

The appendix in such a child may give symptoms because it is kinked, scarred, or is obstructed by some solid material within its lumen. Quite often the appendix may be disappointingly normal in appearance and yet the individual is subsequently relieved of pain. Children with vague and recurring abdominal pain should not be subjected to hasty and lightly considered appendectomy, but in those patients who have undergone adequate studies to rule out other pathologic conditions, this operation, while at times disappointing, will bring relief in a majority of instances.

BIBLIOGRAPHY

1. Botsford, T. W., Hudson, H. W., Jr., and Chamberlain, J. W.: Pinworms and Appendicitis. New England J. Med., *221:* 933, 1939.
2. Bower, J. O.: Acute Appendicitis: A Survey of Its Incidence and Care in Philadelphia. J. A. M. A., *96:* 1461, 1931.
3. Caldwell, E. H.: Appendicitis in Childhood. Surg., Gynec. and Obst., *67:* 169, 1938.
4. Coller, F. A., and Potter, E. B.: The Treatment of Peritonitis Associated with Appendicitis. J. A. M. A., *103:* 1753, 1934.
5. Fine, J., Hermanson, L., and Frehling, S.: Further Clinical Experiences with Ninety-five Per Cent Oxygen for the Absorption of Air from the Body Tissues. Ann. Surg., *107:* 1, 1938.
6. Giertz, K. H.: Twenty-five Years' Experience in the Treatment of Peritonitis. Ann. Surg., *104:* 712, 1936.
7. Gordon, H.: Appendiceal Oxyuriasis and Appendicitis, Based on Study of 26,051 Appendices. Arch. Path., *16:* 177, 1933.
8. Harris, W. H. and Browne, D. C.: Oxyuris Vermicularis as a Causative Factor in Appendicitis. J. A. M. A., *84:* 650, 1925.

9. Hudson, H. W., Jr., and Chamberlain, J. W.: Acute Appendicitis in Childhood. J. Pediat., *15:* 408, 1939.

10. Ladd, W. E.: Immediate or Deferred Surgery for General Peritonitis, Associated with Appendicitis in Children. New England J. Med., *219:* 329, 1938.

11. Miller, E. M., Fell, E. H., Brock, C., and Todd, M. C.: Acute Appendicitis in Children. J. A. M. A., *115:* 1239, 1940.

12. Sperling, L., and Myrick, J. C.: Acute Appendicitis; A Review of 518 Cases in the University of Minnesota Hospitals from 1932 to 1935. Surgery, *1:* 255, 1937.

13. Wangensteen, O. H., and Dennis, C.: Experimental Proof of the Obstructive Origin of Appendicitis in Man. Ann. Surg., *110:* 629, 1939.

15

CHAPTER XVI

ILIAC ADENITIS

Symptoms.—Staphylococcal or streptococcal infection of the perineum, anus, or leg may give rise to inflammation in lymph glands of the iliac fossa. Iliac adenitis manifests itself as an acute process with symptoms primarily of *abdominal pain* or of *restriction in leg movements*. In the first category there is fever, restlessness, and constant abdominal pain which is apt to be more severe in one of the lower quadrants. Nausea and vomiting are minimal and indeed usually absent—a point of some importance in differentiating a right-sided adenitis from acute appendicitis. In the second group the iliopsoas muscle is thrown into spasm by the inflamed nodes which lie upon it, so that a limp or a flexion deformity of the thigh is produced. Not infrequently this latter type of patient comes to the attention of the orthopedist because of an altered gait, which suggests a hip infection, osteomyelitis at the upper end of the femur, or a psoas abscess originating in the spine.

Physical Examination.—Examination of these patients shows deep, lower-abdominal *tenderness* which is most marked just above the inguinal region. If the infection has been of short duration no swelling can be detected, but in later stages there is *edema* and *induration* of the subcutaneous tissues and a palpable mass medial to and below the anterosuperior spine. As the abscess mass increases in size it extends forward toward Poupart's ligament, but obviously does not involve the inguinal canal. By *rectal examination* nothing abnormal may be detected, or a swelling may be felt high on one side of the pelvis—according to the size of the lesion. A *portal of entry* of the infection may be found on the leg or possibly around the anus, but the initial lesion is often healed and not discernible by the time the patient seeks advice for the abdominal pain. In most of the cases the infection has skipped the femoral and inguinal glands and lodges solely in the iliac group. The temperature ranges from 101° to 104° F. The white blood count is elevated to 15,000 or 25,000, but it may be as high as 40,000.

Differential Diagnosis.—Iliac adenitis differs from *appendiceal abscess* in that it usually has no intestinal symptoms, and that its tenderness is closer to Poupart's ligament. It is contrasted to the *psoas abscess* of spinal origin in that it develops more rapidly, there is less flexion deformity of the thigh, and no spinal lesion is demonstrable. It is to be differentiated from *infection of the hip joint* because rotation of the hip is less interfered with and the tenderness or mass is above Poupart's ligament.

Course.—Iliac adenitis will spontaneously disappear in about half of the cases. This subsidence can be aided by bed rest, sedatives, and application of heat to the lower abdomen. In the remaining patients *suppuration* occurs and as much as several hundred cubic centimeters of exudate may become pocketed in the iliac fossa outside of the peritoneum. It is a great rarity for this to break into the general abdominal cavity, but in one case we have

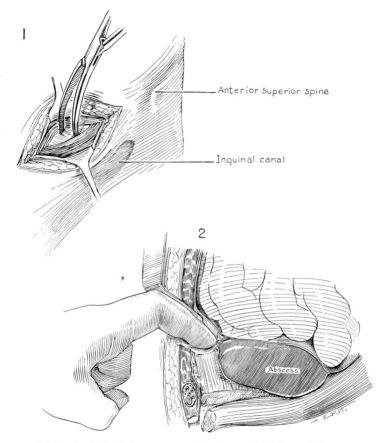

Fig. 130.—Method of draining suppurative iliac adenitis. *1,* The external oblique fascia has been split and retracted. Muscles are being bluntly separated with a half-length clamp. *2,* Parasagittal section showing peritoneum pushed inward with a retractor and finger being passed outside of this to reach the abscess cavity.

seen it force its way around in front of the peritoneum and finally rupture into the urinary bladder. The exudate in most cases tends to dissect along outside of the peritoneum and point at or near the internal inguinal ring. The resulting swelling may be mistaken for a tender, incarcerated, inguinal hernia, but the fever, leukocytosis, duration of the lesion, and absence of intestinal symptoms should exclude this diagnosis.

Surgical Drainage.—When suppuration occurs, surgical drainage must almost inevitably be done. If it is obvious that inflammation is advancing instead of subsiding, the problem arises of choosing the correct time for incision and drainage. It is best to wait until adequate walling off from surrounding structures has taken place, and until the mass has assumed considerable size and pushed the peritoneal fold well above the inguinal canal. At such a time the abscess may be readily opened extraperitoneally without danger of soiling the abdominal cavity. While the dissecting pus can pierce the deeper tissues of the abdominal wall, it is stopped by the external oblique fascia. Hence, fluctuation is almost never found and operation should not be delayed in the hope that it will develop.

Surgical drainage is readily effected through a short *incision* below and medial to the anterosuperior spine (Fig. 130) ; care should be taken to keep the wound above the inguinal canal so that this will not be exposed to the infection. The external oblique fascia is split in the direction of its fibers and the underlying muscles are bluntly separated. When the pyogenic membrane becomes obvious, it is pierced by the tip of a hemostat, the jaws of which are then separated. Purulent material usually gushes out at this stage, and the tip of an exploring finger can be passed extraperitoneally into the abscess cavity in the iliac fossa. When an adequate opening has been made, a soft rubber wick or a cigarette drain is inserted into it and the wound left open.

These patients do extremely well after proper drainage has been instituted. The suppuration rapidly subsides and hospitalization is seldom necessary for more than a week or two. In the Children's Hospital series, eighteen children, ranging in age from one to eleven years, were operated upon, and all of them recovered. Seventeen other children were believed to have iliac adenitis without suppuration which subsided under conservative therapy.

BIBLIOGRAPHY

1. Coutts, W. E.: Acute Inflammation of Deep Iliac Lymph-Nodes. Ann. Surg., *86:* 782, 1927.
2. Frank, L.: Suppurative Adenitis of Iliac Lymph Nodes of Hemolytic Streptococcal Origin. Ann. Surg., *105:* 975, 1937.
3. Hyman, A.: Suppurative Retroperitoneal Pelvic Lymphadenitis. Ann. Surg., *91:* 718, 1930.
4. Irwin, F. G.: Acute Iliac Adenitis; Report of 18 Cases. Arch. Surg., *36:* 561, 1938.

CHAPTER XVII

OMENTAL CYSTS AND MESENTERIC CYSTS

OMENTAL CYSTS

Cysts of the omentum presumably originate in the same manner as do those of the mesentery, namely, by obstruction of an existing lymphatic channel or by growth of congenitally misplaced lymphatic tissue which does not communicate with the vascular system. These cysts are thin walled, rounded or lobulated, and contain serous fluid. Microscopically, they are lined by a flattened layer of endothelial cells. The cysts may be small and embedded within the substance of the omentum, or they may be very large and entirely replace this structure. One specimen we have excised measured $13 \times 8 \times 6$ cm.; a second was larger, and contained more than 1000 cc. of fluid; a third was of such size that it extended from the greater curvature of the stomach down into the pelvis and out into either flank so that it entirely covered the intestines.

Symptoms and Signs.—The symptoms are usually those of a slowly enlarging abdominal mass which gives little or no discomfort. The three patients we have encountered were two eight-year-old girls and a three-year-old boy. *Physical examination* discloses little more than a prominent or protuberant abdomen within which an elastic, nontender, forward-lying mass can be palpated. The rounded or slightly lobulated cyst can often be dislodged from side to side and if it is large, a fluid wave can be elicited.

Diagnosis.—The diagnosis of an omental cyst is usually suggested by the physical findings and the silent nature of the swelling. It may be difficult to differentiate between mesenteric and omental cyst, but the latter diagnosis is suggested if the mass is found to lie in front of the intestines by roentgenologic studies.

Treatment.—This can be easily carried out by simple excision. Large cysts may require amputation of almost the entire omentum. Smaller ones can be dissected out from the surrounding omental fat, which should be saved because of its usefulness in combating infections which might arise in the peritoneal cavity at a subsequent time.

MESENTERIC CYSTS

Cysts may arise in any portion of the mesentery of the small or large intestine. They may reach enormous proportions and because of their slow growth they may give symptoms over long periods of time. The surgical

233

treatment of these lesions is not difficult. Recurrences are almost unknown and benefits accruing from operation are lasting.

Etiology.—Mesenteric cysts could conceivably arise by obstruction of a preexisting lymphatic trunk, but the absence of demonstrable inflammation or other fibrosing lesion in the mesentery of these individuals makes this theory improbable. It is more than likely that mesenteric cysts develop from misplaced bits of lymphatic tissue which proliferate and then accumulate fluid because they do not possess communications with the remainder of the lymphatic system.

Pathology.—Mesenteric cysts are most commonly found in the mesentery of the jejunum or ileum, but in two of our cases they appeared in the trans-

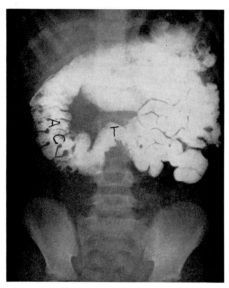

Fig. 131.—Roentgenogram from a gastro-intestinal series on a patient with a large jejunal mesenteric cyst (see Fig. 132). *AC,* Ascending colon. *T,* Terminal ileum. The intestines are all displaced upward. At operation the lower abdomen was filled by the cyst.

verse mesocolon and in the mesosigmoid, respectively. The cysts obviously must pass through a stage when they are quite small, but by the time that they have produced symptoms justifying operation they have usually reached a large size. Not infrequently they are as large as an orange or a grapefruit, and indeed they may fill a major portion of the abdominal cavity. One specimen, Fig. 132, contained 1200 cc. of fluid. The cysts are almost always unilocular, but they may be quite lobulated. In the majority of cases only one cyst is present, but in two of our patients the main cyst was accompanied by several smaller ones in the base of the mesentery.

The cysts lie between the peritoneal leaves of the mesentery (or mesocolon) and may be situated anywhere from its base out to the enteric border. The cysts are usually not tensely filled, and tend to have a flabby consistency. It is common for them to have a dumbbell shape (Figs. 133 and 134) and to project out from either surface of the mesentery, sometimes partly surrounding the adjacent intestine in the form of a saddle. Such a

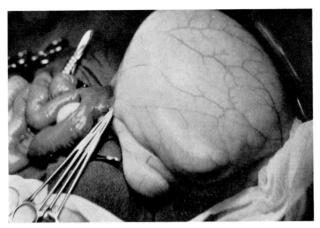

Fig. 132.—Photograph taken at operation. Six-year-old girl (Case 2) with a chylous cyst of the mesentery. The cyst contained 1200 cc. of milky fluid and protruded through on the opposite side of the mesentery as seen at the left.

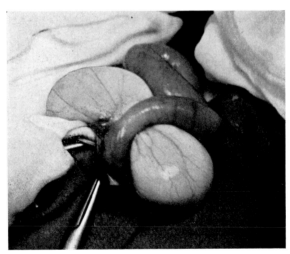

Fig 133.—Operating-table photograph of chylous cyst of jejunal mesentery in a seven-week-old boy (Case 3). The cyst has a dumbbell shape and bulges out on both sides of the mesentery.

saddle-shaped structure can strangle the adjacent loop of intestine and obstruct it. The walls of the cysts are quite thin and rarely more than a millimeter or two in thickness. The inner surfaces are smooth. By microscopic examination the walls are found to consist of connective tissue.

There is no muscular coat or mucosal lining. In well-preserved specimens a layer of flattened endothelial cells can be identified on the inner surface.

Fluid within the cysts may be of two sorts. In most instances it is serous and colorless, but in others it is chylous and has the appearance and consistency of whitish or yellowish-white milk. Of our eight examples five had a *serous* and three a *chylous* fluid. All of the chylous cysts arose from the mesentery of the jejunum, where material draining from the intestinal tract presumably contained a high percentage of fat. Fluid from the serous cyst of the mesosigmoid, shown in Fig. 137, was found by chemical examination

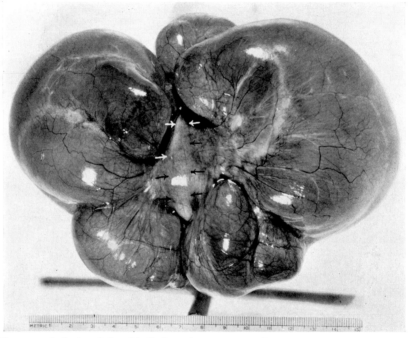

Fig. 134.—Lobulated dumbbell-shaped cyst removed from ileac mesentery of a four-year-old boy. The specimen is viewed from its anterior aspect. The cyst bulged out from both surfaces of the mesentery and ballooned up around the intestine (indicated by arrows) which it partially obstructed.

to contain the following: sodium, 133 milliequivalents per liter; chlorides, 101 milliequivalents per liter; nonprotein nitrogen, 31 mg. per cent; total protein, 4.9 gm. per cent; cholesterol, 68 mg. per cent. The concentration of these substances was approximately the same as that of plasma. Chemical examination of the chylous fluid from the cyst illustrated in Fig. 132 showed: chlorides, 108 milliequivalents per liter; nonprotein nitrogen, 29 mg. per cent; total protein, 2.1 gm. per cent; fat, 1 per cent.

Differential Diagnosis.—There are many descriptions in the literature which confuse true mesenteric (lymphatic) cysts with *enteric* cysts (duplications—see Chapter VII). These two lesions have somewhat similar positions in the mesentery, but it is desirable to distinguish between them because they are pathologically different and because they require different forms of treatment. The *duplication* is a thick-walled structure which has a serous coat, two layers of smooth muscle, and a mucous membrane lining. It usually lies immediately adjacent to the bowel between the folds of the mesentery, and the musculature of the duplication is so intimately associated with that of the intestine that they cannot be separated without injury to the latter. Also, the blood supply of the duplication is the same as that of the intestine to which it is adjacent, so that the duplication cannot be removed without destroying the blood supply to the segment of intestine. The *mesenteric cyst,* on the other hand, is thin walled and has no muscular coat or mucosal lining. While it may lie against the mesenteric surface of

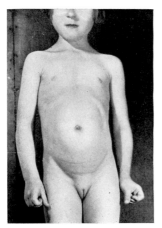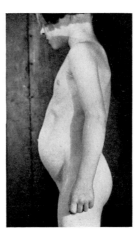

Fig. 135.—Photographs of six-year-old girl with a cyst of the mesosigmoid. Prominence of abdomen noted in lateral view.

the intestine, there is a line of cleavage between the two so that it can usually be excised without injuring the bowel or its blood supply.

Clinical Findings.—Mesenteric cysts are rarely detected in infancy; they are more apt to be found later but yet within the first decade of life. The ages of our eight patients varied from seven weeks to seven years. The symptoms may be of three sorts: (1) In the typical case a painless, slowly *enlarging abdomen* is the only complaint. The progressive enlargement (Fig. 135) is sometimes noted for a year or two before surgical advice is sought. (2) There may be recurring attacks of mild to moderate *abdominal pain* which at times are associated with vomiting. These usually last for a day or two and appear only at infrequent intervals. There may be reduced appetite and poor weight-gain. (3) In occasional patients (*e.g.,* No. 6 of Table 28) the symptoms are those of acute intestinal *obstruction* if the cyst lies at the free border of the mesentery where it can press upon or angulate the gut.

Whether or not a mesenteric cyst can be felt through the abdominal wall depends somewhat upon its size and tenseness. If the child is examined within the first few months of illness, abdominal *palpation* may reveal no abnormality. Indeed, even the largest cysts may elude detection because they are so flabby that their borders cannot be mapped out. However, in most cases a fairly well-defined, fluctuant, soft mass can be palpated. This can be shifted within the abdomen and it is more freely movable in a lateral than in a vertical direction. If the cyst is large, a fluid wave or even shifting dullness may be detected.

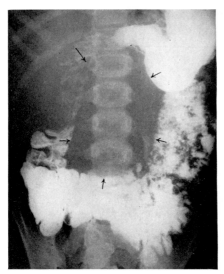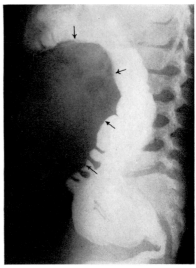

Fig. 136.—Anteroposterior and lateral roentgenograms which outline an intra-abdominal mass (indicated by arrows). At operation this was found to be a cyst of the mesosigmoid, shown in Fig. 137.

Roentgenologic Findings.—Films of the abdomen, with or without a barium meal, often give a valuable lead, for a gasless shadow will be found which displaces intestines into other parts of the abdomen (Figs. 131 and 136). Fluoroscopic study shows that the mass can be pushed into different parts of the abdomen. Since these lesions rarely produce intestinal obstruction, dilated intestine is seldom found.

Treatment.—Surgical treatment can be effected in one of three ways: (1) The cyst and adjacent portion of intestine (if this is unduly adherent) may be *excised* and a side-to-side anastomosis performed. (2) The cyst may be *marsupialized,* but there is little to recommend this form of therapy. (3) The cyst may be *dissected* out from the mesentery. This is the preferred method of treatment.

Excision of a cyst is effected by peeling away the peritoneal leaves of the mesentery from the underlying mass and by displacing the important blood vessels to one side. It is usually not difficult to dissect the sac away from the intestine or colon. The proper cleavage planes are easier to find

TABLE 28

DATA FROM CASES OF OMENTAL AND MESENTERIC CYSTS

Case	Age and Sex	Symptom Duration	Position of Cyst and Type of Fluid in Cyst	Size of Cyst	Operation	Result
			Omental Cysts			
1	3 years, male		Omentum—serous	Filled entire anterior abdomen	Excision	Cured
2	8 years, female	3 months	Omentum—serous	1000+ cc.	Excision	Cured
3	8 years, female	5 days	Omentum—serous	13 by 8 by 6 cm.	Excision	Cured
			Mesenteric Cysts			
1	3 years, male	2 years	Jenunal—chylous	Orange size	Excision with intestinal resection	Cured
2	6 years, female	6 months	Jejunal—chylous	30 by 30 by 15 cm.	Excision	Cured
3	7 weeks, male	12 hours	Jejunal—chlyous	Size of 2 golf balls (dumbbell shape)	Excision. Reduction of a volvulus	Died
4	3 years, male	2 years	Jejunal—serous	Size of 3 fists (dumbbell shape)	Excision	Cured
5	7 years, male	2 years	Ileum—serous	Size of 2 fists (dumbbell shape)	Excision	Cured
6	4 years, male	5 days	Terminal ileum—serous	Lobulated dumbbell shape	Excision with resection of ileum	Cured
7	2½ years, male	1 year	Transverse colon—serous	Size of grapefruit	Excision	Cured
8	6 years, female	5 months	Sigmoid—serous	10 by 8 by 8 cm. 875 gm.	Excision with resection of sigmoid	Cured

if the cyst is not opened or ruptured. When the sac has been removed a considerable rent may be left in the mesentery, which is now repaired with interrupted sutures of fine silk or catgut. If dissection is carefully done the blood supply of the adjacent gut will not be interfered with. If the major portion of a cyst membrane is dissected out, but it appears too dangerous to remove a small bit which remains against an important blood vessel or against the intestine, this can be cauterized with carbolic acid (followed by alcohol) according to the suggestion of Peterson.[10]

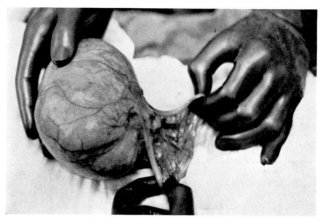

Fig. 137.—Photograph taken during operation. Grapefruit-sized serous cyst of mesosigmoid. See Figs. 135 and 136.

Eight patients with mesenteric cysts have been operated upon at the Children's Hospital. Some data from these cases are summarized in Table 28. The only death was in a seven-week-old baby who also had a volvulus with resulting extensive infarction of the intestine.

BIBLIOGRAPHY

Omental Cysts

1. Berger, L., and Rothenberg, R. E.: Cysts of Omentum, Mesentery and Retroperitoneum; Clinical Study of 18 Cases. Surgery, 5: 522, 1939.
2. Guernsey, C. M.: Primary Tumors and Cysts of Omentum. Proc. Staff Meet. Mayo Clin., 14: 694, 1939.
3. Hall, D. P.: Lymphangiomata of the Great Omentum. Ann. Surg., 111: 605, 1940.
4. Horgan, J.: Cysts of Omentum; Review and Report of Case. Am. J. Surg., 29: 343, 1935.

Mesenteric Cysts

5. Carter, R. M.: Cysts of the Mesentery. Surg., Gynec. & Obst., 33: 544, 1921.
6. Flynn, C. W.: Mesenteric Cysts, With Report of a Case of Cystic Lymphangioma. Ann. Surg., 91: 505, 1930.
7. Gale, J. W., and Keeley, J. L.: Mesenteric Cysts Causing Intestinal Obstruction. Am. J. Surg., 40: 647, 1938.
8. Messer, F. C.: Analysis of Fluid from Chylous Mesenteric Cyst. J. Lab. & Clin. Med., 23: 596, 1938.
9. Peterson, E. W.: Mesenteric and Omental Cysts. Ann. Surg., 96: 340, 1932.
10. Peterson, E. W.: Cysts of the Mesentery. Ann. Surg., 112: 80, 1940.
11. Swartley, W. B.: Mesenteric Cysts. Ann. Surg., 85: 886, 1927.

CHAPTER XVIII

DISEASES OF THE SPLEEN

Much has been written about the physiology and the pathologic states of the spleen in relationship to abnormalities of the blood and circulation. No attempt will be made in this chapter to describe or even list all of the diseases to which the spleen is heir. The following sections are limited to those disorders which can be treated by surgical means with varying degrees of success. *Splenectomy* has been performed in young children with Mediterranean or Cooley's erythroblastic anemia with no beneficial results. In fact, the operation is contraindicated because it may be followed by a more severe anemia. Splenectomy has been undertaken in cases of aplastic anemia, usually with disappointing effects. Occasionally there is a slight improvement in the blood picture and a slight diminution in the frequency of transfusions which are subsequently necessary; there is rarely a remission in the anemia, but this is certainly not the rule and the operation should be employed only as a last resort. Dr. Louis K. Diamond[6] has made extensive clinical studies on the Children's Hospital patients with diseases of the spleen. Many of the observations included in this chapter have been taken from his review.

The conditions for which splenectomy has known therapeutic value are: (1) congenital hemolytic anemia; (2) idiopathic hemorrhagic purpura; (3) Banti's disease; (4) Gaucher's disease; (5) traumatic rupture or torsion of the spleen; (6) cysts and neoplasms of the spleen.

CONGENITAL HEMOLYTIC ANEMIA

Symptoms.—This condition, also known as "familial hemolytic anemia," "chronic hemolytic jaundice," "acholuric jaundice," etc., is characterized by a chronic or recurring type of anemia associated with hemolytic crises, increase in fragility of the erythrocytes, a tendency for many of the red blood cells to be microcytic and spherical, a high percentage of circulating reticulocytes, a mild icterus, increased excretion of urobilin in the urine and stools, and enlargement of the spleen. These children are apt to be retarded in their physical development; they may be somewhat underweight; it is common for them to be smaller in stature than the expected normal (Fig. 138). A suitable investigation often shows that other members of the family have had the same disease, yet a familial incidence is not found in all cases.

The *anemia* may be of moderate or marked degree. The red count ranges between 2,000,000 and 3,000,000, but it has been found as low as 1,000,000 cells per cubic millimeter. Following crises, the red blood count rises slowly. It may reach normal levels, but it is more characteristic for some degree of anemia to persist. It is typical for the disease to have periods of exacerbation and remission. *Hemolytic crises* with fever, abdominal pain, pallor, jaundice, and weakness, occur at varying intervals. At these times there is excessive destruction of red blood cells, as is shown by a falling red count, a rising icteric index, and an increased excretion of urobilin in

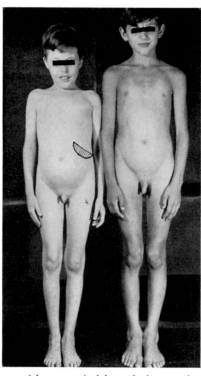

Fig. 138.—Photograph of boy with congenital hemolytic anemia and a normal boy of the same age. Note the retardation in growth. Lower border of spleen is outlined.

the stools and urine. Crises may be of a minor sort, or they may be so severe that the patient dies with profound anemia and anoxemia, in spite of repeated transfusions. The *icteric index* rises to 40 or 50, but it does not increase to the high values observed in most cases of biliary obstruction. A mild *jaundice* may be present most of the time, or it may appear only when there is excessive erythrocyte destruction.

Diagnosis.—A diagnostic feature of the disease is the increased *fragility of the erythrocytes* when placed in varying dilutions of salt solution. Normal red cells will begin to hemolyze in solutions of about 0.42 per cent sodium chloride and the hemolysis will be complete in concentrations of about 0.34 per cent. In contrast, cells from an individual with hemolytic anemia may begin to disintegrate in 0.85 per cent saline and the hemolysis is usually complete in concentrations of 0.40 per cent.

Microscopic examination of the blood shows a tendency for the erythrocytes to be microcytic and globular (so-called *spherocytosis*) —a point of some diagnostic importance. *Reticulocytes* occur in great numbers, and are above what might be expected for the existing degree of anemia. Counts of 20 to 30 per cent are common, but values as high as 90 per cent circulating reticulocytes have been observed. Nucleated erythrocytes may appear in the circulating blood during a crisis. The leukocytes and platelets are within normal limits except with a crisis.

These individuals excrete as much as 30 to 40 times the normal amount of *urobilin* in the stool and urine; this elimination goes hand in hand with the destruction of red cells and liberation of their pigments. Urobilin increases particularly during or immediately after hemolytic crises, at which times the urine may have a dark yellow or orange color. Quantitative determinations of this substance can be made on the stool, but it is easier to study the urine by testing it with Ehrlich's reagent.

Roentgenologic Examination.—Roentgenologic studies may show some relevant changes which, however, are not characteristic of the condition. The epiphyses may show retardation of growth, a point which is best determined by examination of the wrist bones. When the bone marrow is overactive and hyperplastic the medullary substance is expanded so that there is a concurrent thinning of the adjacent cortical bone. These bony readjustments are best observed in the long bones where there is thinning of the cortex or in the skull where there is a striate or fuzzy appearance of the tables. These changes are similar to but not as common or as marked as those which are found with erythroblastic anemia.

Course.—Increased excretion of blood pigments by way of the biliary tract not infrequently leads to development of *gallstones,* even in preadolescent years. These calculi are largely of the pigment variety (Fig. 159), but calcium and cholesterol can also be included in small amounts. The discovery of cholelithiasis in any child should always make one suspect the possibility of congenital hemolytic anemia.

The severity of the anemia, the frequency of the crises, and the ultimate prognosis are all somewhat related to the age at which the disease begins. Individuals whose symptoms first appear in late childhood or early adult life may have but slight disability and exhibit only mild anemia, jaundice and possibly cholelithiasis. When the disease starts in infancy or the first few years of life there is a more fulminating process, and death not infrequently occurs during a crisis, even during the initial one. In such individuals the destruction of blood may be so rapid that repeated transfusions will not tide them over the acute episode. In short, the earlier in life that the disease begins, the poorer is the outlook and the more urgently should splenectomy be advised.

Treatment.—*Splenectomy* is a specific treatment for congenital hemolytic anemia; it gives quick and permanent relief of symptoms. If possible, this should not be done during a crisis. Following splenectomy there is a gradual fall in the reticulocytes and an increase in the number of circulating red

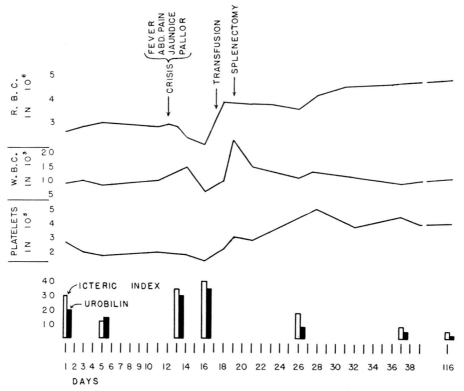

Fig. 139.—Chart showing data from a child with congenital hemolytic anemia who was treated by splenectomy.

blood cells. The erythrocytes still retain their increased fragility but the abnormal destruction of red cells ceases. The changes in red count, white count, platelet count, icteric index, and urobilin excretion before and after operation in an eleven-year-old girl are graphically set forth in Fig. 139.

Postsplenectomy Thrombosis.—After splenectomy there is always some increase in the number of circulating blood platelets. These may reach 600,000 or 700,000 per cu. mm., and counts of 1,000,000 or more are occasionally found. This sharp rise begins within the first week after operation and has usually disappeared by the end of the second or third week (Fig.

140). If the platelets become very numerous, *thrombi* can develop in various parts of the body, particularly in branches of the portal system. Unexplained abdominal pain and fever occurring in the first two weeks after operation should strongly suggest that venous thrombi are forming, particularly if the platelet count is high during this period.

There are two ways to combat such an unfortunate but not rare complication. Deep *x-ray irradiation* over the heart (to affect the circulating blood) will apparently reduce the number of platelets, though the response may be somewhat slower than is desirable under such urgent circumstances. *Heparin* administered intravenously will immediately prolong the bleeding time and will prevent formation of thrombi. Any individual whose platelet

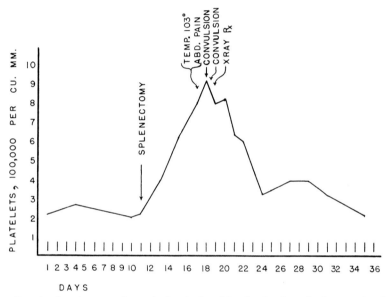

Fig. 140.—Graph showing number of circulating blood platelets during a platelet crisis after splenectomy. From a case of congenital hemolytic anemia.

count has reached 750,000 and is apparently still climbing, should probably receive heparin. Certainly, if the count reaches 1,000,000 heparin should be given without delay and should be continued for four or five days until the danger of thrombosis has passed.

Results of Treatment.—In the Children's Hospital series, twenty-three individuals with congenital hemolytic anemia have been subjected to splenectomy and the results of operation have been most gratifying. There has been a striking improvement in growth and development, when these were previously retarded. In only one case was there a continuation of the hemolytic crises, but even here the attacks were much less frequent and less severe. Two individuals developed venous thrombi and one of them died

16

three weeks after operation with portal obstruction. One child died during operation for cholecystectomy, common duct exploration and splenectomy. This combination of cholecystectomy and splenectomy at one sitting should be avoided because the operative shock is too great. In summary, twenty-one cases have survived operation. One of these has had marked amelioration of symptoms and the other twenty have been completely relieved.

IDIOPATHIC PURPURA HEMORRHAGICA

Idiopathic purpura hemorrhagica (variously known as "idiopathic thrombocytopenic purpura," "idiopathic purpura," etc.) is a disease in which there is a bleeding tendency because of a diminished number of circulating platelets. Blood smears show a paucity of platelets which by actual counts may be depressed to 75,000 or less per cubic millimeter (by the method of Ottenberg and Rosenthal). The bleeding time tends to be prolonged, although it may be normal. The clotting time is not lengthened, but retraction of the clot is delayed and poor. Other than the diminished platelets, the blood usually shows no abnormalities except those which can be attributed to blood loss.

Symptoms.—Idiopathic purpura appears at any age, and may have an acute or a chronic form. There may be spontaneous *oozing* from the mucous membranes from time to time, and indeed such bleeding may be profuse. *Epistaxes* and subcutaneous *extravasations of blood* are particularly common. *Ecchymoses* may be induced by the slightest trauma, but they can also appear without injury. Mild fever may accompany the more extensive lesions. Prolonged oozing may complicate minor surgical procedures. In females, the menstrual periods may be prolonged and the bleeding may be profuse. *Retinal hemorrhages* are frequently encountered. Placement of a tourniquet around a limb usually produces *petechial hemorrhages* in the extremity within a few minutes. The spleen may be somewhat enlarged, particularly in the chronic forms.

Diagnosis.—The diagnosis is usually made without difficulty, and is based on a history of recurring purpuric manifestations, the finding of a low platelet count, and the absence of other diseases which might depress the number of circulating thrombocytes. Conditions which can *secondarily* produce thrombocytopenia are infections, some drug poisonings, aplasia involving all the elements of the hematopoietic system, and leukemia or other neoplastic infiltration which replaces normal bone marrow and thereby crowds out platelet-forming tissue. In a series of more than 200 cases of thrombocytopenic purpura observed on the medical service of the Children's Hospital, only about 15 per cent were finally considered to fall into the idiopathic group.

Treatment.—When the diagnosis of idiopathic purpura has been established, the form of therapy must be decided upon. Symptomatic treatment for bleeding in these cases includes *bed rest,* proper *sedation,* local *control of blood loss* by styptics or thromboplastic substances, and possible *blood transfusions* to increase temporarily the available platelets and to replace blood which has been lost. Transfusion may tide the individual over for a few days, but it has no permanent influence on the course of the disease. *Parathyroid extract* is beneficial in a small percentage of cases.

Splenectomy.—It is generally conceded that splenectomy is valuable in the chronic form of idiopathic purpura hemorrhagica, but most students of this disease advise against splenectomy in the acute type from which the patient often spontaneously recovers. If the symptoms have been severe and have recurred over a long period of time, removal of the spleen has beneficial effects in a high percentage of cases, but it is by no means always curative. It is well to bear in mind that many children have this disease in a mild form and tend to have diminishing symptoms with the passage of years. Therefore, splenectomy should be reserved for those patients whose hemorrhagic tendencies are severe enough to justify the slight but definite dangers of laparotomy.

At the Children's Hospital, ten patients have been subjected to splenectomy after other types of therapy had been unsuccessful. Two of these had only temporary relief which was followed in a few months by lowered platelet levels and return of bleeding tendencies. The remaining children have been completely relieved of their purpuric manifestations and have maintained normal platelet levels.

BANTI'S DISEASE

There are few terms which connote such a multiplicity of lesions to different physicians as does "Banti's disease." It is evident that under this title there have been grouped several more or less associated conditions which have in common certain symptoms or clinical findings. Banti's syndrome usually begins in young, otherwise healthy adults, but it may also arise in children. It is a chronic disease which may prove fatal within a few years, or it may have a course extending over several decades.

Symptoms and Diagnosis.—Banti separated the disease into three *stages:* In the *first,* which usually lasts a variable number of years, there is gradually increasing pallor, weakness, abdominal discomfort, possibly digestive disturbances, and an enlargement of the spleen. During this period a moderate anemia, esophageal varices, and possibly hematemesis can develop. The *second* or intermediary stage is rather a transitory one and is not always clinically recognizable. During this time there are increased digestive disturbances and the liver becomes enlarged and palpable. The *third* or terminal stage is predominated by hepatic disease in which there is cirrhosis,

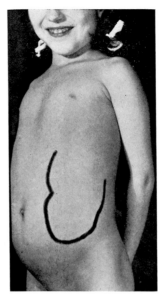

Fig. 141.—Photograph of nine-year-old girl with Banti's disease. The liver was palpable 3 cm. below the costal margin. Outline of spleen is shown. This was known to be enlarged since one year of age. Splenectomy subsequently performed because of bleeding from esophageal varices.

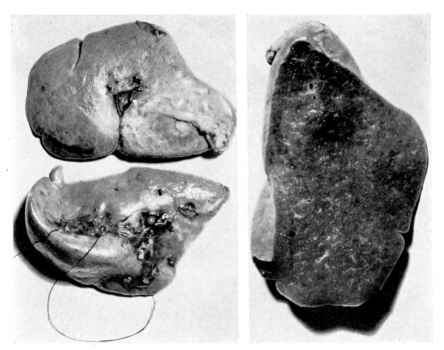

Fig. 142.—A spleen weighing 575 gm. removed from girl shown in Fig. 141. Cross section of the organ shows increased prominence of the fibrous tissue septa.

recurrent painless ascites, increasing anemia, emaciation, possibly jaundice, and an increasing severity and frequency of esophageal hemorrhages. These three stages of Banti's disease may overlap one another and it may be impossible to define them clearly.

Special attention should be directed to a small group of children with symptoms depending upon *obstruction of the splenic vein* or *the portal*

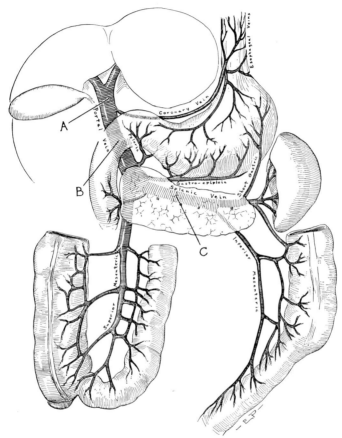

Fig. 143.—Sketch of a typical portal system (some subjects show considerable variation in the way the vessels empty into the splenic and portal veins). Obstruction occurring within the liver produces engorgement of the entire system, enlargement of the collateral channels and development of esophageal varices. Obstruction at *A* will produce the same changes. Obstruction at *B* will probably give the same changes. Obstruction at *C* will usually not lead to development of esophageal varices.

vein before it enters the liver (Fig. 143). It is usually difficult or even impossible to separate these cases clinically from those having portal obstruction because of *cirrhosis of the liver*. These patients have recurring bleeding from gastric or esophageal varices as their outstanding complaint. The blood loss may temporarily produce severe anemia. If the patient is examined during or immediately after a hemorrhage, abdominal palpation shows that the spleen is not palpable or is only barely felt. However, during the ensuing few days the spleen becomes enlarged and remains so until a subsequent hemorrhage occurs and the organ again diminishes in size for a three- or four-day period. These children develop collateral venous channels, principally through the esophageal veins, in the effort to reduce their portal hypertension. Accordingly, bleeding from esophageal veins temporarily reduces the portal engorgement and the spleen shrinks in size—only to

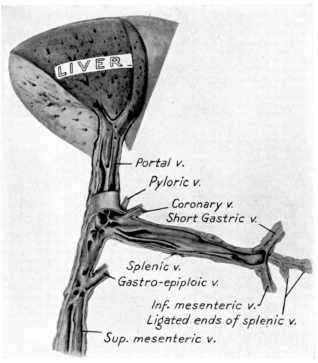

Fig. 144.—Autopsy sketch of portal system from a ten-year-old girl who died of fatal esophageal hemorrhage after splenectomy for Banti's disease. There are old, extensive, and partially recanalized thrombi in the portal, superior mesenteric, and splenic veins, giving rise to extrahepatic venous obstruction. These presumably formed during the multiple severe infections which the child was known to have in the first year of life.

enlarge again in a few days when the patient's blood volume is restored by natural processes or by transfusion.

Extrahepatic obstructions in the splenic vein or other parts of the portal system may result from a number of lesions. Thrombophlebitis can follow regional or distant infections (Fig. 144). An adequate history often reveals an *omphalitis* or other severe infection in early life which was presumably responsible for thrombi within the abdomen. The pathologic studies of Farber indicate that omphalitis during the neonatal period is frequently a contributing factor, since organisms can proceed inward along the vessels of the round ligament and gain direct access to the portal system. Valves are found as normal structures in various portal channels during embryonic and early postnatal life. While they normally disappear, portions of them may persist and partly obstruct the vessels concerned.

Various authors have called attention to this syndrome of portal obstruction and hematemesis *without* cirrhosis of the liver. Warthin[18] gave an excellent description of such cases. Smith and Farber[15] summarized the findings in fifteen patients who had been treated at the Children's Hospital up to 1935, and Dr. Sidney Farber has made subsequent studies on additional postmortem material (*e.g.*, Fig. 144) which form a basis for ideas presented here. Rousselot[13] recorded further examples with clinical studies including bromsulfalein tests, showing that the liver functions were normal. It is important to recognize that such a pathologic process can exist in order to emphasize that many children with a picture of early Banti's disease do not progress to an ultimate stage in which there is cirrhosis of the liver.

For the present discussion it is best to let the term "Banti's disease" include all conditions in which there is anemia or alimentary tract bleeding resulting from portal hypertension (whether this is from hepatic cirrhosis or extrahepatic venous obstruction). Inasmuch as there are somewhat different clinical problems in early and late forms of Banti's disease, it is well to consider these separately, as is done in the following two sections.

Early Banti's Disease.—Children with "early Banti's disease" may manifest this condition in either of two ways: *First,* the picture may be mainly that of portal or splenic vein obstruction with recurring and exhausting hemorrhages from esophageal varices. *Second,* the picture may be one of splenomegaly, hypochromic anemia, leukopenia, possibly thrombocytopenia, with or without esophageal hemorrhages—a complex often referred to as "splenic anemia." Either of these two states may subsequently advance to "late Banti's disease," but some individuals do not develop such serious and terminal changes.

Treatment.—When the diagnosis of early Banti's disease has been made, *splenectomy* is definitely beneficial, regardless of whether anemia or hematemesis has been the outstanding symptom.

At the Children's Hospital, eight children have been operated upon because of *splenic anemia*. In most cases the erythrocytes, hemoglobin, leukocytes, and platelets have returned to normal levels. The fatigue, anorexia, and pallor which were attributable to anemia have disappeared. Some of these patients have been followed as long as twelve years, and only one has acquired signs suggesting hepatic cirrhosis. It is possible that longer periods of observation will show that others will subsequently develop liver disease. Even if such complications do eventually appear, the immediate relief of symptoms has been quite satisfactory and splenectomy has been thoroughly justified.

The Children's Hospital material also includes fourteen patients who were operated upon because of severe *bleeding from esophageal varices.* Splenectomy under these conditions has been performed to diminish the portal engorgement. It has been estimated that closure of the splenic artery reduces by as much as 20 per cent the amount of blood flowing into the portal circuit. In the more recent cases, removal of the spleen has been combined with division of the esophageal branches of the coronary veins (to divert blood from existing esophageal varices) and with establishment of an omentopexy (to provide additional collateral anastomoses between the portal and peripheral systems). The majority of these patients appeared to have considerable relief over a period of many years, while others have continued to have hemorrhages which have even resulted in death. On the whole, the frequency and the severity of attacks have been reduced by these operative procedures. Recently, operation has been supplemented by injection of the esophageal varices with sodium morrhuate through an esophagoscope. It is too early to evaluate definitely the merits of this procedure, but so far they are not very encouraging.

Late Banti's Disease.—In the terminal stages of Banti's syndrome there may be enlargement and cirrhosis of the liver, splenomegaly, hypochromic anemia, increasing emaciation, progressive ascites, and repeated hematemesis. Death usually follows from intercurrent infection or by exsanguination from a ruptured varix. These final developments are more apt to be found in middle adult life, but they are occasionally observed in late childhood.

Treatment.—The therapy is largely confined to *supportive measures.* Rest, sedation, and withdrawal of solid food will help to control episodes of bleeding. Subsequent administration of *iron,* or *transfusions* when necessary, will aid in restoring the red count to normal.

Splenectomy has a rather limited usefulness. If the organ is large and causes abdominal distress, its removal will appreciably increase the patient's comfort. If esophageal hemorrhages are severe or frequent, the removal of the spleen will reduce the amount of blood flowing into the portal channels and thereby diminish the congestion in the esophageal veins. Finally, if there is ascites, the removal of the spleen will usually prevent reaccumulation of fluid, presumably by diminishing the congestion in the portal system. On the whole, splenectomy does not give any brilliant results in treatment of these cases, but there are some studies to indicate that life is slightly prolonged, that ascites is relieved, and that hematemeses are less troublesome. If splenectomy is to be performed, it should be combined with omentopexy and with division of the esophageal branches of the coronary veins.

Splenectomy in such individuals carries several hazards. *First,* there is apt to be postoperative hemorrhage from the operative site, because of the regional venous engorgement. It is therefore imperative to ligate carefully even the smallest vessels which are severed in the field. *Second,* such spleens are apt to be surrounded by numerous and vascular adhesions which complicate the removal of the organ. *Third,* the platelet count may rise to unduly high levels in the first few weeks after operation, and in order to avoid thromboses in various parts of the body, intravenous administration of heparin may be necessary.

GAUCHER'S DISEASE

There are three primary disorders of lipoid metabolism which are closely associated with one another. According to the type of lipoid involved, these may be grouped as: (1) *Schüller-Christian's disease* (generalized xanthomatosis), a cholesterol disturbance; (2) *Niemann-Pick's disease,* a phosphatide (sphingomyelin) disturbance; (3) *Gaucher's disease,* a cerebroside (kerasin) disturbance.

Symptoms and Diagnosis.—Gaucher's disease manifests itself by excessive accumulation of kerasin in cells, principally of the liver, spleen, lymph nodes, and bone marrow. In some instances a marked *splenic enlargement* dominates the picture and there is progressive abdominal distention, discomfort, anorexia, fatigue, and retardation of physical growth. Whenever there is bony involvement there may be local pain, limitation of motion, and even pathologic fracture. The *roentgenologic* picture of localized destruction of bone is often mistaken for osteomyelitis.

If such a lesion should be exposed at operation, removal of some of the yellowish brown material for *histologic examination* should establish the diagnosis. The large, lipoid-laden cells have a wrinkled appearance and do not take the Smith-Dietrich stain as do the lipoid-filled, foamy-appearing cells of Niemann-Pick's disease. The patients with Gaucher's disease may subsequently develop foci in other bones, and it is important to recognize that these are lipoid accumulations, and that operation (for suspected osteomyelitis) is not necessary.

Treatment.—The bone lesions, like those of Schüller-Christian's disease, can be effectively treated by exposure to x-rays. This induces fibrosis, healing, and symptomatic relief. Indeed, such changes may appear spontaneously in some cases, but they are speeded up and advanced by x-ray treatments.

If the spleen is large, its removal has been found to be of definite value. The *indications for splenectomy* are: (1) progressive enlargement of the organ; (2) development of anemia or thrombocytopenia with a tendency toward bleeding; (3) retardation in growth and physical development of the individual. Following splenectomy the abdominal discomfort is relieved, the anemia is improved, and physical growth becomes accelerated.

Results of Treatment.—At the Children's Hospital six splenectomies have been performed on patients with Gaucher's disease with satisfactory results. Particularly impressive has been the rapid increase in growth, so that the retarded child reaches a normal average size for his age within a few years. It might be argued that removal of the spleen would precipitate or accelerate the accumulation of the lipoid in the skeleton, but numerous roentgenologic observations on our cases lead us to believe that such is not the case. Although it may still be too early for final evaluation of splenectomy in this disease, it is our distinct impression that the operation has considerable merit.

TRAUMATIC RUPTURE OF THE SPLEEN

Symptoms.—Abdominal injuries, particularly those resulting from direct violence, such as a blow on the abdomen, a fall from a considerable height, or an impact from a moving vehicle, may rupture various viscera including the spleen. When the spleen is torn the important symptoms are those of *hemorrhage.* The amount of blood lost into the peritoneal cavity naturally depends upon the extent of the splenic lacerations. Whenever there is known abdominal injury, a rising pulse, declining blood pressure, pallor, thirst, air hunger, and a falling red count, there are sufficient indications for *exploratory laparotomy,* provided the blood loss cannot be accounted for elsewhere. Left shoulder *pain* may suggest some pathologic condition below the left diaphragm, but this symptom is not always present. Inasmuch as the violence usually produces some contusion of the abdominal wall, the physician often has difficulty in deciding whether the local *pain* and *tenderness* are due to abdominal wall trauma or to intraperitoneal trauma. To delay operation until shifting dullness has appeared implies waiting until the individual is exsanguinated. It is usually impossible to determine before operation the extent of the injury and what organs have been affected.

Treatment.—When operations of this sort are undertaken, provisions for immediate *transfusion* should always be made. Indeed, it is a wise precaution to place a cannula in the arm or leg vein before opening the abdomen so that blood may be administered during the procedure, if this should be necessary. Not infrequently, more free blood is found in the peritoneal cavity than had been anticipated, and there may be additional loss before the site of hemorrhage can be identified and bleeding can be controlled. The operator's troubles are considerably lessened and the patient's chances for survival are greatly enhanced if transfusion can be given during or immediately after this period.

The average spleen is so friable that once its capsule has been ruptured, fractures into its substance are apt to be deep and difficult to repair. *It is therefore easier and preferable to remove the entire organ.* The vessels of the splenic pedicle should be compressed or ligated as soon as possible to stop the leakage of blood from the ruptured spleen.

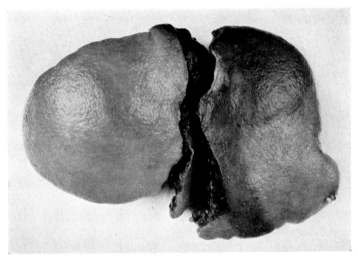

Fig. 145.—Ruptured spleen removed from a five-year-old boy. There had been extensive intraperitoneal hemorrhage.

At the Children's Hospital two boys, five and seven years old, respectively, have been treated for this accident. One was struck in the abdomen with a board and was then knocked down. The other fell 3 or 4 feet onto a stone sidewalk (Fig. 145). Both recovered following splenectomy.

CYSTS AND TUMORS OF THE SPLEEN

Small cysts of the spleen, 1 or 2 cc. in diameter, are occasionally observed at the autopsy table, particularly in conjunction with congenital cysts of the liver or kidneys. Cysts of the spleen which are large enough to be of clinical importance are very rare. Fowler[7] collected reports of 137 nonparasitic splenic cysts and of this group only ten occurred in the first decade of life.

Varieties.—The lesions may be of several sorts: (1) *Thin-walled serous cysts* presumably arise from inclusion of a nest of peritoneal cells so that these become pinched off in a cleft on the splenic surface. From this nidus there develops a small intrasplenic sac which accumulates and retains fluid. (2) *Lymphangiomata* of the spleen have often been described. These are usually multilocular and have a honeycombed appearance. They may be so large that they replace most of the splenic substance. (3) *Epidermoid cysts* are rare, usually do not attain a large size, and do not accumulate hair or sebaceous material. They are lined with squamous epithelium which does not keratinize. (4) *Parasitic cysts* are almost always of echinococcus origin. They may be found in conjunction with similar lesions of the liver, lung, or other viscera, but in some instances they develop solely in the spleen.

Tumors of the spleen are rare, but sarcomas and hemangiomas have been described.

Treatment.—Removal of the spleen for treatment of a cyst is seldom necessary unless it is large enough to cause local discomfort. Neoplasms are extremely rare, but if the mass is felt through the abdominal wall, or if it is discovered during laparotomy for some other condition, removal of the organ is indicated.

TECHNIC OF SPLENECTOMY

The removal of a spleen may be a simple procedure or it may be a most trying abdominal operation. Oozing of blood because of some dyscrasia, difficulty in severing dense and vascular perisplenic adhesions, and inadequacy of exposure may all contribute toward making splenectomy a hazardous undertaking. *Mortality rates* for this operation have often been high, but with improved methods for controlling bleeding by transfusions and with better operative exposures, fatalities have now been reduced to a minimum. In a series of seventy splenectomies at the Children's Hospital there have been four deaths during operation or in the immediate postoperative period. With present surgical care, at least two of these fatalities would now be regarded as avoidable. Since it is impossible to predict in a given case whether operation will be simple or difficult, it is essential that the surgeon be thoroughly prepared for any eventuality before opening the abdomen.

Preoperative Treatment.—This is important. When the patient has a bleeding tendency it is desirable to *transfuse* him within twenty-four hours before operation and to be prepared to repeat this during or immediately thereafter. In those patients with anemias below 3,500,000 or 4,000,000 the red count should be brought up to adequate levels by medication and transfusion. The preparations should include selection of a properly matched, compatible blood donor who will be available during operation if an emergency should arise. Finally, cleansing and *deflation of the stomach and colon* will allow these organs to be more easily packed off in the operative field and will enhance the exposure.

Exposure of the Spleen.—There is some variance of opinion concerning the type of incision which should be employed. If the spleen is large it is easier to approach its pedicle by a *left paramedian* or *rectus muscle-splitting incision.* Likewise, if division of the coronary veins is contemplated, a longitudinal anterior incision gives a better exposure of the subdiaphragmatic region.

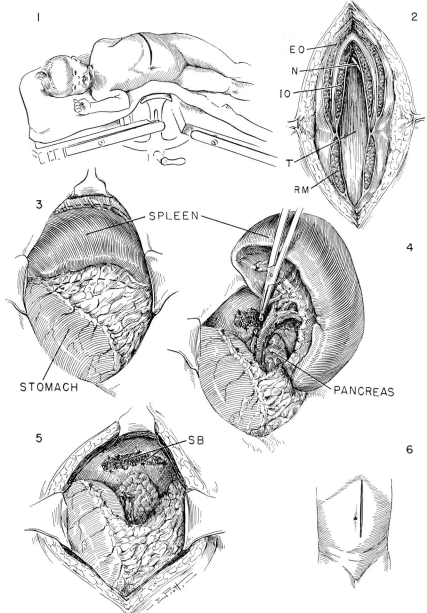

Labels within figure: 1; 2; EO; N; IO; T; RM; 3; SPLEEN; 4; STOMACH; PANCREAS; 5; SB; 6

Fig. 146.—Operative steps for splenectomy. *1*, Position of patient. Incision to be made as indicated. *2*, The external oblique and the internal oblique muscles have been divided, exposing the transversalis muscle on which the tenth nerve is identified. The rectus muscle has been divided. *3*, Abdomen opened and spleen exposed. Tenth nerve pulled to posterior angle of wound by small retractor. Posterior attachments of the spleen to be cut along the dotted line. Anterior omental attachments will be severed along the dotted line to expose the tail of the pancreas and the splenic vessels. *4*, The splenic artery has been divided. The vein will be divided next. *5*, Splenic artery and veins ligated. Bleeding points in the splenic bed have been ligated. *6*, Position of operative incision when anterior longitudinal wound is desired.

EO, External Oblique Muscle   *N,* Tenth Nerve   *IO,* Internal Oblique Muscle

T, Transversalis Muscle   *RM,* Rectus Muscle   *SB,* Splenic Bed

For most splenectomies, a *transverse* or *obliquely transverse incision* running forward from the lateral and lower costal border is much to be preferred (Fig. 146). The spleen is more easily brought into the wound, adhesions can be more easily and safely divided, and the intestines are less disturbed. The incision should not be carried posteriorly beyond the midaxillary line, for to do so may lead to division of the lower thoracic nerves as they course along between the internal oblique and the transversalis muscles. The incision should be carried backward until the tenth nerve is identified and can be protectively held in the posterior angle of the wound with a retractor. If the spleen is small it is not necessary to divide the rectus muscle, but if it is large the rectus can be cut across with impunity, provided its ends are properly joined when the abdominal wound is closed.

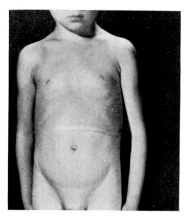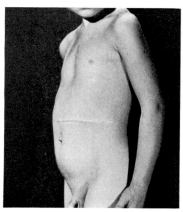

Fig. 147.—Postoperative photographs showing position of transverse wound for splenectomy. There is no bulging or weakness of the abdominal wall.

Transverse incisions heal extremely well. They give a narrow cutaneous scar and are not followed by any weakness of the abdominal wall from division of nerves.

Excision and Wound Closure.—With either incision it is desirable in most instances to make a small opening in the gastrocolic omentum and tie the splenic artery and vein as the first step in the removal of the spleen. In this way the spleen can contract somewhat and can squeeze out blood into the circulation. After this has been done the lienorenal ligament and other attachments can be cut and the spleen removed. When this order of procedure is adopted a minimum of bleeding takes place.

After the spleen has been removed, a thorough inspection should be made of its bed, so that any bleeding points can be carefully sutured. The abdominal wall is closed in layers, without drainage.

BIBLIOGRAPHY

1. Anderson, N. A.: Traumatic Rupture of Spleen in Children, With Special Reference to Left Shoulder Pain. J. Pediat., *15:* 535, 1939.
2. Andrus, W. D.: Conference on the Treatment of Disorders of the Spleen. J. A. M. A., *115:* 299, 1940.
3. Barg, E. H., and Dulin, J. W.: Splenectomy in the Treatment of Banti's Syndrome. Arch. Surg., *41:* 91, 1940.
4. Dameshek, W.: Rouleaux Formation in Fresh, Unmodified Blood as a Diagnostic Test for Hemolytic Anemia. New England J. Med., *221:* 1009, 1939.
5. Davis, H. H., and Sharpe, J. C.: Splenic Vein Thrombosis Following Splenectomy. Surg., Gynec. & Obst., *67:* 678, 1938.
6. Diamond, L. K.: Indications for Splenectomy in Childhood. Results in 52 Operated Cases. Am. J. Surg., *39:* 400, 1938.
7. Fowler, R. H.: Cystic Tumors of the Spleen. Internat. Abstr. Surg., *70:* 213, 1940.
8. Levine, D. B., and Michelson, H.: Acute Thrombopenic Purpura Treated Successfully With Solution of Parathyroid. J. A. M. A., *115:* 360, 1940.
9. McClure, R. D., and Lam, C. R.: Experiences in Heparin Administration. J. A. M. A., *114:* 2085, 1940.
10. Montgomery, A. H., McEnery, E. T., and Frank, A. A.: Epidermoid Cysts of Spleen. Ann. Surg., *108:* 877, 1938.
11. Ottenberg, R., and Rosenthal, N.: A New and Simple Method for Counting Blood Platelets. J. A. M. A., *69:* 999, 1917.
12. Ravenna, P.: Banti Syndrome (Fibrocongestive Splenomegaly). Definition, Classification, and Pathogenesis. Arch. Int. Med., *66:* 879, 1940.
13. Rousselot, L. M.: The Late Phase of Congestive Splenomegaly (Banti's Syndrome) with Hematemesis but without Cirrhosis of the Liver. Surgery, *8:* 34, 1940.
14. Sherwin, B., Brown, C. R., and Liber, A. F.: Cystic Disease of Spleen. Ann. Surg., *109:* 615, 1939.
15. Smith, R. M., and Farber, S.: Splenomegaly in Children with Early Hematemesis. J. Pediat., *7:* 585, 1935.
16. Thompson, W. P.: The Pathogenesis of Banti's Disease. Ann. Int. Med., *14:* 255, 1940.
17. Vogt, E. C., and Diamond, L. K.: Congenital Anemias, Roentgenologically Considered. Am. J. Roentgenol., *23:* 625, 1930.
18. Warthin, A. S.: The Relation of Thrombophlebitis of the Portal and Splenic Veins to Splenic Anemia and Banti's Disease. Internat. Clin., *4:* 189, 1910.
19. Wintrobe, M. M., Hanrahan, J. M., Jr., and Thomas, C. B.: Purpura Haemorrhagica with Special Reference to Course and Treatment. J. A. M. A., *109:* 1170, 1937.
20. Whipple, A. O.: Splenectomy as a Therapeutic Measure in Thrombocytopenic Purpura Haemorrhagica. Surg., Gynec. & Obst., *42:* 329, 1926.

CHAPTER XIX

CONGENITAL ATRESIA OF THE BILE DUCTS

Until recent years, congenital atresia of the bile ducts was regarded as a pathologic curiosity and a condition which was not amenable to medical or surgical therapy. While it is true that the great majority of these infants have an obstruction of the intrabiliary or extrabiliary tree which is ultimately incompatible with life, there are some of these patients in whom it is possible to anastomose remnants of the bile ducts with adjacent portions of the gastro-intestinal tract. The number of such successful operations is small, but in a condition which is otherwise uniformly fatal, it is best to explore all of these babies in the hope of finding a condition which is amenable to surgical relief.

Congenital obstruction of the bile ducts will always be associated with the name of John Thomson[5] for his careful analysis of fifty cases in 1892. However, it was the detailed study of more than 100 examples of biliary anomalies by Holmes[2] in 1916 that called attention to the fact that many of these babies presented conditions which could be corrected by surgical means. Following the publication of Holmes' work, we began to explore routinely all infants with such pathology. In 1927 operation was first performed successfully (by Ladd) for the relief of congenital atresia of the bile ducts.

It was the contention of earlier writers that relief of the biliary obstruction—when it was possible—would be a futile procedure because the extensive *biliary cirrhosis* which is always present would militate against successful issue. We have now learned, however, that this is not true, for we have followed patients with such cirrhosis and with operative relief of biliary obstruction for periods as long as twelve years and there has been no evidence of hepatic insufficiency. Therefore, considerable evidence has now accumulated to show that a liver has extraordinary powers of regeneration and that, if the biliary obstruction can be relieved, the existing cirrhosis disappears and the individual will possess a normally functioning liver.

In most reports the emphasis in treatment has been placed on the absorption of fats, the digestion of food, and the various other chemical problems that occur as a result of the absence of bile from the intestinal tract. Although such considerations are important, they are now overshadowed by the therapeutic possibilities of operative intervention in some cases.

PATHOLOGY

The extrabiliary ducts are partially or completely represented by fine cords of fibrous tissue possessing no lumina. The obliterative process may involve the hepatic duct, the common duct, the cystic duct, and the gallbladder. Such solid cords of tissue lie in positions which normal ducts would occupy at the porta of the liver and in the gastrohepatic ligament. The extent of such obliteration, of course, determines the operability in each case. In other words, if the atresia exists in the lower part of the hepatic duct or in the common duct, there remains a small bulbous enlargement of the ductal system above this point of obstruction. In a review of forty-five cases from the Children's Hospital which have been studied either at operation or at autopsy (or both) it was found that the hepatic duct alone was patent in three cases; that the hepatic and upper part of the common duct were patent in six patients; that the gallbladder, cystic and common ducts were

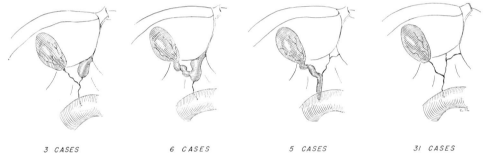

| 3 CASES | 6 CASES | 5 CASES | 31 CASES |

Fig. 148.—Sketch of types of atresia of the extrahepatic bile ducts, as found in surgical exploration of forty-five cases. *1*, Hepatic duct patent and connecting with liver. *2*, Hepatic and part of common duct patent (gallbladder may be atretic or patent). *3*, Hepatic duct atretic. Gallbladder, cystic duct and common duct normal. *4*, Hepatic and common ducts atretic.

patent and connected with the duodenum but the hepatic duct was atretic in five cases; and, finally, that all the extrahepatic ducts were atretic in thirty-one cases (Fig. 148).

Gallbladder.—The gallbladder may be found in one of four pathologic states: (1) It may be completely *atretic* and may be represented by only a cord of fibrous tissue 3 or 4 mm. thick and 2 or 3 cm. in length. (2) It may contain a *lumen,* but yet be so small that it is not more than 8 or 9 mm. in diameter and 2.5 or 3 cm. in length. Such a gallbladder usually contains a little clear mucoid material. (3) It may be quite large and tensely filled with accumulated *secretory products* of its own mucosal glands. Such contents may be described as "white bile." (4) It may be relatively normal in appearance and may contain *bile,* indicating that the obstruction is in the common duct.

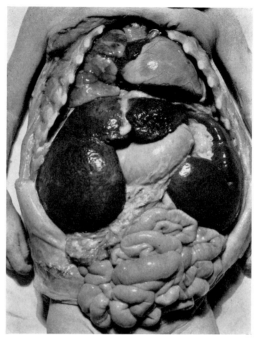

Fig. 149.—Photograph taken at autopsy table to show enlargement of liver and spleen in a baby who died with inoperable atresia of the bile ducts.

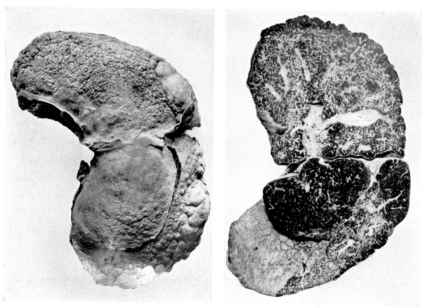

Fig. 150.—Photographs of liver with typical cirrhosis from a patient who died with atresia of the extrahepatic bile ducts. The liver was dark green in color because of biliary stasis. *Left,* External view to show the pebbly surface. *Right,* Cut surface showing increased fibrous tissue in periportal zones.

Liver.—The liver always shows a well advanced portal *cirrhosis* of the obstructive type. The organ is two or three times its normal size. It is very firm, and is stained a *dark-green color* by the accumulation of bile pigments. The surface is diffusely nodular (Fig. 150). In the depressions between these nodules there is a firm, grayish, fibrous substance representing an increased amount of interlobular connective tissue. The cut surface of the liver shows further evidence of extensive cirrhosis. There is diffuse destruction of liver substance and evidence of regeneration. The intense green color is strikingly contrasted to the light gray connective tissue which abounds in the periportal regions. Macroscopic enlargement of the ducts within the liver is rarely seen, in spite of the complete obstruction which has existed for many months. Presumably the ducts are kept small in size by the dense fibrous tissue which surrounds them.

Microscopic examination shows widespread degeneration of hepatic lobules and distortion of lobular architecture, accompanied by active liver-cell regeneration. In the periportal zones, there are usually large numbers of small bile ducts with considerable ductal regeneration and proliferation. This network of ducts is embedded in a dense fibrous tissue. There may be mild inflammatory cell reaction in these periportal zones, but this is not a striking feature. Biliary stasis is shown by the marked accumulation of pigments within the ductal lumina and within liver-cell cytoplasms.

Spleen.—The spleen may be slightly enlarged (Fig. 149)—a change presumably dependent upon portal obstruction which is set up by the biliary cirrhosis. Further evidence of portal obstruction is exhibited by the collection of fluid within the abdominal cavity.

ETIOLOGY

Numerous theories have been proposed to explain the origin of congenital atresia of the bile ducts. It was once thought that *fetal peritonitis* produced local inflammatory reactions which were responsible for this obliterative process. The absence of adhesions or of inflammatory lesions in other parts of the abdomen in most cases tends to discredit this view.

Congenital *syphilis* has often been listed as the etiologic factor. The absence of histologic evidence of syphilis and the finding of a negative Wassermann reaction in both child and mother in most cases makes it clear that congenital obliteration of the bile ducts is not the result of luetic infection.

Ylppö has pointed out that the extrahepatic bile ducts are always patent in early fetal life, but that under normal conditions they afterward lose their lumina by epithelial concrescence, and then become patent again at a later time. It is highly probable that an *arrest of development* during the solid stage is the true explanation for congenital atresia of the bile ducts.

Certainly this view explains the pathologic observations far better than any other theory does.

SYMPTOMS

The outstanding symptom in congenital atresia is *jaundice* of a high degree. It is usually present at birth or shortly thereafter. Not uncommonly, however, two or three weeks will elapse before there is sufficient staining of the skin or scleras with bile pigments to make the jaundice conspicuous. After jaundice once appears, it is persistent unless operative relief is possible. Furthermore, the intensity of the color never abates, a point which is helpful in ruling out several other diseases.

The presence of obstruction in the extrabiliary tree implies that bile pigments are absent in the intestinal tract. Therefore *the stools are always clay-colored or white from birth,* even though jaundice may not be noticed until the second or third week of life. As the condition progresses and as the child reaches an older age, there is an increasing saturation of the blood

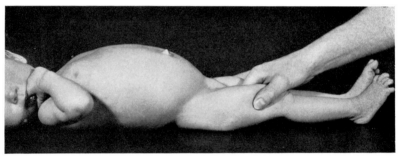

Fig. 151.—Photograph of six-months-old infant with obliteration of all the bile ducts, to demonstrate the good general physical condition which can exist with complete exclusion of the bile from the alimentary tract. (Icteric index was 150.)

plasma and various organs of the body with biliary pigment. Some of this is excreted in small amounts by glands of the intestinal tract and colon, so that a faint yellowish tint may be imparted to the stools. Pigments which are excreted in the stool by this route have a low concentration; hence the stool is puttylike in consistency and predominantly white in color. The persistence of light-colored stools from birth onward contrasts the condition to the other forms of biliary obstruction described in the two succeeding chapters.

The *nourishment* of these babies is usually better than might be expected. The absence of bile in the intestinal tract may cause some difficulty with absorption of fats. Hence, there is usually a history that the formula has been changed on several occasions and often a fat-free or low-fat mixture has been administered and better tolerated. Taken as a whole, these babies are somewhat below par in their physical development, but yet nutrition may be fairly good if the child is not more than three or four months of age. This is illustrated in Fig. 151, which is a photograph of a baby six months of age who had complete obstruction of the bile ducts and an icteric index of 150.

An abnormal *bleeding tendency* may be observed, but our cases showed a striking rarity of this symptom in the babies who were less than six months old. The ages when these babies have been referred to the hospital varied from one week to eleven months, with an average just under three months.

PHYSICAL FINDINGS

The salient finding is *jaundice,* the degree of which may be appreciated by the average icteric index of 125 in our cases. The lowest icteric index we encountered was 50 and the highest was 325. When the jaundice is deep, even the tears and saliva may be yellow. The general nutrition of the child is usually fairly good, but the subcutaneous fat may be reduced in amount. These babies tend to be somewhat lethargic and slow in their physical movements and mental reactions.

Examination of the *stool* is important, for it is strikingly whitish in color, and has a pasty or puttylike consistency. The urine is highly colored and gives a positive test for biliary pigments.

Fullness of the *abdomen* is produced by enlargement of the liver and by accumulation of ascitic fluid. The presenting liver edge may extend well down toward the umbilicus. The spleen may be slightly enlarged. In two cases there was a situs transversus of all the thoracic and abdominal viscera.

The *blood* findings are usually not remarkable. There may be a slight anemia with a red cell count rarely below 3,500,000 or 4,000,000. The clotting time may be increased to six or seven minutes, but rarely longer. Examination of the blood for prothrombin in two of our cases showed a normal value in one and a depression to 60 per cent of normal in the other.

DIFFERENTIAL DIAGNOSIS

Icterus neonatorum can usually be ruled out without difficulty. The jaundice usually diminishes by the end of the second week of life and has certainly disappeared by the end of the first month. Such an infant does not have enlargement of the liver, acholic stools, or heavily pigmented urine, which are all found in cases of biliary atresia.

Erythroblastosis foetalis, sometimes classified under the name of *icterus gravis* or *erythroblastic anemia,* may present a clinical picture simulating that of biliary obstruction. The jaundice may be of like intensity and the liver may be of equal or greater size. In this condition it is common to have an associated splenomegaly. A golden-colored vernix caseosa and a hyper-trophied placenta should make the obstetrician suspect the presence of erythroblastosis. The finding of an increased number of erythroblasts on successive blood examinations is an important factor in recognizing the disease. Because the condition is associated with a very high mortality in the first few days or weeks of life, the chance of confusing it with malformation of the bile ducts becomes progressively less as the age of the baby increases.

The *jaundice of hemolytic sepsis* may resemble that which is due to biliary obstruction. While the hemolytic jaundice resulting from a bacteremia may be deep, there are usually signs which point to the presence of infection, such as fever, leukocytosis, or progressive anemia. It is important to point out that an overwhelming infection in a small infant may show no febrile reaction, yet such babies have a profound toxicity which is not found in individuals with biliary obstruction. Patients with hemolytic sepsis do not have acholic stools or bile-stained urine.

Congenital syphilis may be mentioned in the differential diagnosis, but it is rarely a source of confusion. A careful maternal history, a Wassermann test on the mother and child, and roentgenologic studies of the long bones usually give sufficient data to rule out syphilis as a cause of the hepatic enlargement and jaundice.

As a general rule, it may be stated that if one delays in making a final diagnosis of congenital biliary obstruction until the infant is four to six weeks old, the chance of error is not great. Except for particular indications, it is better not to operate in cases of biliary obstruction before the end of the first month. Nothing is lost by this delay, and the assurance of a correct diagnosis is gained. Delay beyond the first month will not contribute further evidence in arriving at a correct diagnosis; and since these jaundiced infants have a low resistance to infections, they may die if the operation is deferred too long.

SURGICAL TREATMENT

Preoperative Measures.—If any anemia exists before operation, *transfusions* should be given to put the baby in the best possible condition for the operative procedure. One or two small infusions of blood are indicated for all cases prior to operation. Recently *vitamin K* has been administered in the hope of further diminishing any bleeding tendency. For many years these children were fed *ox-bile salts,* with the purpose of improving the digestion, but there is probably little to recommend this procedure.

Anesthesia.—Operation in all of our cases has been performed under *ether* narcosis given by the drop and open mask method. There has been only one death during or immediately following the operative procedure which might in any way be attributed to the anesthetic. In this fatal case the extent of the operative manipulations was probably sufficient to explain the death on the basis of shock without blaming the anesthesia as a contributing factor. Great relaxation of the abdomen is necessary for a generous exposure, and this cannot be obtained with local anesthesia of the abdominal wall.

Exploration of Biliary System.—A long *incision* is made from the costal margin well down below the umbilicus, separating the fibers of the right rectus muscle. Great care must be taken to *ligate all bleeding points.* It is surprising to find how rarely oozing of blood is a troublesome factor. The enlarged liver is retracted upward, and the extrabiliary system examined. The gallbladder is usually small and deeply embedded in liver substance which has mounded up around it. The peritoneal covering of the gastrohepatic ligament is carefully opened, to expose the region of the common and hepatic ducts. Great care must be exercised in the subsequent dissection in order to avoid injury to the small vessels in the gastrohepatic ligament, hemorrhage from which will impede the operation. The position and size of the ducts are now carefully estimated. Should the hepatic and common ducts appear to be atretic, one must turn attention to the gallbladder itself.

If the gallbladder possesses a lumen, its tip is now opened. The presence of bile in the bladder implies that the hepatic and cystic ducts are patent, even though they might not appear so by external examination. If the gallbladder contains clear fluid a small catheter is tightly sewed into its fundus, so that it can be distended with salt solution. By this irrigation a lumen may be detected in the hepatic and common ducts which might otherwise elude detection.

After this examination, which perforce will require considerable time and delicacy, the operator must decide which procedure will give most satisfactory operative relief, provided there is some structure connecting with the liver which can be joined to the gastro-intestinal tract. As a general rule, it is much better to anastomose the hepatic or common duct, rather than the gallbladder, with the duodenum, in spite of the fact that the latter is technically easier to do.

Hepaticoduodenostomy.—In three cases there was an atresia of most of the extrabiliary system, with only a small nubbin of *hepatic duct* presenting at the porta of the liver. In each instance this duct was but 3 to 5 mm. in diameter, yet it could be anastomosed directly to the duodenum (Figs. 152 and 153). This is best accomplished by placing several silk ligatures to anchor the mobilized duodenum to the presenting nubbin of duct before opening the hepatic duct and duodenum. A small piece of No. 8 or 10 catheter about 1.5 cm. long is then threaded up into the hepatic duct and also down into the duodenum. With this tube left in place, an anterior row of sutures is placed so as to anchor the anterior wall of the duct to the duodenum and complete the union. With so small a duct and with such limited exposure one can rarely place more than a single row of interrupted sutures around such a line of anastomosis. It is imperative to use silk, to insure fixation of the two adjoining structures until proper healing has taken place.

It is important to make the anastomosis over a *small piece of tubing,* to prevent constriction of the lumen during the operative procedure. If the tube is too long, it may not pass spontaneously into the intestine (Fig. 154). In one case a tube 7 to 8 cm. in length was employed, which did not move during the following two months when observed by x-ray examination. This child subsequently died of peritonitis—presumably from pressure necrosis and perforation of the opposite wall of the intestine. Following this disastrous experience we have always employed a short piece of tubing— 1.5 to 2 cm. in length—and have found that this always spontaneously passes several days after operation.

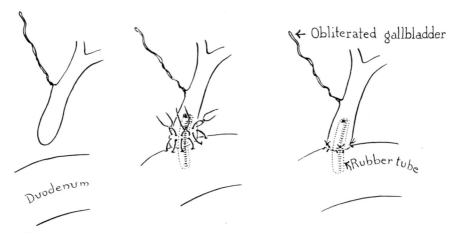

Fig. 152.—Sketch of method of anastomosis of common (or hepatic) duct with the duodenum. The union is made over a short piece of urethral catheter which is threaded into the duct and also into the duodenum. Anastomosis is made with interrupted silk sutures.

When atresia exists at the *lower end of the common duct,* three procedures are available (Fig. 153):

1. **Cholecystostomy.**—If the child is beginning to show evidence of shock, and if the cystic duct and gallbladder are patent, a tube can be quickly inserted into the gallbladder to establish external biliary drainage. This is done in the hope of performing a second operation at a later time when direct anastomosis of the intestinal tract and the biliary tree can be done.

2. **Cholecystoduodenostomy.**—If the common duct is so small that there will be great technical difficulty in anastomosing it to the intestine, the gallbladder—if it connects with the biliary tree—may be freed from its bed, turned over, and anastomosed to the duodenum or stomach.

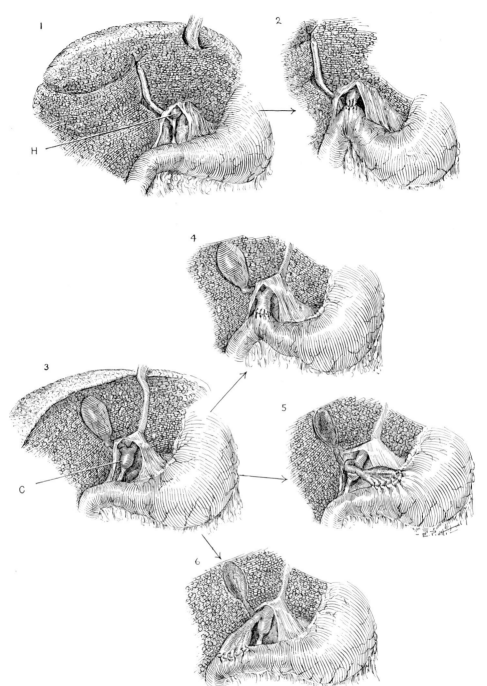

Fig. 153.—Types of operative relief which have been effected for atresia of bile ducts. *1*, Atresia of hepatic duct treated by hepaticoduodenostomy, as shown in *2*. *3*, Atresia of the common duct treated by choledochoduodenostomy, cholecystogastrostomy and cholecystoduodenostomy, as shown in *4*, *5*, and *6*, respectively. Choledochoduodenostomy is believed to be a better procedure than cholecystogastrostomy or cholecystoduodenostomy.

H, Blind end of hepatic duct. *C*, Blind end of common duct.

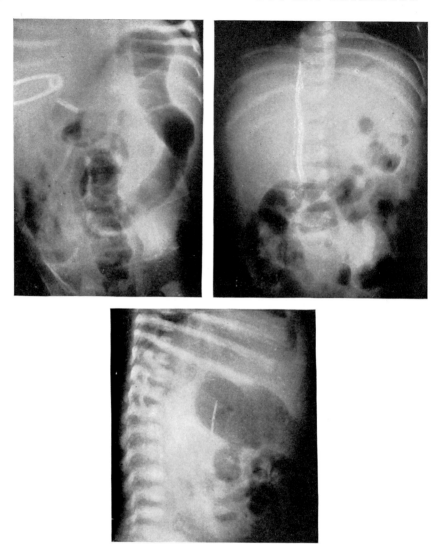

Fig. 154.—*Above, left,* Roentgenogram of patient with atresia of common duct following choledochoduodenostomy, to show piece of rubber tubing over which the anastomosis was made. (Tubing was subsequently passed spontaneously.) *Above, right,* Roentgenogram of another patient showing tubing in place following a hepaticoduodenostomy for atresia of the hepatic duct. This tube was too long, and its failure to pass into the intestine led to pressure necrosis, perforation, and fatal peritonitis. *Below,* Piece of ureteral catheter in a choledochoduodenostomy. Common duct would barely admit this small diameter catheter. Tubing spontaneously passed within eight days. Baby completely recovered from biliary obstruction.

3. **Choledochoduodenostomy.**—If the common duct can be mobilized, choledochoduodenostomy is the operation of choice and has proved most successful in our hands. The actual technic employed depends upon the size of the presenting common duct. If the duct is large enough, a double layer

of sutures may be placed, using an external row of interrupted silk and an internal continuous suture of very fine catgut to join the mucosal edges of duct and duodenum. However, the duct is usually only a few millimeters in diameter and one is rarely able to insert more than a single row of sutures.

These anastomoses should always be made over a piece of *catheter* to insure that the lumen at the anastomotic site is not constricted during placement of the last sutures. In one case the cystic and common ducts were large enough to permit passage of a catheter down the gallbladder, through the cystic and common ducts, through the anastomosis, and into the duodenum. After the anastomosis had been performed, the catheter was withdrawn through the gallbladder. The small size and the tortuosity of the cystic duct does not often permit the employment of a catheter in this way.

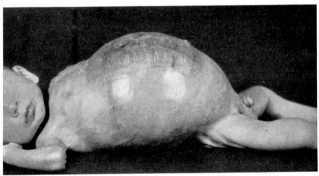

Fig. 155.—Photograph of six-months-old infant following operation for inoperable atresia of the bile ducts, showing the marked abdominal distention which is apt to follow these explorations.

Postoperative Disruption of Wound.—Great care must be taken in closing the abdominal wall, because these patients are very apt to have disruption of the wound and evisceration during the postoperative course. Postoperative distention is troublesome because of accumulated peritoneal fluid and because of paralytic ileus—a combination which is particularly common (Fig. 155). A second factor which leads to disruptions of these wounds is the poor healing power of the individuals. It has therefore always been our practice to employ silk in the reconstruction of the abdominal wall and in later years we have added through-and-through silkworm-gut sutures to give the wound additional support.

RESULTS AND PROGNOSIS

Prior to 1916 these children were not explored; and a review of our autopsy material corroborated the teaching of others that occasional cases might have been relieved by operation. We have not considered any of these earlier cases in the following statistics. Since 1916 all cases have been subjected to surgical *exploration,* except in a few instances when the child entered the hospital in extremis or had some other serious malady which contraindicated operation. There have now been forty-five cases in which exploration has been done. In this group nine patients were found to have a patent hepatic duct or common duct connecting with the intrahepatic ductal system, but not with the duodenum. In other words, 20 per cent of the cases were operable (Table 29).

In three patients the hepatic duct was the only patent structure connecting with the liver. In each of these patients *hepaticoduodenostomy* was performed; one of these died and two recovered.

In six patients the atresia was limited to the lower end of the common duct. *Choledochoduodenostomy* was performed four times, and was fol-

TABLE 29

RESULTS OF TREATMENT IN OPERABLE CASES OF ATRESIA OF EXTRABILIARY SYSTEM (CHILDREN'S HOSPITAL SERIES)*

Treatment	Died	Recovered
Atresia of lower end of hepatic duct:		
Hepaticoduodenostomy.	1	2
Atresia of lower end of common duct:		
Choledochoduodenostomy.	1	3
Cholecystoduodenostomy.		1
Cholecystostomy.	1	
Totals.	3	6

* Forty-five patients with atresia of the biliary system were explored. Nine of these were found to be operable, giving an operability of 20 per cent.

lowed by one death and three survivals. *Cholecystoduodenostomy* was performed once and was successful. *Cholecystostomy* was performed once with fatal issue. In this last case a second procedure was planned to unite the biliary and alimentary systems, but the child did not live long enough to undertake the additional step.

The six individuals who have survived have been in excellent general health, and have had no symptoms suggesting cholangitis or hepatitis. These children have been followed twelve years, eight years, seven years, five years (2 cases), and four years respectively since operation. In all of them the jaundice has disappeared and has not reappeared at any subsequent date. In none has there been any accumulation of abdominal fluid. As each patient has grown there has been diminution in the relative size of the liver, so that now the liver appears to be of a size which is normal for the age of the individual. In short, the livers have all shown remarkable evidence of regeneration, and in no case has there been any hepatic insufficiency.

In the individuals who were found to be inoperable, the average age at subsequent death was five months. One child lived to be twelve months old. In most instances death followed a downhill course, characterized by progressive jaundice and inanition, usually terminated by superimposed infection and in a few cases by fatal hemorrhage.

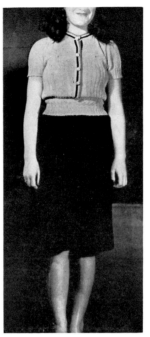

Fig. 156.—Photograph of a patient twelve years after choledochoduodenostomy for atresia of the bile ducts. Jaundice has entirely disappeared and there have been no symptoms of ascending biliary infection or of hepatic insufficiency at any time.

BIBLIOGRAPHY

1. Donovan, E. J.: Congenital Atresia of the Bile Ducts. Ann. Surg., *106:* 737, 1937.
2. Holmes, J. B.: Congenital Obliteration of the Bile Ducts: Diagnosis and Suggestions for Treatment. Am. J. Dis. Child., *11:* 405, 1916.
3. Ladd, W. E.: Congenital Atresia and Stenosis of the Bile Ducts. J. A. M. A., *91:* 1082, 1928.
4. Ladd, W. E.: Congenital Obstruction of the Bile Ducts. Ann. Surg., *102:* 742, 1935.
5. Thomson, John: On Congenital Obliteration of the Bile Ducts. Edinburgh Med. Jr., *37:* 523, 1892.

CHAPTER XX

OBSTRUCTIVE JAUNDICE FROM INSPISSATED BILE OR MUCUS IN THE BILIARY PASSAGES

A chapter on congenital obliteration of the bile ducts should be followed by a presentation of material relating to jaundice in infancy which results from plugging of the bile passages by inspissated mucus or bile. In these two conditions the clinical pictures are similar, but the prognoses are quite different. We have encountered only eight cases of obstructive jaundice from inspissated bile or mucus, but the high degree of success following operation for the condition makes it desirable to recognize this entity so that surgical relief can be instituted.

PATHOLOGY

Within the common duct, hepatic duct, or indeed within the larger radicles of the intrahepatic passages, small *concretions* of inspissated, sticky, firm material may be found. These plugs may extend along several of the ducts or else there may be a small globular concretion which obstructs the duct at only one level. The origin of this plug of material is not clearly understood. In several newly born babies we have found similar accumulations of sticky material in the intestine or colon which have caused obstruction. A consideration of these cases along with those in which there are inspissated plugs in the bile passages suggests that these conditions might have a common etiology. Such plugs in the biliary passages can produce important obstruction, and, indeed, can completely impede the flow of bile into the intestinal tract. With this degree of obstruction, one finds in the liver most of the changes which are associated with congenital obliteration of the bile ducts. The liver is *enlarged,* quite *cirrhotic,* and is deeply *stained* with retained bile pigments. This hepatomegaly may induce partial portal obstruction which manifests itself clinically in the accumulation of abdominal ascitic fluid and enlargement of the spleen.

SYMPTOMATOLOGY

Infants with obstruction of the biliary passages from inspissated mucus or bile have *jaundice* which appears in the first few weeks of life and which may be present at birth. The jaundice may reach a high intensity. Nutrition is usually well maintained, but there may be some slight intolerance to fat. The *stools* are clay-colored or white, and have a puttylike consistency. The *urine* is deeply colored with pigments. Some *bleeding tendency* may be in evidence, though this is not the rule.

The general history in these cases is practically the same as in those with congenital obliteration of the bile ducts, and, indeed, in several instances the history made us feel that obliteration of the bile ducts was actually present. In a few cases, however, there has been a suggestion that the jaundice has changed in intensity from time to time, and that on some occasions there was a faint green or yellow color to the stools. Therefore, a history of *jaundice of varying degree,* particularly when associated with *intermittent* appearance of bile pigments in the stool, is at once suggestive of intermittent or partial obstruction of the ducts by inspissated mucus or bile plugs. However, it must be emphasized that a history of intermittent symptoms is not always obtained in these cases.

PHYSICAL FINDINGS

The age of these infants when presented at the clinic varied from one week up to three months of age, with an average slightly under two months. In all of them the outstanding feature was a marked *jaundice.* The lowest recorded *icteric index* was 85, and the highest was 120, with an average of about 100. Thus, the intensity of the jaundice cannot be used as a factor to differentiate this condition from congenital obliteration of the bile ducts. In each case there was an *enlarged liver,* usually associated with accumulation of some intra-abdominal fluid, and in three cases the *spleen* was palpable. In all eight of these babies the *stool* was acholic at the time of hospitalization.

DIFFERENTIAL DIAGNOSIS

All of the conditions listed under "Differential Diagnosis" in the preceding chapter on Obliteration of the Bile Ducts must be considered and the same differentiating points might be listed here. The only thing which should be added is the differentiation from congenital obliteration of the bile ducts itself. This can be done only if there is a history or clinical findings suggesting *intermittency* of the obstruction.

TREATMENT

Fluoroscopic Introduction of Cholagogue.—In one case not listed in Table 30, a three-month-old female with this condition was successfully treated with the placement of a duodenal tube, under fluoroscopic control, and then the injection of 25 per cent *magnesium sulfate* into the duodenum by way of this tube. This cholagogue stimulated the flow of bile sufficiently to dislodge material from the common duct which had previously been obstructing it. Subsequent to this procedure, bile appeared in the stool, the jaundice disappeared, and there has been no recurrence of symptoms. While the treatment in this case proved to be highly successful, we have not had such good fortune when attempting this therapy in other individuals. The failure to repeat this successful treatment apparently implies that the ducts in most cases are too tightly plugged to be cleared by the action of chola-gogues.

Surgical Treatment.—Except for rare cases in which the above medical therapy is successful, surgical treatment should always be instituted, because of the high percentage of success which follows operative measures.

Exploration is made through a long right upper-quadrant *incision,* to allow adequate exposure of the subhepatic fossa. The peritoneal covering of the gastrohepatic ligament is then opened and the common and hepatic ducts are brought carefully into view. This procedure alone may be all that is required to relieve the obstruction. If it does not, two things can be at-tempted. First, *actual manipulations* of the ducts in the gastrohepatic liga-ment may successfully dislodge an obstructing plug. Second, irrigation of the ductal system with saline introduced by way of the gallbladder will dilate the ducts and wash downward any foreign material. It is well to supplement the manipulations routinely with these irrigations. If a catheter is sewed into the gallbladder and warm physiologic saline is introduced under pressure from a syringe, it may at first be found that the fluid will not run freely, but then as the common duct obstruction is relieved there is a free passage of the liquid into the duodenum.

In several of our cases the hepatic and common ducts (as seen at the operating table) were small and an obliteration of the ducts was thought to exist. Hence, we were agreeably surprised to find that the biliary obstruc-tion was completely relieved after operation. These few patients, who pre-sumably had hopeless obliteration of the bile ducts and who subsequently completely recovered, made us conclude that obstruction of the ducts by inspissated material cannot be always recognized either clinically or even at the operating table. We have therefore adopted the attitude that babies who have been explored for biliary obstruction and who are thought to have an unrelievable condition should always have *supportive treatment* for several weeks after operation, because it is never known when obstruction might have been due to unrecognized ductal plugs which were unwittingly dis-lodged during the operator's manipulations in the region.

RESULTS OF THERAPY

In one case treated by medical therapy, the introduction of concen-trated magnesium sulfate into the duodenum produced a flow of bile which was quickly followed by the appearance of bile in the stools and rapid dis-appearance of the jaundice. In eight other cases treated by surgical means and listed in Table 30 the obstruction could be relieved by manipulation

TABLE 30

SURGICAL TREATMENT IN CASES WITH JAUNDICE AND DUCTAL OBSTRUCTION FROM INSPISSATED BILE
OR MUCUS

Treatment	Died	Recovered
Exploration and manipulation of extrabiliary system...................	1	3
Exploration of extrabiliary system and irrigation of ducts via gallbladder.	1	3
Totals..	2	6

or by irrigation of the ducts by way of the gallbladder. Of these eight individuals who were operated upon, six survived and have had no recurrence
of symptoms, and two died shortly after the procedure, one of operative
shock and the other of evisceration on the fourth postoperative day.

18

CHAPTER XXI

IDIOPATHIC DILATATION OF THE COMMON BILE DUCT

Cystic dilatation of the common bile duct is a congenital lesion characterized by unusual enlargement of this part of the biliary system without significant mechanical obstruction. In some cases there is a demonstrable stenosis, angulation, or valvelike fold in the ampulla of Vater or in the lower part of the common duct, but in other well-studied specimens the outlet of the common duct shows no apparent abnormality. The dilated duct may be as large as an orange or a grapefruit and in exceptional cases it has been even bigger. Once the "cyst" has appeared, it tends to become even larger because its weight makes it hang to one side and thus angulate the inferior end in such a way that stasis and further obstruction follow. Excellent reviews of this subject have been made by Judd and Greene,[3] Zinninger and Cash,[7] and others. Gross[2] reviewed a series of 52 cases observed in childhood, and 130 cases in all age groups have been studied by Blocker, Williams, and Williams.[1]

PATHOLOGY

Dilatation of the common duct is the characteristic finding and takes the form of a spherical enlargement of a part or of the whole of the ductus choledochus. This distention may involve only the common duct proper, or it may also include the junction of the cystic, hepatic, and common ducts. Thus, there may be only one duct entering the cyst (the upper part of the common duct), or the hepatic and cystic ducts may enter the cyst separately and their orifices may be 2 or 3 cm. apart (Fig. 157). In either instance, the cyst is connected to the duodenum by the lower part of the common duct. In rare cases the enlargement may involve such a low portion of the common duct that the pancreatic duct opens directly into the choledochal cyst.

This *localized* dilatation of the biliary system is unique and is to be differentiated from enlargements which obtain in purely obstructive lesions of the lower common duct, such as those found with carcinoma at the head of the pancreas in the adult. Dilatations which result solely from obstruction tend to extend through the entire biliary tree, and in such cases the common duct is seldom larger than a loop of small intestine. Also, in the obstructive lesions, the gallbladder is markedly dilated. Contrary to such conditions, a true choledochal cyst represents a localized dilatation, primarily of the common duct, and the gallbladder is rarely enlarged.

The *dimensions* of such a cyst may be very great, especially when one considers the size of the patient in whom the abnormality exists. Many of the cysts have had a capacity of 1 or 2 liters, and frequently they are described as being the size of a "fist," or the size of a "child's head." The size is seldom related to the duration of the symptoms. There is no constant correlation between the size of the cyst and the age of the patient, although the larger ones tend to be found in older individuals.

The *cyst wall* is quite firm and varies from 2 to 4 mm. in thickness. This structure is composed of a dense connective tissue in which elastic tissue and

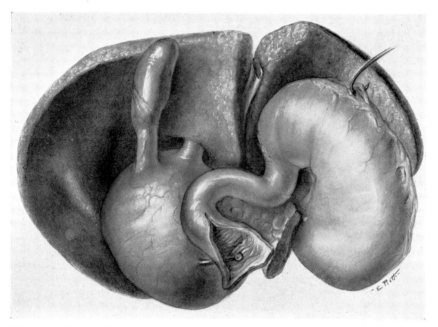

Fig. 157.—Cystic dilatation of the common bile duct, as found in a three-year-old girl. Cystic and hepatic ducts are somewhat dilated and enter the "cyst" separately. Lower portion of the common duct is normal in caliber and normally enters the ampulla of Vater. The dilated portion of the common duct measured 7 cm. in diameter and 12 cm. in length.

smooth muscle are often lacking. Epithelium has usually disappeared from the lining of the cyst, which is commonly represented by only a dense layer of connective tissue. The inner surface may be roughened and irregular, may be covered by heavy deposits of bile pigment, and occasionally there is a purulent exudate indicative of severe secondary infection. Microscopically, the cyst wall generally has evidence of some inflammatory reaction.

At the *outlets* of these cysts there are a great variety of findings. Valve-like folds have been described in a small number of cases. Stenosis of the lower part of the common duct has been observed, but is by no means a universal finding. The common duct below the dilated portion may be normal in size and appearance, and in a few cases has actually been abnormally large—a fact which dispels the idea that obstruction is the sole factor in the causation of the choledochal cyst. In some cases it was noted that the lower part of the common duct was angulated, but could be probed.

The cystic duct, hepatic duct, and gallbladder may have minor degrees of dilatation, but these changes are minimal when compared to the great size of the common duct.

The *liver* is frequently enlarged and cirrhotic. In a minority of cases the intrahepatic ducts are grossly dilated. Microscopically, there is often a cirrhosis with increased periportal connective tissue, proliferation of the bile capillaries, and rarely some bile stasis. Infection is common, and leukocytic infiltration of the portal areas may be marked. Cholangitis may reach an advanced stage, and intraductal suppuration has been seen.

ETIOLOGY

Many hypotheses have been advanced regarding the underlying cause for the production of this malady and the following include some of the leading views:

1. An anomalous direction of the common duct through the duodenal wall kinks the duct and produces obstruction to biliary flow.

2. A congenital stenosis of the lower part of the common duct causes back pressure sufficient to produce dilatation.

3. The dilatation may be due to an achalasia, namely, a failure of Oddi's sphincter to relax at the proper time, which would cause obstruction by a neuromuscular incoordination.

4. The cyst represents a developmental anomaly which is present before birth, and is primarily due to weakness of the common duct wall which allows dilatation under normal intraductal pressure. The condition has been compared to a congenital idiopathic hydronephrosis or hydro-ureter, and, similar to this renal condition, there may be no demonstrable obstruction.

5. The common duct wall lacks contractile elements and balloons out locally following obstruction in the lower portion of the duct. Some writers support this theory and claim that the obstruction is due to valve formation from redundant membrane of the duct secondary to cholangitis. Others postulate the congenital weakness of the duct wall, but believe the obstruction to be due to fibrosis of the lower part of the duct from a preceding cholangitis.

6. The cyst is of "congenital origin" and represents a malformation of the duct, while the valve formation is entirely secondary. Thus, a cyst will be displaced downward (because of its size and weight), and the resulting

angulation will lead to a valve formation. Such a valve, after it is once formed, may give obstruction and aggravate the symptoms, but it is not the primary cause of the ductal dilatation.

7. The cystic dilatation may arise from an abortive diverticulum of the common duct similar to the diverticulum which gives rise to the ventral pancreas.

With such a multiplicity of explanations it is entirely possible that we are dealing with a heterogeneous group of lesions which may be produced in several ways, for while many of the theories are plausible, no one explanation fulfills the conditions found in all cases.

In review, the most feasible theory is that which accepts a congenital weakness of the duct wall, a weakness not in itself producing dilatation unless there is a second factor of obstruction with resultant increased intra-ductal pressure. Such obstruction in various cases has been caused by duct angulation, valve formation, inflammation, stenosis of the lower portion of the common duct, or by achalasia.

SYMPTOMS AND SIGNS

The outstanding clinical feature of the choledochal cyst is the triad of abdominal pain, abdominal tumor, and jaundice.

Pain is observed in a large majority of cases. It is usually located in the epigastrium or in the right upper quadrant, but in some instances it is referred to the umbilicus. It may be of a colicky type, but more often it is of a "dragging" nature, or is described as pressure or a vague fullness. The pain is usually not very severe, and while it may cause considerable discomfort, it is rarely sufficient to make the patient "double up" or cry out. Pain is occasionally accompanied by nausea, but vomiting has occurred in only a few instances. There is no correlation between the size of the cyst and the severity of the pain.

Abdominal tumor is found in about 90 per cent of the cases. Hence, the presence of an intra-abdominal mass, either as given in the history or as found by physical examination, is a very important observation. In about half of the cases a well-defined and circumscribed mass has been palpated just below the liver edge, but there may be only a resistance to palpation in the right upper quadrant. When the cyst can be felt, it is often farther to the left than might be expected, because an enlarged liver can push the dilated common duct over beyond the midline of the body. In occasional cases the mass has been designated as "definitely cystic," "elastic," "tensely cystic," or some such term which indicates its physical nature, but not infrequently it has been so tense that it has been described as firm or solid. Hence, the clinician may have the impression that it represents a neoplasm or an enlarged lobe of the liver.

The size and tenseness of the cyst may vary from time to time, depending upon varying obstructions at the cyst outlet or quantitative changes in the production of bile. It is quite likely that this is a sign which has been present more often than recorded.

Jaundice is a prominent symptom and is seen in about 90 per cent of the cases. Acholic stools and highly colored urine have been noted from time to time in about one third of the patients.

Fever is occasionally found, and is probably a reflection of cholangitis or hepatitis. The temperature range is usually to 101° or 102° F., but has been recorded as high as 104° F.

The order of appearance of pain, tumor, and jaundice, etc., varies in different cases. Thus, any one of these symptoms may occur first, may exist alone, or may persist in combination with the others. One of these may exist for a long period of time before additional ones are evident. The *duration of symptoms* before the condition is recognized varies over a wide range, but the chronicity of complaints is noteworthy. The average duration of symptoms is about three years before the underlying condition is found, but in some cases it is much longer than this. The severity of symptoms bears no constant relationship to the duration of complaints.

The *intermittency* of symptoms should be emphasized. When it is stated that symptoms are "intermittent," it is meant that the general course of the illness has been one of exacerbations and remissions, even though one or more of the symptoms may be persistent.

The condition is about four times as common in females as it is in males. In 128 cases collected from the literature,[1] the *ages* of the patients at time of hospitalization were as follows: forty-four from birth to ten years; thirty-one from eleven to twenty years; thirty-two from twenty-one to thirty years; eleven from thirty-one to forty years; and ten over forty years.

The *diagnosis* of choledochal cyst is rarely made preoperatively. However, a review of individual case reports gives rise to the impression that a correct diagnosis usually could have been reached if the possibility of idiopathic choledochal cyst had been entertained as a cause of the patients' complaints.

DIFFERENTIAL DIAGNOSIS

Echinococcus cyst of the liver may give symptoms and physical findings similar to those of a choledochal cyst, but more often there is a palpable tumor of the liver which causes little disturbance to the patient's health. The swelling is usually of long standing and is the only complaint; but if suppuration occurs, there are additional indications of infection, and if the tumor is very large, there may be associated jaundice. An echinococcus cyst is stationary or progressive in size, whereas the choledochal cyst tends to vary in size, especially following the ingestion of food. A hydatid cyst of the liver moves with respiration and rarely produces pain. The presence of echinococcus cysts in other organs is of aid in detecting the parasitic infection. The geographic location of the patient in countries where the disease is rare, the absence of these parasites in dogs of the community, and the lack of intimate contact with dogs, all tend to exclude echinococcus cysts as a probable diagnosis. Where facilities are available, negative complement-fixation tests or precipitation reactions should rule out the possibility of echinococcus infection.

Cholelithiasis is rare in children and its exclusion should be made with ease. x-Ray studies may aid in indicating the presence of stones. Furthermore, gallstones in children usually result from some blood dyscrasia in

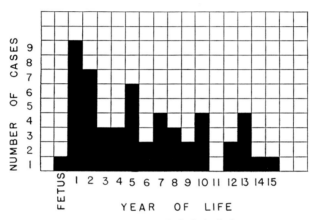

Fig. 158.—Ages of fifty children at onset of choledochal cyst symptoms. The number of patients in each group is indicated by the height of the columns. (One case occurring in a fetus is also indicated.)

which there is an abnormal hemolytic process. The absence of such hematologic disorders makes the diagnosis of cholelithiasis unlikely in most cases.

Abdominal neoplasms in childhood, without treatment, run a rapidly progressive and fatal course. Thus, if a child has had symptoms from an abdominal mass for a year or more and still maintains fair nutrition and vitality, neoplasm as a causative agent is unlikely. Therefore, when this differential diagnosis is in question, a long duration of symptoms should tend to exclude malignancy. Neoplasms may certainly be excluded if the subhepatic mass has been found to vary in size.

Congenital atresia of the bile ducts should give no difficulty, chiefly because of the different age groups into which the two classes of patients fall. The average age of patients with congenital atresias of the extrahepatic ducts is from one to three months when first seen. In those cases not amenable to operative relief, the expectancy of life is a matter of a few months.

In contrast, only about 5 per cent of the patients with a choledochal cyst have symptoms before six months of age. Thus, the older age incidence of patients with choledochal cysts sharply differentiates the two conditions. Figure 158 indicates the age at onset of symptoms in a group of fifty-two children with cystic dilatation of the common duct.

TREATMENT

The results of operation have depended in large measure upon the time when the nature of the cystic lesion was first recognized. In many cases exploration has been continued unduly long so that therapeutic procedures had to be curtailed because of onset of surgical shock. It is therefore pertinent to emphasize that *the surgeon must be familiar with the pathology of this condition,* for only then can he quickly recognize the lesion and rapidly promote drainage of the biliary system into the intestine which has proved to be so efficacious in curing these individuals. Thus, even if the diagnosis is not made preoperatively, the probabilities of a cure are high if the condition is recognized at the operating table and proper treatment is immediately instituted.

In a number of patients the dilated common duct has been *drained externally* in the hopes of joining the ductal system and intestine on a later occasion. Such external drainage of the choledochal cyst has been followed by an exceedingly high mortality rate.

Without question, the treatment of choice is to perform a *primary anastomosis* between the biliary system and the intestinal tract at one operation. The gallbladder may be united to the stomach or duodenum, but the best treatment of all is to anastomose the cyst directly to the duodenum. If desired, a cystostomy may be established in addition as a temporary outlet to relieve tension on the suture line of the choledochoduodenostomy. While this extra step may be omitted, it doubtless has some merit as an additional safety factor.

Excision of the cyst should never be attempted, for it is unnecessary and is productive of dangerous surgical shock. There has been ample opportunity to demonstrate the potentiality of the cyst to shrink to small dimensions when adequate drainage is instituted. Abdominal *tapping* is to be avoided, because of the danger of producing a leak from the cyst into the abdominal cavity, and because of the possible injury to other viscera.

RESULTS OF TREATMENT

In a group of fifty-two childhood patients originally collected and studied by Gross[2] the total mortality was 69 per cent, but in those treated by primary anastomosis of biliary tract and intestine, the mortality was 9 per cent. These findings are summarized in Table 31.

TABLE 31

RESULTS OF TREATMENT IN FIFTY-TWO CASES OF CHOLEDOCHAL CYST IN CHILDHOOD (COLLECTED FROM THE LITERATURE)

Treatment	Died	Recovered
1. No operation	9	0
2. Type of operation not stated	1	0
3. External drainage of the biliary system:		
(a) Drainage of choledochal cyst	15	1
(b) Drainage of gallbladder	1	0
(c) Drainage of hepatic duct and excision of cyst	3	0
(d) Drainage of gallbladder and excision of cyst	1	0
4. Drainage of cyst at first operation, and anastomosis to intestine at second operation	5	5
5. Anastomosis of biliary system and intestine at one operation:		
(a) Hepatico-enterostomy with cholecystectomy and excision of choledochal cyst	0	1
(b) Cholecystenterostomy	0	2
(c) Choledocho-enterostomy	1	7
Totals	36	16

We have treated six children with various types of operation (Table 32). Five of these survived and were restudied nineteen, sixteen, fourteen, eleven, and six years respectively after operation, to determine their general health and the condition of their biliary systems. One of them, sixteen years later, is still having recurring cholangitis and jaundice. Since this anasto-

TABLE 32

RESULTS OF TREATMENT IN IDIOPATHIC DILATATION OF THE COMMON BILE DUCT (CHILDREN'S HOSPITAL SERIES)

Treatment	Died	Recovered
Choledochoduodenostomy	0	2
Cholecystoduodenostomy	0	2*
Cholecystogastrostomy	0	1
Dilated common duct excised; hepatic duct externally drained	1	0
Totals	1	5

* One of these patients (in whom anastomosis was performed with a Murphy button) has recurring cholangitis.

mosis had been performed with a Murphy button, we believe that the poor clinical result was dependent upon the establishment of too large a communication through which intestinal contents could regurgitate into the biliary tract. In each of the other four patients who had anastomoses by direct suture, the follow-up study has shown excellent physical development in each and biliary disease in none.

BIBLIOGRAPHY

1. Blocker, T. G., Jr., Williams, H., and Williams, J. E.: Traumatic Rupture of a Congenital Cyst of the Choledochus. Arch. Surg., *34:* 695, 1937.
2. Gross, R. E.: Idiopathic Dilatation of the Common Bile Duct in Children. J. Pediat., *3:* 730, 1933.
3. Judd, E. S., and Greene, E. I.: Choledochus Cyst. Surg., Gynec. and Obst., *46:* 317, 1928.
4. McWhorter, G. L.: Congenital Cystic Dilatation of the Bile and Pancreatic Ducts. Necropsy Thirteen Years after Hepaticoduodenostomy. Arch. Surg., *38:* 397, 1939.
5. Swartley, W. B., and Weeder, S. D.: Choledochus Cyst with a Double Common Bile Duct. Ann. Surg., *101:* 912, 1935.
6. Wright, A. D.: X-ray Appearances Produced by Congenital Cystic Dilatation of the Common Bile Duct. Brit. J. Radiol., *8:* 227, 1935.
7. Zinninger, M. M., and Cash, J. R.: Congenital Cystic Dilatation of the Common Bile Duct. Arch. Surg., *24:* 77, 1932.

CHAPTER XXII

CHOLECYSTITIS, CHOLELITHIASIS, HEPATIC TUMORS, ANOMALIES OF THE GALLBLADDER, INJURY TO THE EXTRAHEPATIC BILE DUCTS

CHOLECYSTITIS

Cholecystitis and cholelithiasis in childhood have been assuming increasing importance in recent times, for it is evident that these conditions are not as rare as was once taught. Nearly 450 cases of gallbladder disease have been recorded in the literature, and the number which are discovered each year appears to be steadily growing. While cholecystitis and cholelithiasis are admittedly uncommon, the present-day success in treating these lesions by surgical means makes it important to recognize them.

Symptoms.—The symptoms of acute cholecystitis in the child vary but little from those in the adult. They consist of severe, poorly localized, right upper-quadrant *pain, nausea, vomiting,* and *fever.* The general picture of abdominal pain, vomiting, and *distention* often leads to a diagnosis of intestinal obstruction. Hence, the presence of biliary disease may not be suspected until the abdomen is opened.

Treatment.—In adults cholecystitis is commonly initiated by irritation from a stone or by blockage of the cystic duct with a calculus, whereas in children it is more apt to be a bacterial inflammation unaccompanied by stones. Hence, in a child the process will often subside without resort to surgical means, and the treatment can be more conservative than that generally employed in adults. If the diagnosis appears to be fairly clear, the individual can be tided over the acute episode with sedation, application of heat to the abdomen, a fat-free diet, and gentle saline purging.

If the fever and white blood count are rising and the local symptoms are advancing, exploration is advisable to arrest the spread of infection. Under these circumstances *cholecystectomy* is the procedure of choice. If edema around the neck of the gallbladder prevents easy isolation and ligation of the cystic duct and cystic artery, *cholecystostomy* is safer and preferable.

CHOLELITHIASIS

Symptoms.—Cholelithiasis, though rare, is more common than acute cholecystitis in children. Stones tend to remain in the gallbladder and the symptoms are largely those of recurrent upper abdominal *pain, nausea,* and *vomiting.* Calculi may enter the diminutive cystic and common ducts and produce intermittent biliary obstruction with resulting *jaundice* and more severe vomiting. It is rare for a child to complain of the back pain or shoulder pain which is so frequently found in the adult.

The most common cause of cholelithiasis in children is related to the excessive excretion of pigments during a *hemolytic anemia*. In fact, the association is so frequent that cholelithiasis in childhood should always arouse one's suspicions concerning a *blood disorder*. The four patients (ages three, four, nine, and fourteen) we have operated upon for cholelithiasis were studied in this regard and three were shown to have had a hemolytic anemia. Cholelithiasis should never be treated without due regard for the blood picture, for not only must the stones be removed, but the reason for their formation must be corrected.

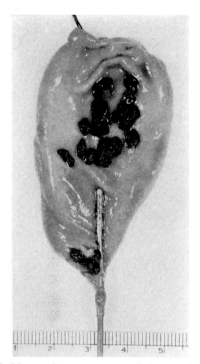

Fig. 159.—Gallbladder and stones removed from a four-year-old boy.

Diagnosis.—Gallstones in children are composed mostly of pigment, but sufficient calcium may be precipitated to cast positive shadows on x-ray films of the abdomen. When this is not true, *cholecystography* will show negative shadows in the dye-filled gallbladder.

Children with *congenital hemolytic anemia* have recurring bouts of jaundice due to temporary saturation of the blood stream with liberated pigments. If biliary obstruction is superimposed on this picture, it may be quite difficult to decide whether the jaundice depends upon a hemolytic crisis or a common duct stone. A higher icteric index, particularly when associated with abdominal pain and vomiting, is more suggestive of biliary obstruction.

Clinical evidence of extrahepatic bile duct obstruction in children does not necessarily imply that there is a common duct stone. In two individuals we have found *lymph nodes* pressing on the common duct. In six others there was an *idiopathic dilatation* of the common duct (see Chapter XXI), the angulation and displacements of which produced intermittent bile stasis. Indeed, biliary obstructions from an enlarged lymph node and from idiopathic dilatation of the common duct (totaling eight cases) have been more common than obstruction from stone (four cases) in our experience.

Treatment.—When the diagnosis of cholelithiasis has been confirmed by roentgenologic means or by unequivocal signs of biliary obstruction, exploration and removal of the stones is in order. If the calculi lie wholly within the gallbladder *cholecystectomy* can be done, but if the bladder wall is not thickened *cholecystostomy* and removal of the stones may be all that is necessary. This is particularly true if the individual has congenital hemolytic anemia which has been corrected or is going to be corrected by splenectomy. Under these circumstances the chances of future formation of stones is minimal and the gallbladder can be saved with impunity. If there has been obstructive jaundice the common duct must be thoroughly explored for any small calculi it might contain.

In the individual with both congenital hemolytic anemia and cholelithiasis the question arises of whether it is preferable to correct the hemolytic process or to remove the biliary calculi first. This decision must necessarily depend upon the conditions in any given case. In general, *it is better to perform the splenectomy first, and then remove the calculi at a subsequent operation.* If, however, the patient has a high-grade common duct obstruction, the operator must explore the common duct first and leave the splenectomy for a subsequent time. In no case should cholecystectomy (or common duct exploration) be combined with splenectomy, because this combination carries too high a risk of severe and even fatal shock.

HEPATIC TUMORS

Pathologic Types.—Neoplasms of the liver are rare, but several pathologic types have been described. Primary liver-cell *carcinoma* is the most common of the malignant forms and carries the worst prognosis. This lesion grows at a rapid rate, replaces a large part of the normal hepatic tissue, and ultimately has widespread metastases. Small *hemangiomas* of the liver are not infrequently listed as incidental findings at autopsy. They are seldom large enough to be of clinical significance. *Hamartomas* of the liver are rare, but it is important to recognize them because surgical removal can be followed by a fairly good prognosis. These are really not neoplastic growths; they should be regarded rather as development of abnormally placed liver tissues which are attempting to form liver substance but yet not attaining the complete pattern of the normal organ (Fig. 160). Hence, the mass contains imperfectly formed hepatic lobules, biliary ducts, and possibly blood vessel networks in a purposeless arrangement. Mitotic figures are rare, there is no tendency to invasion of the surrounding tissues, and metastases do not occur. The mass may be encapsulated or it may merge widely with adjacent liver substance.

Symptoms and Signs.—The symptoms and signs of a liver tumor depend upon the size of the lesion, the site at which it appears in the liver, and the rapidity of the growth. *Abdominal discomfort, nagging pain,* and a *palpable mass* are the rule. If the liver tissue is largely replaced, or if intrahepatic bile ducts are pressed upon, varying degrees of *jaundice* are encountered. The nutritional state of the patient may be good or there may be advanced *cachexia.*

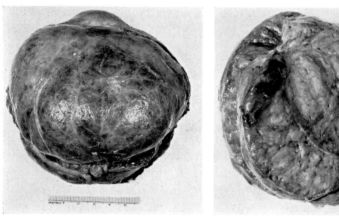

Fig. 160.—Hamartoma of the liver successfully removed from an eight-month-old baby. Specimen weighed 400 gm. (normal liver of a baby at this age weighs 260 gm.).

Prognosis.—In the Children's Hospital material there are nine patients with tumors of the liver. Six of them (five under one year and one at six years of age) had primary carcinomas. One (eight months old) had a large adenoma of the liver. One (one month old) had a large hemangioma. One (eight months old) had a large hamartoma which was removed (Fig. 160). While the prognosis for liver tumors in general is bad, all such patients should be explored, because an occasional benign growth will be found which can be resected.

CONGENITAL ANOMALIES OF THE GALLBLADDER

Anomalies of the gallbladder are rare, but the surgeon and roentgenologist should be familiar with them. In 1936 Gross[11] reviewed 148 cases of such abnormalities which had been previously recorded in the literature.

Histologic studies on these specimens were usually lacking and notes on the blood supply to these organs were very poor. The various conditions which might be briefly described are: double gallbladder, bilobed gallbladder, diverticulum of the gallbladder, floating gallbladder, anomalous position of the gallbladder, and absence of the gallbladder.

Double Gallbladder.—The term "double gallbladder" is used to describe twenty-eight examples of duplication of the vesica fellea in each of which

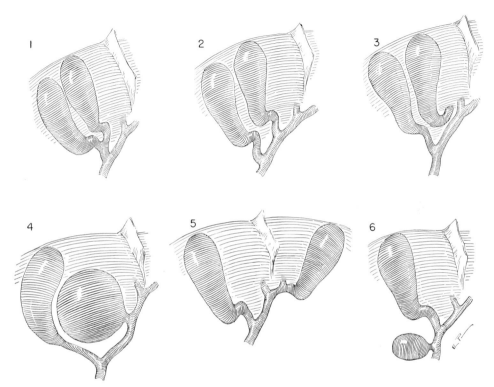

Fig. 161.—Types of double gallbladder, showing positions of the accessory organ and the distribution of its cystic duct. *1*, In the normal fossa with Y-shaped cystic duct. *2*, In the normal fossa with a separate cystic duct. *3*, In the normal fossa with cystic duct directly to the liver. *4*, Partially embedded in the liver (see Fig. 162) with cystic duct entering main hepatic duct. *5*, Under the left lobe of liver and communicating with left hepatic duct. *6*, In the gastrohepatic ligament and emptying into the common duct.

there were two separate bladder cavities and two separate cystic ducts (Fig. 161). The paired cystic ducts either join as a V-shaped structure or else open separately into the extrahepatic bile ducts. The accessory gallbladder may be alongside of the normal one or it may rest in some unusual location, for instance, under the left lobe of the liver or along the gastrohepatic ligament. In one case (Fig. 162) the accessory bladder was globular and was largely embedded within the right lobe of the liver. The accessory bladder usually is about the same size as the normal one, but it may be much larger or it may be diminutive.

Duplicate gallbladders have been discovered *roentgenologically* in a few cases, either by observing two rows of positive shadow gallstones or by finding two distinct shadows of dye by cholecystography.

These patients do not have any characteristic *symptoms or signs* which might make the physician suspect the presence of congenital anomaly before operation or autopsy. When the accessory organ is the seat of inflammatory

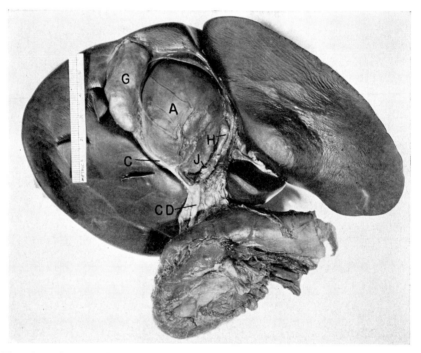

Fig. 162.—Photograph of liver and accessory gallbladder from a three-year-old boy.

A, Accessory Bladder	*G,* Normal Gallbladder
C, Normal Cystic Duct	*H,* Hepatic Duct
CD, Common Duct	*J,* Junction of Accessory Gallbladder to the Hepatic Duct

change or stone formation, the symptoms and signs are indistinguishable from those occurring with cholecystitis or cholelithiasis in a normally formed organ.

Whether or not an accessory organ is more likely to be involved by *disease* is difficult to state, but the fact that most of these anomalies have been found at the operating table and only a few at postmortem examinations tends to show that the accessory structure is more likely to have pathologic changes than is a normally formed one.

Bilobed Gallbladder.—A bifid or partially divided gallbladder, which is so common in many of the higher vertebrates, is seldom encountered in the human. About six examples have been described. Included in this category are those specimens which have two cavities, both of which are drained by a single cystic duct. *Two types* are found (Fig. 163). In one, the bladder has a normal external appearance, but contains an internal longitudinal

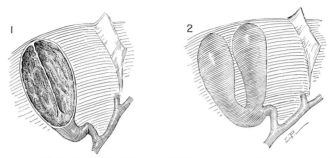

Fig. 163.—Forms of bilobed gallbladders. *1*, With an internal septum. *2*, Paired at the fundic portion and joined at the bladder neck.

septum which divides it into two chambers. In the other type there is a complete division of the fundic portions and a fusion of these at the bladder neck.

Diverticulum of the Gallbladder.—A diverticulum may be found anywhere along the free surface of the bladder from the fundus to the neck (Fig. 164). In the ten cases studied, the diverticula varied from ¼ to 1½

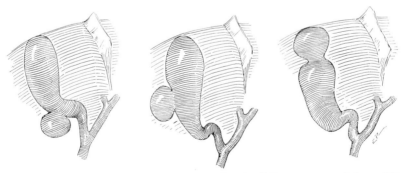

Fig. 164.—Forms of congenital diverticula occurring in different parts of the gallbladder.

inches in diameter. Only a small number have been observed at operation, but they are occasionally recognized by cholecystography as incidental findings. A calculus may form in such a pouch.

Floating Gallbladder.—The bladder may hang from the liver on a sort of "mesentery" (Fig. 165). The peritoneal fold may run the entire length of the gallbladder and cystic duct, or it may support only the cystic duct

19

and allow the gallbladder to hang free and movable. Gallbladders with this type of attachment are fairly common. It is not difficult to foresee the clinical significance of this anomaly, because an organ which is so freely movable is apt to become twisted, and infarction will supervene from impairment of its blood supply. Cases of this sort have been frequently listed in the literature (mostly occurring in adults).

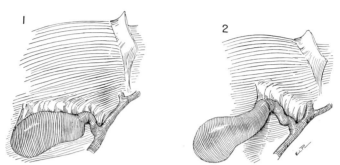

Fig. 165.—Floating gallbladders—suspended by a "mesentery." *1,* Mesentery supporting both bladder and cystic duct. *2,* Mesentery supporting only the cystic duct, allowing the bladder to hang freely.

The *symptoms* are those of severe local pain, nausea and vomiting, collapse, and even fatal peritonitis if the gallbladder ruptures.

Anomalous Positions of the Gallbladder.—These are rare, but at least three locations (Fig. 166) should be mentioned because of the interest they

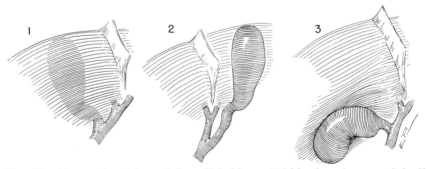

Fig. 166.—Abnormal positions of the gallbladder. *1,* Within the substance of the liver. *2,* Under the left lobe of the liver. *3,* On the posterior-inferior surface of the right hepatic lobe.

have had for surgeons and the technical difficulties they have sometimes presented at operation. These are respectively: *intrahepatic, left-sided,* and *retrodisplaced* positions.

Absence of the Gallbladder.—More than 200 cases of atresia of the extrahepatic bile passages have been recorded in the literature, and about one sixth of these had an associated absence of the gallbladder. In addition to these, no less than thirty-eight cases have been reported in which the hepatic and common ducts were normal and the congenital absence of the gall-bladder was the only abnormality noted. As far as could be determined from the reports, the absence of the bladder did not in any way impair the health or digestive functions of these persons. The absence of the gall-bladder, per se, was rarely accompanied by any compensatory dilatation of the hepatic or common ducts.

TRAUMA TO THE GALLBLADDER AND BILE DUCTS

The gallbladder of a child is relatively small, is rather well protected beneath the inferior surface of the liver, and rarely sustains important trauma. The extrahepatic bile ducts in the gastrohepatic ligament are less well protected and may be lacerated or even completely severed during severe abdominal injuries.

A *rupture of the gallbladder* is easily treated by cholecystectomy.

A *transection* or *extensive laceration of the common or hepatic ducts* should be repaired if possible by end-to-end suture or by suitable plastic reconstruction over a piece of small catheter to insure the continuity and patency of the ductal lumen. If the common duct is extensively damaged the gallbladder can be anastomosed to the duodenum, but it is always preferable to reestablish the continuity of the common duct if this is at all feasible.

The only two instances of injury to the extrabiliary passages that we have encountered were in girls four years of age. In one of these the child fell to the ground and was then struck in the abdomen by a falling board. The hepatic duct was torn but not severed. It was impossible to suture the torn edges accurately, so an abdominal drain was merely inserted to this region. Copious amounts of bile escaped through the drain for some weeks, but the sinus then spontaneously closed and the continuity of the biliary passage was presumably spontaneously reestablished, since the child became and remained symptomless.

In the second case the child's abdomen was crushed by the bumper of an automobile and the common duct was completely divided. A large amount of bile escaped into the abdomen, which was greatly distended. Hemorrhage, edema, and disruption of tissue in the gastrohepatic ligament made a repair of the lacerated common duct extremely difficult. Subsequent stenosis appeared at this point, and to relieve the biliary obstruction a cholecystoduodenostomy was performed. However, this child developed re-curring cholangitis, cirrhosis, and bleeding esophageal varices, from which she died eight years later.

As a commentary on these cases of *extravasation of bile into the ab-domen,* it is to be noted that bile—as long as it is *sterile*—seems to be comparatively innocuous. This material in the abdomen causes little discomfort or pain and there is rarely more than a degree or two of fever. If the bile has been concentrated in the gallbladder before it escapes into the abdominal cavity, its relatively high osmotic pressure may draw forth a considerable amount of fluid from the various peritoneal and intestinal tissues, and in this way produce a greater accumulation of fluid than can be accounted for purely on the basis of extravasated bile.

The results of our meager experience with these cases tend to show the same conclusion as does a review of the literature; namely, that ductal injuries are usually best treated by merely *draining* the damaged area. This form of therapy appears to be the preferable one unless a duct has been completely severed, in which case a plastic procedure or a short-circuiting operation must be resorted to.

BIBLIOGRAPHY

Cholecystitis and Cholelithiasis

1. Hamilton, H. B., Rich, C. O., and Bisgard, J. D.: Cholecystitis and Cholelithiasis of Childhood. J. A. M. A., *103:* 829, 1934.
2. Penberthy, G. C., and Benson, C. D.: Surgery of the Biliary Tract in Infants and Children. Am. J. Surg., *40:* 232, 1938.
3. Potter, A. H.: Biliary Disease in Young Subjects. Surg., Gynec. & Obst., *66:* 604, 1938.
4. Seidler, V. B., and Brakeley, E.: Gallstones in Children. Report of a Case Diagnosed by Roentgen Examination and Confirmed at Operation. J. A. M. A., *114:* 2082, 1940.
5. Swing, A. T., and Bullowa, J. G. M.: Acute Cholecystitis Complicating Scarlet Fever. Am. J. Dis. Child., *55:* 521, 1938.

Liver Tumors

6. Montgomery, A. H.: Solitary Nonparasitic Cysts of the Liver in Children. Arch. Surg., *41:* 422, 1940.
7. Schmelling, J. W.: Rare Case of Congenital Multiple Tumors of Liver (Hamartomas) in Infant 4 Months Old. Nederl. tijdschr. v. geneesk., *78:* 3566, 1934.
8. Wilens, G.: Adenoma of Liver. Am. J. Dis. Child., *55:* 792, 1938.

Anomalies of the Gallbladder

9. Boyden, E. A.: The Accessory Gall-Bladder: An Embryological and Comparative Study of Aberrant Biliary Vesicles Occurring in Man and the Domestic Animals, Am. J. Anat., *38:* 177, 1926.
10. Eisendrath, D. N.: Anomalies of the Bile Ducts and Blood Vessels. J. A. M. A., *71:* 864, 1918.
11. Gross, R. E.: Congenital Anomalies of the Gallbladder. A Review of 148 Cases, with Report of a Double Gallbladder. Arch. Surg., *32:* 131, 1936.
12. Murray, J. F.: Torsion of the Gall Bladder. Brit. J. Surg., *20:* 687, 1933.
13. Schachner, A.: Anomalies of the Gall Bladder and Bile Passages. Ann. Surg., *64:* 419, 1916.

Injury to Biliary Passages

14. Ladd, W. E.: Toxicity of Bile, with Report of an Unusual Case. Boston M. & S. J., *168:* 166, 1913.

15. Rudberg, H.: Traumatic Rupture of Common Bile Duct. München. Med. Wchnschr., *68:* 1650, 1921.
16. Walters, W.: Strictures and Injuries of Bile Ducts; Study of Results of Operations in 80 Cases. J. A. M. A., *113:* 209, 1939.
17. Waugh, G. E.: Traumatic Rupture of the Common Bile-Duct in a Boy Six Years Old. Brit. J. Surg., *3:* 685, 1916.

CHAPTER XXIII

RARE CONDITIONS OF THE UMBILICUS AND ABDOMINAL WALL

The most common lesions of the navel of surgical significance are omphalocele, omphalitis, and umbilical hernia. All of these will be discussed in following chapters. Four other conditions of the abdominal wall which are rarely seen, but which deserve brief mention, are *cyst of the umbilical cord, patent urachus and urachal cyst, persistent vitelline duct,* and *neoplasms* of the abdominal wall.

CYST OF THE UMBILICAL CORD

Within any portion of the cord, and particularly toward its attachment at the abdominal wall, there may be a large collection of *Wharton's jelly* which locally distends the structure and gives rise to a cyst (Fig. 167). This

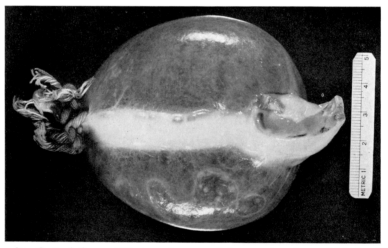

Fig. 167.—Cyst of the umbilical cord removed from a three-hour-old baby. The cord had been divided and ligated at the left; the cyst had been attached to the abdominal wall at the right.

may be large enough to interfere with descent of the baby through the birth canal. If it appears at the very base of the cord, there is no space between the cyst and the abdominal wall for proper placement of the ties by the obstetrician. When this occurs the ligatures must be applied distal to the cyst and the latter must then be surgically removed from the abdominal wall—a dissection which can be done with little difficulty. Inasmuch as the cyst wall has a poor blood supply, there is a tendency to rapid necrosis and sloughing; hence surgical removal should be done within the first twenty-four hours of life.

PATENT URACHUS AND URACHAL CYST

A patent urachus may give rise to considerable annoyance because of recurring umbilical discharge of urine, and a urachal cyst can be a source of real danger if it should become infected. Fortunately, these complications can be avoided by recourse to surgery.

Pathogenesis.—The urachus is derived from the superior part of the allantois. In embryos of 10 to 24 mm. the bladder normally extends up to the umbilical region, but subsequently it descends along the anterior abdominal wall. During this downward migration its upper portion becomes

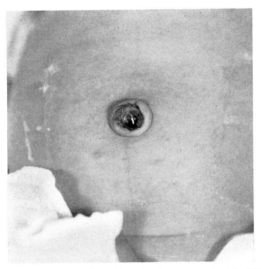

Fig. 168.—Photograph of patent urachus. Navel of one-month-old child from which urine intermittently discharged.

more and more attenuated to form the narrow, tubelike *urachus* which subsequently becomes obliterated. If this entire tract persists, the urinary bladder retains an opening at the navel in postnatal life. If only a segment of the tract remains, a cyst (lined by transitional epithelium similar to that of the bladder) develops external to the peritoneum somewhere between the umbilicus and the superior surface of the bladder.

Symptoms and Diagnosis.—*Patent Urachus.*—Patent urachus manifests itself by an *intermittent escape of variable amounts of urine* at the umbilicus. If the cutaneous opening is tiny there is little more than a recurring moisture of the navel, but if the orifice is large a great deal of urine is emitted by this route. The visible part of the opening is lined by skin or by a pouting and reddened mucous membrane (Fig. 168).

A patent urachus must be differentiated from a *granulating umbilicus* (which readily yields to local applications of silver nitrate) and from a *persistent vitelline duct*. The latter usually communicates with the intestinal tract and the character of the umbilical discharge should suggest the proper diagnosis. Furthermore, gentle injection of lipiodol into the presenting tract before taking lateral roentgenograms will quickly tell whether the connection is with the intestine or the bladder. A cystogram, made by injecting iodide solution through the urethra, will visualize any urachal tract running forward and upward to the navel (Figs. 169 and 171).

Urachal Cyst.—Urachal cyst manifests itself as a deep, midline *swelling* below the navel which has a definite and broad attachment to the internal part of the abdominal wall. This may appear in infants or children, but it

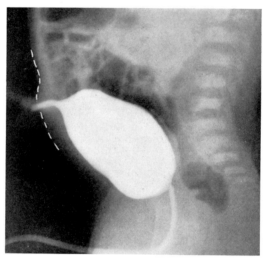

Fig. 169.—Patent urachus (same case as Fig. 168). Cystogram shows the narrow tract running upward through the umbilicus. Dotted line indicates position of abdominal skin.

occasionally escapes notice until adult life. The three in our series were 2 to 5 cm. in greatest dimensions, but larger ones have been described. Not infrequently the mass arises very quickly—a fact which depends upon the sudden closing off of a tiny opening which previously existed between the urachal tract and the bladder proper.

Urachal cysts are apt to become infected and when they do so the clinical features are those of a deep, midline *abscess* of the lower abdominal wall. In one of our cases, a *calculus* formed in this pouch above the bladder.

Lateral *roentgenograms* can aid in making the diagnosis of urachal cyst. No intestines will be found interposed between the mass and the anterior abdominal wall. Furthermore, a cystogram will show the mass to abut directly against the upper surface of the bladder (Fig. 173).

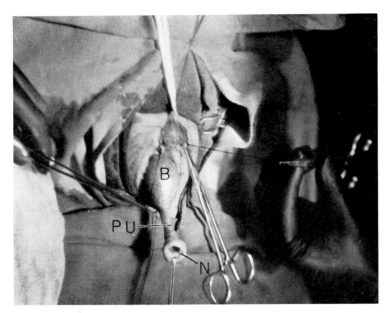

Fig. 170.—Operating room photograph of dissection of patent urachus which was excised along with the umbilicus (same case as Figs. 168 and 169).

B, Bladder. N, Navel, which has been cut away from the abdominal wall. PU, Patent urachus.

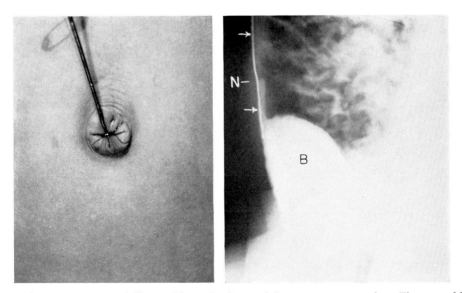

Fig. 171.—*Left,* Umbilicus with probe inserted into a patent urachus. Five-year-old girl with umbilical discharge of urine since birth. *Right,* Roentgenogram showing probe (indicated by arrows) which has been passed through navel (N) down into the iodide-filled bladder (B).

Treatment.—Removal of a urachal cyst or a patent urachus is not difficult if operation is performed *before infection occurs.* The possibility of

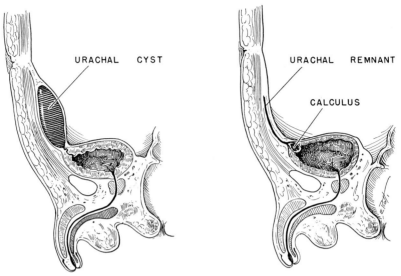

Fig. 172.—*Left,* Sagittal view of a urachal cyst which connected with the bladder by a pinhole opening. *Right,* Sketch from seven-year-old boy with calculus in lower end of a urachal tract. Enuresis cured by excision of the tract and stone.

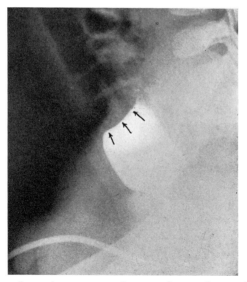

Fig. 173.—Urachal cyst. Lateral cystogram shows a flattened superior border (outlined by arrows) made by a cyst butting down against the bladder.

superimposed infection is so great that surgical excision should always be done as soon as the diagnosis is made. These operations should be done in such a way that the peritoneum is not opened, for if this precaution is heeded the dangers of peritonitis are largely avoided.

Operative Technic.—A midline incision below the umbilicus, separating the rectus muscle bellies, gives an excellent exposure, and with gentleness the lesion can be freed up (Fig. 170) and then peeled away from the peritoneum which is its sole posterior covering. The dissection is continued superiorly so that connections with the umbilicus can be severed, and it is then carried inferiorly to allow separation from the bladder. If an opening is made in the bladder, this is closed with an inverting suture, and an inlying suprapubic or urethral catheter is left in place for about a week to allow the bladder to heal.

Results of Treatment.—In the Children's Hospital there have been four patent urachuses, and three urachal cysts. The four sinuses were excised; one child died of peritonitis and the other three recovered. Two of the cysts were infected and required incision and drainage. Sepsis fortunately destroyed their linings so that no further removal was necessary. The third one contained a calculus and the entire structure was successfully dissected out.

PERSISTENT VITELLINE DUCT

Pathogenesis.—The vitelline duct, extending as it does between the ileum and the yolk sac in the base of the umbilical cord, may remain as a *sinus* after the cord has been separated from the abdominal wall. In this way the intestine may attain an opening at the navel by way of a small mucosa-lined channel several inches in length. If a segment of this vitelline duct becomes closed off, a *cyst* forms which has an attachment to the lower intestine and also to the internal aspect of the anterior abdominal wall. The persistent duct is occasionally the seat of inflammation, but it is more apt to be bothersome because of a disagreeable and malodorous *discharge* at the navel.

Diagnosis.—The proper diagnosis can be readily suspected by local examination and by judicious probing. It can be established beyond doubt if injection of lipiodol into the tract shows a communication with the intestine by fluoroscopic or film studies.

Treatment.—The entire tract (including the umbilicus) must be *excised;* it must be detached from the ileum, and a suitable closure then made of the intestinal wall. If care is taken in cleansing the abdominal skin and in walling off the peritoneal cavity, little soiling results and the dangers of peritonitis are minimal.

NEOPLASMS OF THE ABDOMINAL WALL

Tumors may appear on any portion of the anterior abdominal wall and are found in infants as well as older children. The *prognosis* in any given case varies with the rate of cell growth, and with the size of the neoplasm when treatment is undertaken. Benign growths are more numerous than malignant ones, yet a localized swelling in the abdominal parietes should not be regarded lightly. Any mass, particularly if it has been notice-

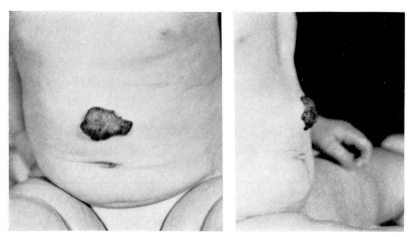

Fig. 174.—Hemangioma in abdominal wall of an eleven-month-old girl.

ably increasing in size, should be immediately and widely removed. Only in this way can the malignant neoplasms be picked up and treated while in an operable stage.

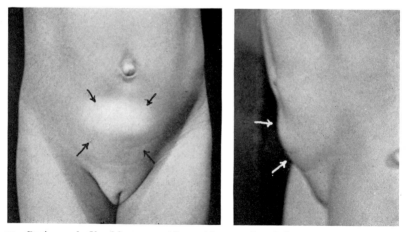

Fig. 175.—Perineural fibroblastoma (desmoid tumor) of lower abdominal wall in a twenty-one-month-old girl.

Hemangioma.—Hemangioma is the most common tumor of the abdominal wall. The rounded, flat, discoid varieties are relatively numerous; they often appear in conjunction with similar cutaneous lesions in other parts of the body. They can be readily treated with applications of carbon dioxide

snow. Less common and more important to the surgeon are those hem-
angiomata which are bulky and which extend through most of the abdominal wall. These usually have some hemangiomatous tissue showing on
the skin surface (Fig. 174) which makes the diagnosis obvious, but they
may reside in the deeper structures of the abdominal wall without involving the skin. The vast majority of blood vessel tumors are capillary and
cavernous hemangiomas, and are entirely benign; an occasional one shows
the more rapid growth of a hemangioendothelioma. In either case total
excision of the mass and suitable fascial repair of the abdominal defect is
the treatment of choice.

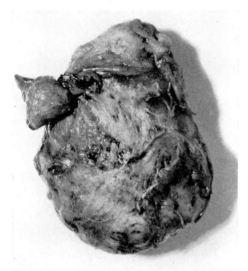
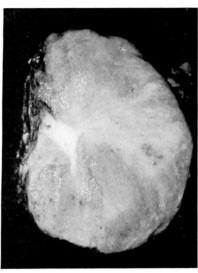

Fig. 176.—External and cross-section views of perineural fibroblastoma (desmoid)
removed from lower abdominal wall (see Fig. 175). Specimen measured 7 by 7 by
3.5 cm.

Lipoma.—Lipomas of the anterior and lateral abdominal wall are not
uncommon. They may reach quite large proportions; they may be accompanied by some similar fatty tumors in other parts of the body. They can be
readily treated by simple excision.

Desmoid Tumors.—Desmoids have been observed in childhood (Figs.
175 and 176). They tend to occur in the midportion of the abdomen, particularly below the umbilicus. They are hard, painless, nontender, flattened
growths with poorly defined borders and with an obvious wide attachment
to the rectus fascia or muscle. Some pathologists believe that desmoid
tumors are perineural fibroblastomas, and the histology in one of our specimens (Fig. 176) strongly suggested such an origin, in spite of the fact that
the mass seemed to arise from the anterior rectus fascia. These neoplasms
tend to recur locally, and hence every effort should be made to remove a

thin layer of normal tissue around the entire tumor, to insure a complete removal. Failure to do this in one patient resulted in a recurrence which necessitated a subsequent and more difficult dissection.

Teratoma.—Teratomas of the abdominal wall are rare. They may carry a poor prognosis if some of their elements are rapidly growing. The specimen shown in Fig. 177 was removed from an eight-day-old baby, but this child unfortunately died at a subsequent time from congenital heart disease.

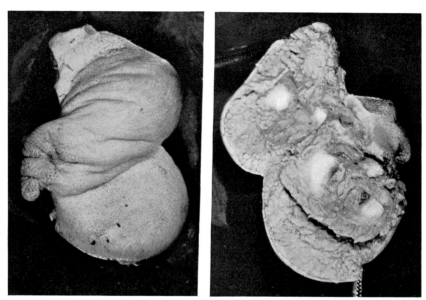

Fig. 177.—Photographs of teratoma removed from abdominal wall of an eight-day-old baby.

In another year-old boy a growth of the upper abdominal wall, which was largely a myxofibroma, was excised on two occasions only to recur and extend locally into the abdomen so that death ensued from intestinal obstruction.

BIBLIOGRAPHY

Cysts of Umbilical Cord

1. Haas, H.: Beitrag zur Lehre von den Cysten der Nabelschnur. Beitr. z. Geburtsh. u. Gynaek., *10:* 483, 1906.

Patent Urachus and Urachal Cyst

2. Begg, R. C.: The Urachus and Umbilical Fistulae. Surg., Gynec. and Obst., *45:* 165, 1927.
3. Dudgeon, H., Jr.: Treatment of Patent Urachus. Surg., Gynec. and Obst., *71:* 302, 1940.
4. Garvin, E. J.: Patent Urachus. J. Urol., *42:* 463, 1939.
5. Kantor, H. I.: Cysts of Urachus; Report of 2 Cases. Ann. Surg., *109:* 277, 1939.
6. Mahoney, P. J., and Ennis, D.: Congenital Patent Urachus. New England J. Med., *215:* 193, 1936.

7. Wyatt, G. M., and Lanman, T. H.: Calculus in a Urachus. Report of a Case with Enuresis. Am. J. Roentgen. and Radium Therapy, *43:* 673, 1940.

Persistent Vitelline Duct

8. Hudson, H. W., Jr.: Meckel's Diverticulum in Children. New England J. Med., *208:* 525, 1933.
9. Ratnayeke, M.: Umbilical Fistula Caused by Patent Meckel's Diverticulum. Brit. J. Surg., *24:* 402, 1936.

Neoplasms of the Abdominal Wall

10. Klot, B.: Bauchdecktumoren. Beitr. z. klin. Chir., *123:* 28, 1921.
11. Meade, W. H., and Brewster, W. R.: Tumefactions of the Abdominal Wall. Am. J. Surg., *45:* 419, 1939.
12. Pfeiffer, C.: Die Desmoide der Bauchdecken und ihre Prognose. Beitr. z. klin. Chir., *44:* 334, 1904.

CHAPTER XXIV

OMPHALITIS

Continued improvements in the care of newly born babies have greatly reduced the incidence of umbilical infections in recent years, yet omphalitis and its sequelae are still frequent enough to merit the attention of obstetricians, pediatricians, and surgeons. Inflammation around the navel in the first two months of life is exceedingly dangerous because bacteria can readily progress inward through the abdominal wall and give rise to regional or distant infections which are a serious menace to life.

ANATOMIC CONSIDERATIONS

The umbilicus has certain anatomic features which have an important bearing on the routes along which infections may spread from this region. The *umbilical vein* pierces the abdominal wall and continues inward at the inferior edge of the falciform ligament. It then branches and communicates with the portal system, and also with the inferior vena cava (via the *ductus venosus*). After birth, the ductus venosus becomes obliterated and forms the ligamentum venosum and the anterior portion of the umbilical vein becomes obliterated and forms the ligamentum teres. Portions of these channels may retain a lumen for some weeks after delivery of the child and it is obvious that bacteria which enter them may have easy access to the portal and peripheral venous systems.

The two *umbilical arteries* pass through the abdominal wall, and then course downward, as the paired *hypogastric vessels,* between the transversalis fascia and the peritoneum, to join the internal iliac arteries in the pelvis. They pass along the inner surface of the anterior abdominal wall on either side of the bladder. While they normally become obliterated soon after birth, a lumen has been known to persist for several weeks. Like the venous channels, these degenerating arteries are able to serve as pathways through which, or along which, bacteria from the umbilicus can reach the blood stream or give rise to suppuration on the inner aspect of the abdominal wall.

Since the hypogastric arteries and the umbilical vein are separated from the abdominal cavity only by a layer of peritoneum and thin areolar tissue, it is at once evident that infection can easily spread from these vessels to the peritoneal cavity and can set up a fatal peritonitis.

The *lymphatic drainage* of the umbilical region is of some importance. The cutaneous channels run downward and outward toward the inguinal nodes, but the deeper ones drain upward and fan out over the pectoral regions. Infections which affect the internal structures of the navel have a tendency to spread along these deep lymphatics and the fascial planes and thus involve the upper abdominal and the lower thoracic wall (Fig. 179).

ETIOLOGY

Contamination of the umbilical cord may occur even before delivery of the child, if there has been premature rupture of the membranes. Organisms may also gain access to the cord during descent of the baby in the birth canal, particularly if vaginal examinations have been made by the attending physician. Most umbilical infections probably begin when the cord is tied and severed or when insufficient care is used during subsequent dressings.

In most cases of omphalitis, the organism concerned is a *hemolytic streptococcus*. Next in importance is the *Staphylococcus aureus,* while the *colon bacillus* or mixed bacteria are the responsible agents in a minority of cases. Particularly troublesome are the *anaerobic* or *microaerophilic* organisms which may give rise to extensive undermining and sloughing of skin.

PATHOLOGY

Granulation tissue frequently persists in the navel several weeks or months after the cord stump has fallen away. Droplets of serous or even purulent fluid may appear on the surface of such granulations from time to time. These lesions rarely give rise to any important sequelae, and they

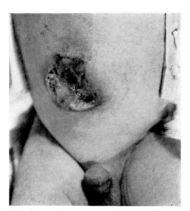

Fig. 178.—Severe omphalitis in a three-week-old baby. There were abscesses extending down along both hypogastric arteries which required incision and drainage. Staphylococcus aureus infection. Subsequent recovery.

can be quickly treated by application of silver nitrate to the exuberant granulations. The resulting raw area will then be rapidly closed over by the surrounding proliferating skin.

In distinct contrast to the benign, weeping or granulating umbilicus just discussed is the *periumbilical cellulitis* or *abscess,* which must be regarded as a serious problem. Infections of this sort are usually limited to

20

the first few weeks of life. Redness and induration may appear in the surrounding skin or pus may exude from the folds of the umbilical depression.

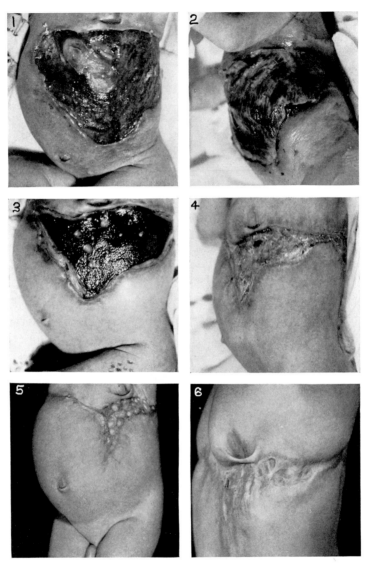

Fig. 179.—Omphalitis followed by infection spreading along the fascial planes or lymphatics, leading to extensive necrosis and sloughing of the upper abdominal and thoracic wall. *1,* Four weeks of age. *2,* Six weeks of age. *3,* Ten weeks of age. Pinch grafts have been taken from the thigh and placed on the granulating area. *4,* Four months of age. *5,* Six months of age. *6,* Four years of age. A portion of this scar was subsequently excised.

Severe omphalitis may take four different courses: (1) The infection may remain locally. An *abscess* may form in the abdominal wall, along the

falciform ligament, or particularly along the hypogastric arteries (Fig. 178).
(2) Inflammation may extend along the fascial planes or lymphatics of the
abdominal wall, so that a *necrotizing lesion* ultimately resulting in extensive
sloughing appears over the epigastrium or lower chest wall (Fig. 179). It
is not uncommon for the infection to burrow beneath the immediate periumbilical skin and leave this intact while destroying the skin of the upper
abdomen. (3) There may be a *blood stream invasion*. When this occurs the
individual manifests a bacteremia by developing multiple foci of suppuration in divers parts of the body, including the hands, feet, subcutaneous
tissues, meninges, lungs, and occasionally the skeleton. (4) Infection may
pass inward through the umbilicus and directly produce a spreading
peritonitis.

CLINICAL FINDINGS

The clinical findings in a case of omphalitis will depend upon which
of the above four conditions exists.

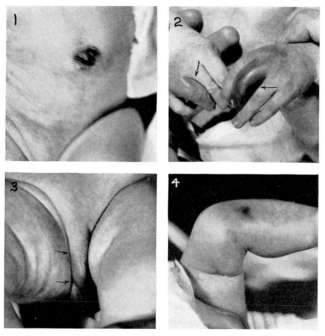

Fig. 180.—Manifestations of bacteremia (hemolytic streptococcus) in a three-week-
old infant. *1*, Omphalitis, from which the pyemia began. *2*, Septic fingers, indicated by
arrows. *3*, Abscess of labium. *4*, Beginning abscess of leg. Child subsequently died from
overwhelming infection.

1. If there is only *regional* infection, then local edema, reddening, tenderness, and serous discharge are the rule. Gentle pressure above or below
the umbilicus may express a droplet or two of purulent exudate, and thus

indicate that there is an abscess adjacent to one of the major extraperitoneal blood vessels.

2. When a *cellulitis* extends along the lymphatics or fascial planes, then edema, tenderness, redness, or duskiness appears in the upper abdominal skin. Subsequent examinations show a deeper red or purplish color indicative of an impaired blood supply and within a few days actual necrosis may begin. When sloughing has once started, it has a tendency to extend with great rapidity. The cutaneous edges become widely undermined and melt away. The musculature and fasciae of the abdominal and thoracic walls are thus directly exposed, and subsequently become covered by granulation tissue (Fig. 179).

3. When *bacteremia* exists, dactylitis, deep-tissue abscesses, high fever, jaundice, or severe toxicity may overshadow what appears to be a minor umbilical infection (Fig. 180).

4. In those individuals with *peritonitis,* the usual complaints include vomiting, marked abdominal distention, high fever, and either diarrhea or constipation. The white blood count may range from 20,000 to 40,000.

TREATMENT

The treatment of omphalitis and its complications depends somewhat upon the conditions which are present.

1. Application of hot, wet boric acid compresses will help to clean up the local infection. If gentle pressure on the abdominal wall expresses purulent material from the navel, a deep-lying *abscess* should be suspected. To investigate this possibility, a probe can be gently passed inward through the tiny umbilical opening. If a sinus leads downward along the course of either hypogastric artery, then a grooved director can be inserted into this tract and the full thickness of the abdominal wall (anterior to the director) is laid open with scissors or scalpel. Extreme delicacy must be exercised to avoid perforation of the thin areolar tissue and peritoneal layer which alone protect the abdominal cavity.

2. Extensive *ulcerations* of the abdominal wall are best treated with large, warm, wet boric acid compresses. Changing of the pack every hour or two will carry away loose débris and will rapidly clean the wound. If there is undermining of the cutaneous edges, application of a zinc peroxide paste followed by a sufficiently airtight dressing will allow slow liberation of nascent oxygen which retards the growth of anaerobic and microaerophilic organisms. Dressings of this type can be changed at daily intervals. It is essential to employ a zinc peroxide powder which has been dried in an oven at 140° C. for four hours, and to prepare the paste freshly just before it is applied to the wound.

3. Infants with a *bacteremia* will require local applications of heat in the various sites of metastatic infection and possibly incision and drainage of these if suppuration occurs.

4. The treatment of the *peritonitis* cases is a disappointing procedure from the first, because of the extremely grave prognosis. However, proper drainage of the umbilicus should be instituted if there is any suspicion that an abscess is pointing inward rather than out through the skin. If there is an appreciable collection of peritoneal exudate, simple incision and insertion of a drain may reduce the individual's toxicity. Supportive measures in the form of a gastric suction, abdominal heat, Fowler's position, parenteral fluids and transfusion should all be undertaken.

At the Children's Hospital there have been a large number of minor umbilical infections which were treated in the outpatient department or which were incidental findings during hospitalization for some other illness. In sixty other cases an omphalitis or its complications was the primary illness for which hospitalization was advised. Of these sixty babies, twelve may be classified as having a local infection; all of them recovered. Five had extensive ulceration of the abdominal wall; four survived and one died. Thirty-seven developed a bacteremia; six of them survived and thirty-one died. Six had an omphalitis and peritonitis; all of them succumbed. The majority of these sixty babies were treated prior to the time when chemotherapeutic agents were available. The death of thirty-eight (63 per cent) doubtless does not reflect the therapeutic results which should be expected today. The more severe forms of omphalitis, particularly when associated with bacteremia or peritonitis, should now have the benefit of *sulfathiazole* or *sulfanilamide,* depending upon the type of organism which is recovered.

The most promising treatment of omphalitis lies in its *prophylaxis.* Adequate precautions should always be used in severing the cord and in subsequent cleansing of the stump with mild antiseptics, such as 70 per cent alcohol. Proper care in this regard by the attending physician or nurse can usually prevent this disastrous type of infection in early life.

Bibliography

1. Adair, F. L.: Care of the Umbilical Stump. A Bacteriologic Study. J. A. M. A., *61:* 537, 1913.
2. Chamberlain, J. W.: Omphalitis in the Newborn. J. Pediat., *9:* 215, 1936.
3. Creadick, A. N.: The Frequency and Significance of Omphalitis. Surg., Gynec. and Obst., *30:* 278, 1920.
4. Hunt, A. B.: Diseases of Umbilicus of Newborn Infant. S. Clin. North America, *17:* 1187, 1937.
5. Siddall, R. S.: The Significance of Inflammation of the Umbilical Stump. Am. J. Obst. and Gynec., *14:* 192, 1927.
6. Weitzman, C. C.: Omphalitis of the Newborn. Am. J. Obst. and Gynec., *26:* 117, 1933.

CHAPTER XXV

OMPHALOCELE (UMBILICAL EVENTRATION)

Umbilical hernia is a weakness of the abdominal wall which is frequently encountered in childhood. The rectus fascia is deficient and permits a small, forward protrusion of peritoneum between the bellies of the rectus muscles, so that this layer is covered solely by fat and by skin. Akin to this is the rather rare malformation, *omphalocele,* which has a very large peritoneal sac which is not covered by skin. An omphalocele consists essentially of a herniation of abdominal viscera into the base of the umbilical cord so that the resulting pouch is a thin translucent structure which consists only of peritoneum internally and amniotic membrane externally. These two layers become fused and make a delicate wall which is less than a millimeter in thickness. It is evident that this latter type of abnormality is totally different from the usual umbilical hernia and that the surgical problems of the two conditions are quite distinct.

This malformation has been designated by many names, such as "funicular hernia of the umbilicus," "hernia into the umbilical cord," "umbilical eventration," "amniotic hernia," "exomphalos," or *omphalocele.* We have chosen to employ the latter term, attempting thereby to set this lesion apart from the usual type of umbilical hernia.

EMBRYOLOGY

From the sixth to the tenth weeks of fetal life the *celomic cavity* has a forward expansion into the base of the umbilical cord, which contains loops of intestines. Such an anatomic arrangement presumably takes place because the abdominal viscera have grown at a greater rate than has the peritoneal cavity itself. After the tenth week the abdomen enlarges at an accelerated pace and the organs are withdrawn into it.

If, for any reason, there should be a permanent disparity in size between the viscera and the abdomen, the intestines or a portion of the liver may continue to remain out in the base of the umbilical cord. Such a disproportion could arise if the liver or intestinal tract is abnormally large, or if the abdominal parietes have a retarded development. The impression is gained from the study of our patients that the latter explanation is the correct one in most instances.

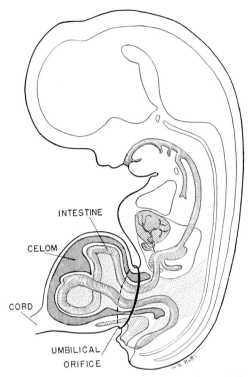

INTESTINE

CELOM

CORD

UMBILICAL
ORIFICE

Fig. 181.—Sketch of a section from a 17 mm. human embryo (after Mall and Prentiss). The celomic cavity normally extends out into the expanded base of the umbilical cord in this early period.

CLINICAL FINDINGS

Physical Characteristics.—An omphalocele sac has a translucent or transparent membranous wall which has very much the same appearance and physical characteristics as the fetal membranes which normally surround the baby. Through this thin structure the intestines, liver, and possibly other abdominal organs are directly exposed to view—as if they were exhibited in a closed showcase.

The omphalocele may be several centimeters in diameter or may be as large as a grapefruit. An average one is from 6 to 8 cm. in cross dimensions. The stump of the cord is attached to the apex of the sac, over which the three umbilical blood vessels course to enter the abdominal wall. The defect in the abdominal wall has no direct relationship to the size of the presenting mass. The fascial opening is usually 4 or 5 cm. in diameter, but indeed it may be twice this large. The abdominal skin usually stops just at the base of the omphalocele, but in some cases it reaches up a centimeter or so beyond this. Loops of small intestine are almost always extruded into the sac, while portions of the stomach, spleen, pancreas, and the urinary bladder may also be displaced. The transverse colon is dislocated in about a third of the cases, and some part of the liver passes out through the abdominal opening in almost half of them. In the first twenty-four hours of life the sac wall is moist and pliable. After this time it tends to become

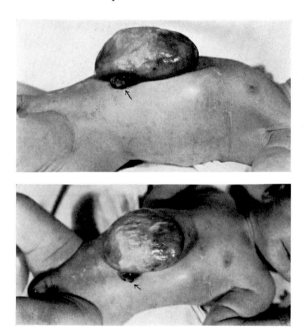

Fig. 182 (Case 9).—Omphalocele in a two-day-old boy. Arrow points to the umbilical cord stump.

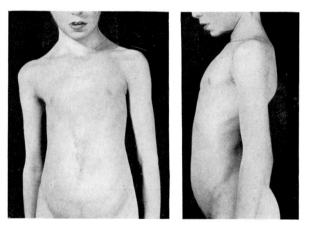

Fig. 183.—Same patient as Fig. 182, nine years after removal of omphalocele. There is no weakness of the abdominal wall.

shriveled, opaque, dried, and somewhat friable. During the first day it will stand a certain amount of gentle handling, but subsequently it is apt to rupture. Such an accident is followed by evisceration and fatal peritonitis.

The membrane, even if unbroken, has a very low resistance to bacterial invasion. These tendencies of the sac to undergo necrosis or become infected are presumably related to its extremely poor blood supply.

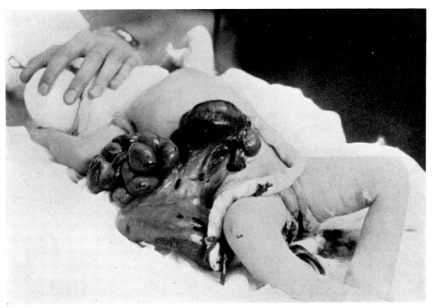

Fig. 184 (Case 11).—Baby with omphalocele which had ruptured prior to hospitalization. Evisceration resulted in fatal peritonitis.

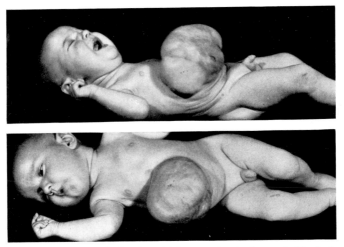

Fig. 185 (Case 13).—Large omphalocele which contained almost half of the abdominal viscera.

Symptoms.—During the first twelve or eighteen hours these babies rarely show any discomfort or altered physiology from the displacement of viscera and the possible exposure of them to a lower temperature. It is rare to find respiratory difficulties or signs of intestinal obstruction. In no instance has jaundice been observed in spite of dislocation of the liver and distortion of

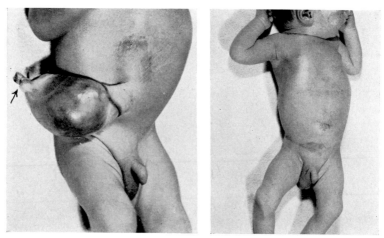

Fig. 186 (Case 14).—*Left,* Three-hour-old baby with omphalocele containing small intestines. Arrow points to stump of cord. *Right,* Same patient eleven days after operation.

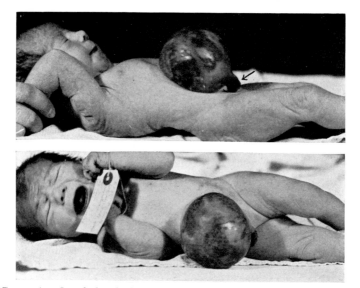

Fig. 187 (Case 15).—Omphalocele in a two-day-old girl. Arrow points to stump of cord. A portion of the liver protruded into the sac.

biliary passages in some subjects. Indeed, the omphalocele appears to act as a compensatory mechanism which permits the baby to be quite comfortable.

Associated Anomalies.—Congenital anomalies in other parts of the body occur with more than coincidental frequency. In five among twenty-two patients, we observed clubfeet, imperforate anus, harelip, or hydrocephalus.

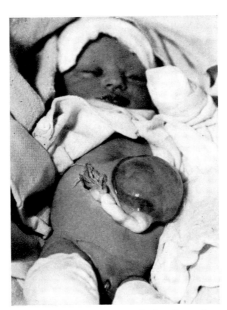

Fig. 188 (Case 17).—Four-hour-old girl with omphalocele and a portion of the umbilical cord.

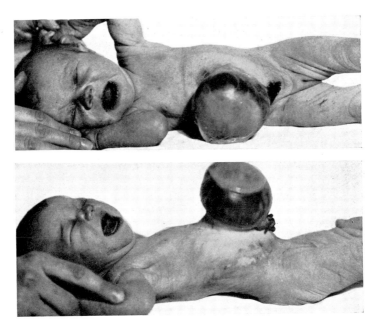

Fig. 189 (Case 19).—Two-day-old girl with an omphalocele which was successfully excised.

Other less serious abnormalities such as Meckel's diverticulum, inguinal hernia, and undescended testicles have also been found. However, the great majority of these babies are well developed except for the umbilical defect.

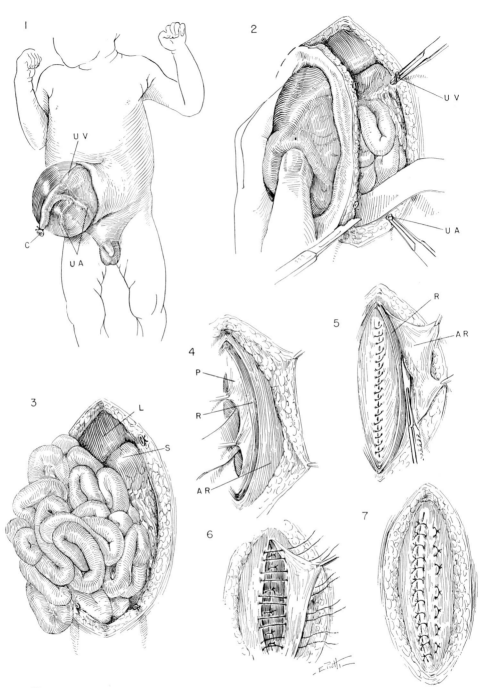

Fig. 190.—Method of surgical removal of an omphalocele. *1*, Preoperative appearance. *2*, Cutting away the sac; removing a narrow rim of the adjacent skin and abdominal wall to freshen their edges. The umbilical vein and arteries are clamped to avoid bleeding. *3*, Sac removed. Umbilical vein and arteries ligated. *4*, Intestines replaced in abdomen.

TREATMENT

Radical and Immediate Operation Is Indicated.—Treatment by any means other than immediate operation exposes the child to the risk of a fatal rupture of the thin sac or a spreading infection of the abdominal wall. Without operation the mortality is extremely high, and most infants succumb within a few days. In one of our cases the skin of the adjacent abdominal wall had started to grow up over the margins of the sac, and we were encouraged to believe that this would continue until the whole structure was covered. Operation was therefore deferred, but infection supervened in the second month and the baby died. There is now quite general agreement that radical and immediate operation offers practically the only hope for continued life. The surgical repair should be performed on the first day, and preferably within the first few hours. Indeed, it has been aptly said that the baby should pass from the obstetrician's hands onto the operating table. Early operation is advantageous because the stomach and intestine are not yet distended by food and gas, and hence the abdominal opening can be closed with less difficulty.

Technic of the Operation.—The plan of operation need not be a set one. The procedure consists essentially of replacement of the various viscera, excision of the sac, and suitable closure of the abdominal wall (Fig. 190). In cutting away the sac it is best to freshen the edges of the presenting ring to obtain the strongest postoperative healing of the wound. Particular attention must be paid to the two umbilical arteries and the umbilical vein, each of which must be carefully ligated. It is not always possible to free up muscle and fascial layers around the ring, but if this is done a better repair can be effected. The peritoneum and posterior rectus sheath should be closed by a continuous suture. The rectus muscles should be mobilized so that they can be approximated in the midline. Likewise, the anterior rectus fasciae should be dissected out and then joined or overlapped with interrupted stitches. It is preferable to repair these last two layers with silk to insure continued tensile strength until adequate fibrous union has taken place.

The *closure of the abdominal wall* is the most difficult part of the operation. The viscera, having forfeited their right of domicile in the abdominal cavity, are difficult and at times impossible to replace. If a satisfactory closure of the wall is obtained, the tension within the abdomen may be so great

Peritoneum freed up. 5, Peritoneum closed. Rectus muscles and anterior rectus fasciae are cleared. 6, Rectus muscles have been approximated. The anterior rectus fasciae are brought together with interrupted silk mattress sutures. 7, Imbrication of rectus fascia.

AR, Anterior Rectus Fascia	*R*, Rectus Muscle
C, Cord	*S*, Stomach
L, Liver	*UA*, Umbilical Artery
P, Peritoneum	*UV*, Umbilical Vein

that respiratory and circulatory embarrassments occur. Considerable judgment must be exercised in determining how perfect a closure should be
attempted. If it is necessary, the peritoneum and posterior rectus fascia can
be left unapproximated. Indeed, in some cases it is wise to leave the peritoneum, fasciae, and muscles completely unsutured and to close only the
subcutaneous fat and skin. While this results in a temporary bulging and
hernia, it does provide adequate coverage and protection for the intestines.
During the ensuing week the muscles and fasciae will stretch, and a secondary closure of the deeper layers of the wound can then be done (Fig.
205). We have adopted this *two-stage* closure on several occasions with
success.

Postoperative Complications.—The operative shock imposed by repair of
an omphalocele is usually minimal, but the postoperative condition of the
baby may be precarious. If viscera are unwittingly squeezed into the abdominal cavity, three serious complications are apt to arise. *First,* the
diaphragm is displaced upward so that respiratory disturbance, severe cyanosis, and death rapidly appear. *Second,* pressure on the inferior vena cava
impedes the return of blood from the lower abdomen and legs, so that
death follows from circulatory collapse. *Third,* pressure on the stomach and
intestines may bring about partial or temporary obstruction. These various
complications are of such a nature that death, when it occurs, follows within
twelve to thirty-six hours. Indeed, it may be stated that if a child lives for
forty-eight hours after one of these procedures the chances of a successful
outcome are excellent.

RESULTS OF TREATMENT

In a series of twenty-two cases at the Children's Hospital, two patients
were not operated upon and both died. In the twenty surgically treated
babies there were ten deaths and ten survivals. Two of the ten living patients had a subsequent weakness in the central portion of the abdominal
wall requiring secondary surgical repair. The great majority of the operative deaths were in the earlier part of the series and were largely due to
injudicious crowding of viscera back into the abdomen. Doubtless some of
these babies could have been saved by the present methods of closing only
the skin and then repairing the deeper layers of the abdominal wall five
or six days later.

The *contents* of the sac have some prognostic value. *Extruded liver* is
a bad sign. It implies that the peritoneal cavity is unusually small and that
there will be difficulty in reducing the omphalocele and closing the abdominal wall. Eight of our patients had some part of the liver in the sac; six of
them died. On the other hand, if the sac contains only small intestines, the
prognosis is excellent.

The *size* of the omphalocele has some prognostic significance. In our patients with a sac less than 8 cm. in diameter, there were 75 per cent sur-

TABLE 33

DATA FROM TWENTY-TWO CASES OF OMPHALOCELE OBSERVED AT THE CHILDREN'S HOSPITAL

Case	Age	Sex	Diameter of Om-phalocele	Contents of Omphalocele				Treat-ment	Result
				Intes-tine	Colon	Liver	Other Viscera		
1	3 days	F.	15 cm.	+	+	+	Pancreas	Excision	Died
2	3 hours	F.	10 cm.	+	0	+		Excision	Died
3	31 hours	?	?	+	+	0		Excision	Cured
4	4 hours	M.	4 cm.	+	0	0	Meckel's di-verticulum	Excision	Cured
5	1 hour	F.	5 cm.	+	+	0	Bladder and tube	Excision	Died
6	2 days	M.	8 cm.	+	0	0		Excision	Died
7	6 days	F.	8 cm.	0	0	+		Excision	Died
8	2 days	F.	7 cm.	0	0	+		Excision	Died
9	2 days	M.	5 cm.	+	0	+		Excision	Cured
10	2 days	F.	15 cm.	+	+	+	Spleen	Excision	Died
11	2 hours	M.	8 cm.	+	+	0	Bladder	Excision	Died
12	2 hours	M.	8 cm.	+	0	0		Excision	Cured
13	4 months	M.	15 cm.	+	+	+		Excision	Died
14	3 hours	M.	6 cm.	+	0	0		Excision	Cured
15	2 days	F.	8 cm.	+	0	+		Excision	Died
16	6 days	M.	5 cm.	+	0	0		Excision	Cured
17	36 hours	F.	10 cm.	+	+	+		None	Died
18	19 days	M.	8 cm.	+	0	0		None	Died
19	2 days	F.	8 cm.	+	0	+		Excision	Cured
20	5 hours	M.	4 cm.	+	+	0		Excision	Cured
21	6 hours	M.	10 cm.	+	0	0		Excision	Cured
22	24 hours	F.	5 cm.	+	0	0		Excision	Cured

vivals. When the sac was greater than 8 cm. in diameter, there were but 15 per cent survivals.

The *age* of the individual at operation is of some importance because delayed operations are apt to be followed by infections of the operative wound. If this once occurs there is a high probability of a subsequent fatal peritonitis.

BIBLIOGRAPHY

1. Arey, L. B.: Developmental Anatomy: a Textbook and Laboratory Manual of Embryology (Fourth Edition). Philadelphia: W. B. Saunders Co., 1940.
2. Bardeen, C. R.: Critical Period in the Development of the Intestines. Am. J. Anat., *16:* 427, 1914.
3. Cullen, T. S.: Embryology, Anatomy and Diseases of the Umbilicus. Philadelphia: W. B. Saunders Co., 1916.
4. Cutler, G. D.: Prolapsus of the Bowel through a Patent Omphalomesenteric Duct Opening on the Side of the Umbilical Cord: Report of a Case with Operation. Boston M. & S. J., *190:* 782, 1924.
5. Dott, N. M.: Clinical Record of a Case of Exomphalos, Illustrating Embryonic Type and its Surgical Treatment. Tr. Edinburgh Obst. Soc., *39:* 105, 1932.
6. Gross, R. E., and Blodgett, J. B.: Omphalocele (Umbilical Eventration) in the Newly Born. Surg., Gynec. & Obst., *71:* 520, 1940.
7. Herbert, A. F.: Hernia Funiculi Umbilicalis; With Report of Three Cases. Am. J. Obst. and Gynec., *15:* 86, 1928.
8. Jarcho, J.: Congenital Umbilical Hernia. Surg., Gynec. & Obst., *65:* 593, 1937.
9. Keibel, F., and Mall, F. P.: Manual of Human Embryology (Vol. 2). Philadelphia: J. B. Lippincott Co., 1912.
10. Stein, J. L., and Gerber, A.: Congenital Omphalocele. J. Pediat., *14:* 89, 1939.
11. Watson, L. F.: Hernia (Chapter XXIV) (Second Edition). St. Louis: C. V. Mosby Co., 1938.
12. Williams, C.: Congenital Defects of the Anterior Abdominal Wall. S. Clin. North America, *10:* 805, 1930.

CHAPTER XXVI

UMBILICAL HERNIA

Pathology.—Umbilical hernia is extremely common in young children. It results from muscular and fascial defects of the abdominal wall at the point where this has been pierced by the blood vessels of the umbilical cord. The forward-projecting peritoneum is covered only by subcutaneous fat and skin. The hernial ring has an edge of firm connective tissue which represents the fused posterior rectus, anterior rectus, and transversalis fasciae. While the separation of the muscle bellies is usually confined to the periumbilical region, it not infrequently extends upward, even as far as the ensiform process, as a diastasis recti. Umbilical hernias are about twice as common in girls as they are in boys—a fact possibly related to the less well-developed musculature of the female. Most of these weaknesses can be detected in the early months of life, but they may escape attention until the child assumes an erect posture and the bulging becomes more marked.

Physical Findings.—The *size* of an umbilical hernia depends upon the extent of the fascial defect and upon the length of time that the sac and overlying skin have been stretched. In infants under one year, the bulge is rarely more than 1½ cm. in diameter. In older children hernias 3 to 4 cm. in cross dimensions are often encountered, and larger ones are sometimes seen. The pocket rarely contains more than omentum or a single knuckle of small intestine. Adhesions seldom form between these viscera and the sac wall.

Symptoms.—In most cases the patient's or the parents' complaints are concerned with the *swelling* which becomes larger and more tense during crying, standing, straining, or other exercise which raises the intra-abdominal pressure. There may be a mild, local discomfort of a vague sort. *Cramps* may appear if a loop of small intestine enters the hernia and becomes partially obstructed. Omentum is sometimes caught in the hernial ring, but intestine is rarely incarcerated. These findings are in distinct contrast to the frequency of incarceration with inguinal hernias in childhood.

TREATMENT

Adhesive Strapping.—Before initiating any measures for treatment of an umbilical hernia, it is well to remember that about half of them will be *spontaneously cured* as the individual grows older and the rectus muscles constrict and finally obliterate the hernial orifice. Thus, small hernias often disappear if the child is observed over a period of several years. This nat-

21   325

ural tendency for small hernias to vanish can be augmented by proper adhesive strapping during the early months of life. This should be done in such a way that the lateral tension of the abdominal wall is diminished and the hernial ring is allowed to shrink. Furthermore, the sac must be kept empty so that nothing interferes with its collapse and obliteration. These

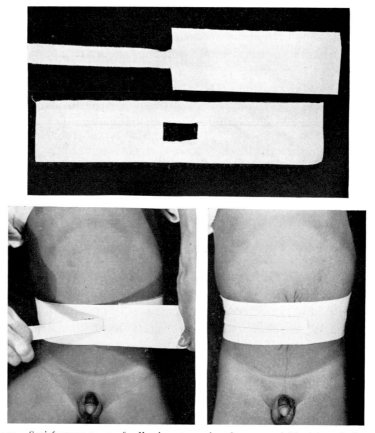

Fig. 191.—Satisfactory type of adhesive strapping for an umbilical hernia in an infant. The adhesive straps are 2 inches wide. One has a hole and the other a tongue, as shown. The two straps are applied to the lateral parts of the abdominal wall and then interlaced with each other. Pulling on the free ends relieves the abdominal wall tension at the umbilicus. When the umbilical skin becomes wrinkled, the free ends of the straps are stuck down.

qualifications are not fulfilled by strapping a metal coin over the protruding navel. Neither are they met by spring trusses or rubber belts fitted with a small projection which is intended to press into the hernial opening.

The most satisfactory support for a small umbilical hernia is the strapping portrayed in Fig. 191. Two pieces of 2-inch adhesive tape are cut, one with a hole and the other with a tongue, so that they can be subsequently interlaced. The abdomen is painted with tincture of benzoin to enhance the sticking qualities of the tape and to protect the skin from ulceration. The straps are placed on either side of the abdomen, as shown, and the narrow tongue is threaded through the hole of the opposite piece. The free ends are then grasped and pulled in a forward and outward direction until the skin becomes lax and wrinkled in the umbilical area. If necessary, an assistant can simultaneously push the hernia inward with the tip of a finger. While the pull is still maintained, the free ends of the adhesive straps are stuck down. If this has been done properly, the umbilical skin will still have longitudinal wrinkles.

The strapping is renewed every week or two. Continued support must be maintained for a period of several months. If no appreciable improvement is noticed by the end of six months, it is useless to continue this form of treatment. A great deal can be accomplished with strapping during the first six months of life, but after this time it has a diminishing value. It has practically no merit for a baby more than a year old.

Umbilical Herniorrhaphy.—Many umbilical hernias cause little nuisance except for the slight disfigurement and the worry to the parent. After the first year of life a swelling which is 1 cm. or less in size should cause little concern, particularly if the palpable fascial ring is less than 7 or 8 mm. in diameter. Such a small sac will often become obliterated as the child grows. Hernias 1.5 to 4 cm. or more in cross dimensions should be repaired, particularly if there has been recurrent discomfort or a tendency to increase in size. Umbilical herniorrhaphy in a child is a rather minor procedure. Operation is seldom an urgent matter and it can usually be deferred until the age of one and a half or two years to make sure that nature is not going to care for the situation without a surgeon's aid.

Technic.—Operative repair should always restore the normal navel depression. To do so does not appreciably complicate the technical procedure and it gives an appearance to the abdominal wall which is more natural and pleasing.

If the hernia is large, the method of repair illustrated in Fig. 192 will be found satisfactory. A *semicircular cutaneous incision* is made below the bulge so that the skin of the navel is turned upward and an adequate exposure of the region is obtained. The undersurface of this skin flap is freed, the peritoneal sac is cleared, and the two are then separated from one another. The redundant peritoneum is imbricated; if the sac is large it is trimmed away and the edges are brought together with a transverse running suture. By blunt dissection the fascial surfaces are now separated from the underlying peritoneum, are overlapped in a transverse direction, and are imbricated. The skin flap is now sutured back into place. A suitable dressing should include a small wad of cotton pressing into the umbilicus. The re-

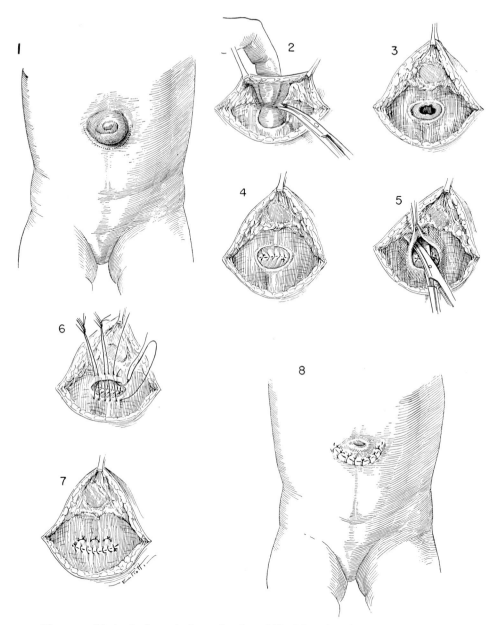

Fig. 192.—Method of surgical repair of umbilical hernia with a curvilinear incision below the bulge. *1,* Incision to be made along the dotted line. *2,* Skin flap dissected up. Inverted umbilical skin is cut free from the presenting peritoneal sac. *3,* Cutaneous flap completely freed up. Opening usually made in the peritoneal sac. *4,* Peritoneum is closed with a transverse running suture. *5,* Undermining and freeing fascial layer from peritoneum. *6,* Mattress sutures in fascial layer. *7,* Mattress sutures tied. Imbrication of fascia with a running suture. *8,* Skin flap replaced and wound closed.

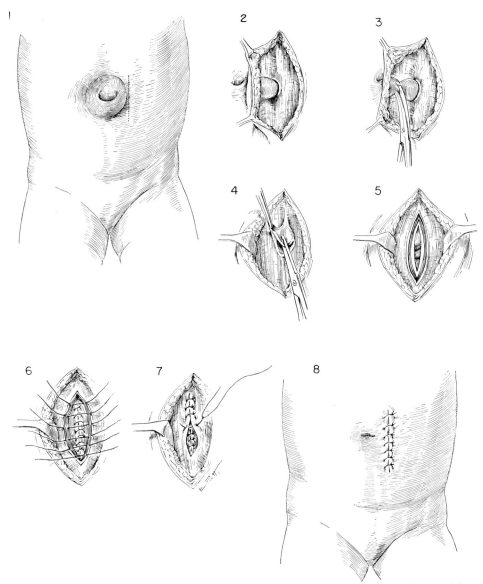

Fig. 193.—Method of umbilical herniorrhaphy with a vertical paramedian incision. *1,* Position of incision. *2,* Skin flap raised and hernial sac identified. *3,* Navel skin is severed from sac. *4,* Sac is being opened. *5,* Fascia, rectus muscles, and peritoneal edges have been identified and freed. *6,* Peritoneum (including transversalis fascia) has been closed with a continuous suture. Interrupted sutures have been placed in the rectus muscle. *7,* Muscles approximated. Fascia being closed with interrupted sutures. *8,* Closure of skin.

sulting cutaneous scar is not unsightly, provided the subcutaneous fat and the cutaneous edges have been carefully approximated so that one margin of the wound is not depressed in relation to the other.

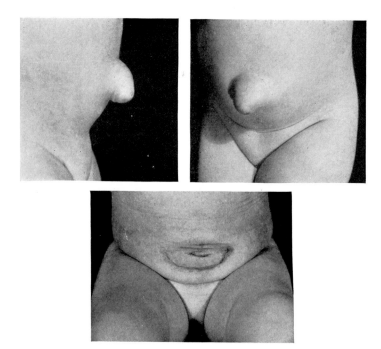

Fig. 194.—*Above,* Photographs of umbilical hernia in a fifteen-month-old girl. *Below,* Photograph ten days after operative repair with a semicircular incision.

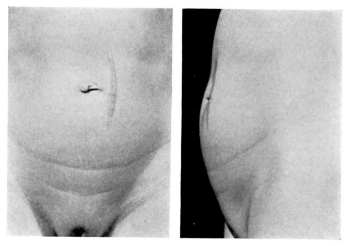

Fig. 195.—Postoperative photographs following umbilical herniorrhaphy with a paramedian incision.

A second method of repair which has been very useful (Fig. 193) employs a *vertical, straight, paramedian incision* to the right or left of the hernia. The umbilical skin is undermined and the peritoneal sac dissected away from it. The edges of the hernial ring are split so that the anterior and posterior rectus fasciae as well as the muscle bellies are defined and freed. The peritoneum is closed with a continuous suture and the remaining layers are then approximated, preferably with interrupted silk. The vertical incision gives an insignificant scar which on the whole heals somewhat better than does the semicircular one. It is particularly desirable for those patients with a separation of the recti when the operator may want to extend the wound upward for repair of the diastasis.

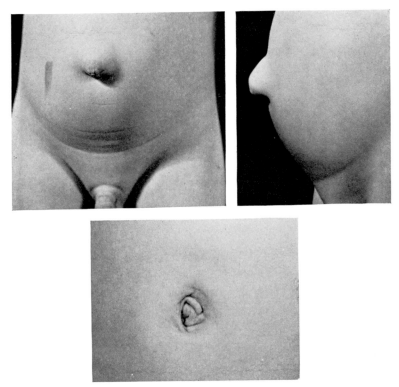

Fig. 196.—*Above*, Photographs of umbilical hernia in a three-year-old boy. *Below*, Photograph after herniorrhaphy with incision which lies in the umbilical folds.

Results of Treatment.—At the Children's Hospital more than 1500 umbilical hernias have been observed during the twenty-five-year period from 1915 through 1939. Most of these were the primary reason for admission to the outpatient department or the house service; others were insignificant and were discovered during routine examination for some other condition. Many of the smaller hernias in babies were cured by strapping. Out of the entire number, 360 were operated upon, and three recurrences have been noted. There was one death, which occurred on the fourth postoperative day from pneumonia.

BIBLIOGRAPHY

1. Barrington-Ward, L. E.: The Abdominal Surgery of Children. London: Oxford University Press, 1937. P. 25.
2. Blodgett, J. B.: Transumbilical Repair of Congenital Umbilical Hernia. Surg., Gynec., and Obst., *72:* 632, 1941.
3. Gorelow, M. A.: Zur Anatomie des Nabelkanals. Arch. f. klin. Chir., *181:* 395, 1934.
4. Herzfeld, G.: Hernia in Infancy. Am. J. Surg., *39:* 422, 1938.
5. Power, R. W.: Preservation of Umbilicus in Radical Cure of Umbilical Hernias in Children. Brit. M. J., *2:* 353, 1934.

CHAPTER XXVII

CONGENITAL HERNIA OF THE DIAPHRAGM

In a book on abdominal surgery of infancy and childhood it is appropriate to include a consideration of congenital diaphragmatic hernia because this defect can be treated best by a transabdominal operation. Diaphragmatic hernia is a not uncommon lesion in the newly born. It can be easily detected by physical examination and roentgenologic study. It can be satisfactorily and permanently cured by properly executed surgical procedures. The recovery of eleven of the last thirteen patients we have treated indicates that diaphragmatic defects can be successfully repaired in babies in spite of the previously reported high mortality rates.

An extensive literature has accumulated on the general subject of diaphragmatic hernia, but relatively little attention has been paid to the condition as it occurs in the first few weeks or months of life. During these age periods the therapeutic problems pertaining to such defects are quite different from those encountered in older children or adults. It is therefore impossible to employ the same surgical measures which have proved to be so effective in repair of acquired (traumatic) diaphragmatic hernia of adults. Various authors have stressed the fact that congenital diaphragmatic hernia is a serious lesion which menaces the life of the individual. In 1931 Hedblom[4] reviewed the literature and found that 75 per cent of patients with the congenital form died before the end of the first month. In a review of the literature up to 1940 we are able to find but thirty-one cases treated by operation in the first year of life, and in only seventeen of these did the patients survive. To this list of operative cases may be added our own series. While the total number of survivors is small, certain principles are now formulated which should insure recovery of 85 to 90 per cent of these individuals.

EMBRYOLOGY

In the young embryo the thoracic and abdominal portions of the body cavity communicate freely with each other. The ventral part of the diaphragm is formed from the septum transversum which separates the heart from the abdominal viscera. This septum is joined posteriorly by a proliferation of mesodermal cells at the upper end of the dorsal mesentery to make a bridge across the celomic cavity from front to back, but openings are left in both posterolateral parts of the diaphragm which are known as the pleuroperitoneal canals. These canals are later closed by a double-layered membrane, consisting of peritoneum on one side and pleura on the other. Striated muscle then develops between these two serous coats to complete and strengthen the partition between the peritoneal and pleural cavities.

The formation of the diaphragm is sufficiently complicated so that there is little wonder that congenital defects are apt to appear. If arrest in development occurs early in embryonic life, the child is born (as is typical of most cases) with a free communication between a pleural cavity and the abdomen. If arrest of development occurs after pleural and peritoneal membranes have closed the defect, but before the muscle has appeared, the child is born with a thin hernial sac which covers the upward protruding intestines.

PATHOLOGY

Congenital hernia may occur in one of three parts of the diaphragm: (1) In either *posterolateral portion,* along the old pleuroperitoneal canal

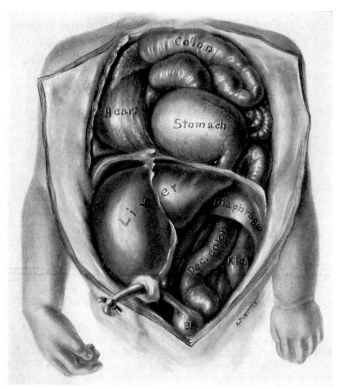

Fig. 197.—Drawing made at postmortem examination on a baby with a left diaphragmatic hernia. Four hours following delivery the child died, after severe cyanosis and respiratory distress. Like most congenital diaphragmatic herniae, there is no sac surrounding the extruded abdominal viscera.

(the foramen of Bochdalek). This is by far the most common site. Hernias appearing here are three or four times more common on the left than on

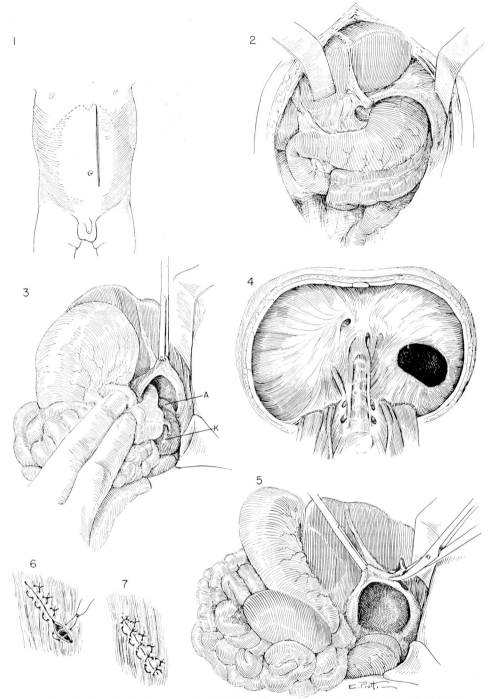

Fig. 198.—Method of repair of a left-sided hernia. *1*, Position of abdominal incision. *2*, View on opening the abdomen. The small intestines, spleen, and portions of the stomach and colon are herniated up into the left pleural cavity. *3*, Abdominal viscera withdrawn from the diaphragmatic opening and pulled out upon the abdominal wall. *A*, Adrenal. *K*, Kidney. *4*, Sketch of diaphragm showing posterolateral position of the hernial opening. *5*, Denuding the edges of the hernial ring. *6*, Approximation of the diaphragmatic edges with mattress sutures of silk. *7*, Closure of peritoneal edges with interrupted silk sutures.

the right. (2) At the *esophageal hiatus*. (3) In the *retrosternal area* (the foramen of Morgagni). This is the least common site.

Hernias which appear at the esophageal hiatus always have a *sac* which partially limits the upward progression of abdominal viscera. Hernias at the foramen of Morgagni may or may not possess a sac. Hernias at the foramen of Bochdalek possess a sac in only about 10 per cent of the cases, whereas the remaining 90 per cent have no such covering.

When a posterolateral hernia has a sac, its superior border may extend into the superior third of the pleural cavity (Fig. 206). When no sac is present, the affected pleural cavity is filled with collapsed lung, most of the intestines, the major portion of the stomach and colon, and either the spleen or liver, according to the side of the defect (Figs. 201 and 202). The great *displacement of viscera* in these cases is facilitated by a rudimentary attachment of the mesentery to the posterior abdominal wall. It is exceedingly rare to find adhesions between these viscera and the intrathoracic surfaces—a situation which is quite different from that found in acquired (traumatic) hernia. The prenatal displacement of abdominal viscera into the chest implies that they have "forfeited their right of domicile" and accordingly the peritoneal cavity is smaller than normal.

CLINICAL FINDINGS

Symptoms.—Diaphragmatic hernia may give findings referable to the respiratory, circulatory, or digestive systems, and the severity of symptoms depends upon the number of abdominal viscera which are displaced into the thorax. A newly born infant who exhibits *cyanosis, dyspnea,* or *vomiting,* should be studied with diaphragmatic hernia in mind.

Cyanosis may be evident immediately after delivery. It may be transient and may appear only during nursing or crying, but in some cases it is so severe that constant use of an oxygen tent is necessary to sustain life. It can be occasionally relieved by turning the baby so that the side of the hernia is downward. In this position the mediastinum falls toward the affected side and gives better expansion of the other lung.

Vomiting may be only occasional, or it may follow most of the feedings. In patients who survive for a month or two, it is common to find poor weight gain and even weight loss.

Physical Examination.—On physical examination, respiratory and pulse rates are found to be increased. By *inspection* the affected side of the chest is seen to move less than the normal side. *Percussion* of the chest on the side of the hernia may give a dull or tympanitic note, depending upon which viscera are residing in the pleural cavity and whether the trapped intestines contain fluid or air. The heart is displaced away from the affected side. By *auscultation* the breath sounds are distant or absent. If intestinal gurgles are heard instead of breath sounds, the correct diagnosis should be suspected at once. When the major part of the alimentary tract is in the thorax, tympany is lacking on abdominal percussion, and the abdomen is scaphoid.

ROENTGENOLOGIC EXAMINATION

Roentgenologic studies quickly confirm the diagnosis and afford a rough method of estimating what abdominal viscera are herniated into the pleural cavity. Film or fluoroscopic examination without the use of contrast media will usually give all the information that is required. Feeding of barium increases the chances of vomiting and aspiration pneumonia. If a contrasting mixture is employed, it should be quite thin.

The *chest findings* may be very bizarre. The unaffected side has a poorly expanded lung because the mediastinum and heart are shifted in this direction. The affected pleural cavity contains viscera which are continuous with those of the abdomen. Thus, a liver or stomach shadow may extend above and below a level where the diaphragm should be, or else the colon can be traced from the abdomen into the chest. If a hernial sac is present, some lung tissue can be seen in the upper part of the chest and the intestines will not extend the entire way up to the apex (Fig. 206). If, however, there is no hernial sac, abdominal viscera can be seen to the very top of the pleural cavity (Figs. 201 and 202).

It is important to emphasize that examination of the *gastro-intestinal tract* with barium should be omitted if possible. This is rarely necessary to establish the diagnosis, and while it is interesting to determine accurately what viscera are in the chest and what is the position and size of the diaphragmatic defect, such information has little practical value. It does not alter the operative approach or procedure and the obtaining of such data may be dangerous for the baby. The only cases in which barium studies are advisable are those with a hernia at the esophageal hiatus. In such patients it is important to know the length of the esophagus and size of the diaphragmatic opening when one is considering the desirability of surgical treatment.

TREATMENT

Importance of Immediate Operation.—There can be no question that surgery is the treatment of choice in all these patients, except the occasional ones with a small esophageal hernia. There is sufficient evidence, from our own failures and from the literature, to show the futility of expectant or medical measures. The general condition of the patient may be temporarily improved thereby, but no enduring improvement can be expected and the risks are great. The policy of waiting until the child is older and stronger is responsible for the loss of a great many lives which might be saved by an early operation. We are convinced that operation should be undertaken as soon as the diagnosis is made.

On a theoretical basis, an operation performed *in the first forty-eight hours* of life is very advantageous, and we have had the opportunity of proving this in two cases. It is our experience that infants in the first forty-eight hours of life stand major surgical procedures extremely well—in fact, far better than they do at the end of a week or ten days. Within the first two days the operator has the added advantage of dealing with an intestine

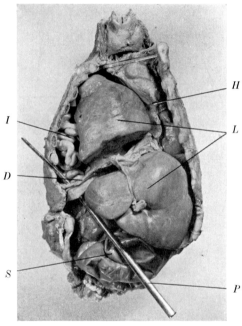

Fig. 199.—Photograph of a postmortem specimen from a newly born child who died with a right-sided diaphragmatic hernia. The liver has a deep fissure where it protrudes through the diaphragmatic opening.

D, Diaphragm	L, Liver
H, Heart	P, Probe through the Diaphragmatic
I, Intestine	Defect
	S, Stomach

which is not yet distended. This can easily make the difference between the possibility or impossibility of replacing intestines into the abdominal cavity.

Preoperative Measures.—The preoperative treatment should be directed toward attainment of proper hydration and toward deflation of the alimentary tract. This latter can be accomplished by enemata, by gastric suction, and by placing the infant in a tent with 90 to 95 per cent oxygen.

Anesthesia.—The anesthetic of choice is *cyclopropane*. It is justifiable to assume the slight risk of explosion which its use entails, because it gives a gaseous mixture with a maximum content of oxygen. This is highly important for a baby whose respiratory apparatus is so seriously handicapped and it also facilitates the operation by decreasing the respiratory excursions of the chest and diaphragm.

Whatever anesthetic is employed, there must always be provision for giving *positive-pressure anesthesia* if the need should arise. Ochsner[15] and others have pointed out that some humans have an anterior mediastinal communication between the two pleural cavities. Hence, the opening of one pleural cavity to atmospheric pressure will permit *both* lungs to collapse, if positive pressure cannot be supplied by the anesthesia machine. It is not necessary or desirable to use an intratracheal catheter because a positive-pressure anesthesia can be easily given through a tightly fitting face mask. The small respiratory exchange of a baby will not produce a flow of gas through the large and long rubber tubes which connect the face mask to the flap-valve chamber of the average gas machine. It is therefore necessary to have an attachment, such as that shown in Fig. 204, whereby the soda lime chamber is brought close to the infant's face mask. With this closed apparatus, the single tube has only a one-way flow and brings oxygen or cyclopropane from the gas machine.

Preliminary Crushing of Phrenic Nerve.—It is not essential, but it is desirable for three reasons, to paralyze the phrenic nerve temporarily on the affected side before proceeding with operative repair of the diaphragm: (1) It is easier to work on the diaphragm if it is at rest. (2) A high and relaxed diaphragm will give more room in the abdominal cavity for the intestines. (3) A resting diaphragm will pull less on its suture line and will promote healing. In one of our cases the phrenic nerve was crushed at an initial operation with the intention of performing the herniorrhaphy four or five days later, but the infant died before that time. It is therefore our present practice to crush the phrenic nerve through a small transverse incision above the clavicle and then immediately proceed with the repair of the hernia. This crushing with a hemostat paralyzes the diaphragm for five or six weeks.

Technic of Operative Repair.—*Abdominal Approach.*—The thoracic approach is probably the best one for exposure and treatment of diaphragmatic hernias in the adult, but the abdominal approach is far superior in babies and young children. In infants, the problem of adhesions between intestines and pleural structures is extremely rare. In the absence of adhesions, it is much easier to pull the abdominal contents out of the chest from below than it is to push them down from above. In fact, in most infant cases it would be impossible to reduce the hernia through a thoracic wound, because the abdominal cavity is too small to receive all of its viscera.

The abdominal incision may be a vertical one through the rectus mus-

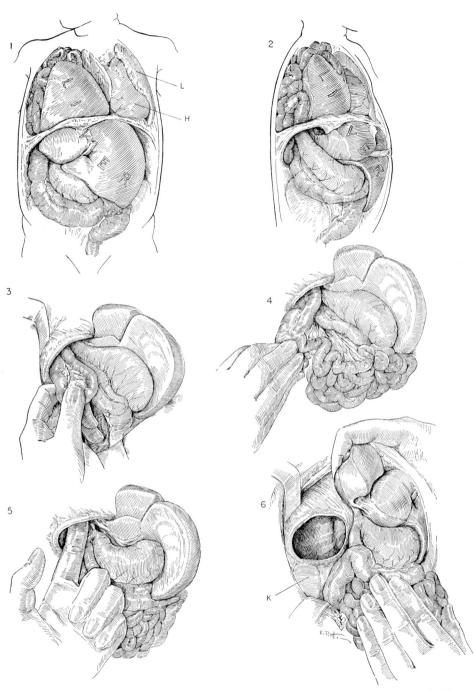

Fig. 200.—Operative reduction and repair of a right diaphragmatic hernia by a transabdominal approach. *1*, Orientation sketch showing position of the viscera in the abdominal and right pleural cavities. Half of the liver is above the diaphragm. *H*, Heart, *L*, Left lung. *2*, Lateral sketch showing position of the liver in the pleural cavity

cle on the affected side, or else a subcostal one—either gives a satisfactory exposure. We have used the *rectus incision* (Figs. 198 and 200), as it destroys less of the nerve supply to the abdominal wall.

Withdrawal of Abdominal Viscera from Thorax.—After the peritoneum is opened one may see at once what viscera are in the peritoneal cavity and deduce, of course, what is in the thorax. A blunt instrument or a rubber catheter is introduced through the hernial ring so that air can enter the thorax. If this is not done the intestines will be sucked back into the chest as fast as the operator pulls them out. After the abdominal viscera are withdrawn from the thorax they are placed outside of the abdominal wall where they are wrapped in warm, moist gauze.

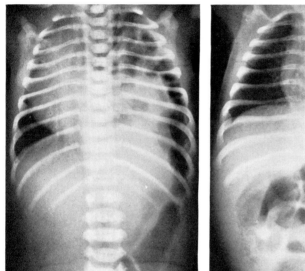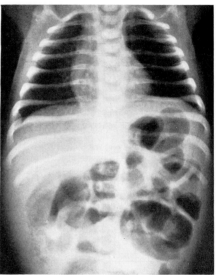

Fig. 201.—Roentgenograms of a baby with left diaphragmatic hernia (Case 8, Table 34). *Left,* Preoperative film. *Right,* Film four weeks after operation.

If the hernial ring is small, it will be found easier to withdraw the abdominal viscera if a definite procedure is followed. For example, in a *left-sided* hernia, the stomach is first brought down, then the small intestine, then the cecum, ascending and transverse colon, and finally the splenic flexure and spleen. In dealing with a *right-sided* hernia when the liver is partly or wholly in the pleural cavity, attempts should not be made to withdraw this most anterior and presenting organ first, for it will be found

in front of the intestines. *3,* Starting reduction by withdrawing loops of small intestines. *4,* Small intestines delivered, colon being pulled out. *5,* Finger passed up into the pleural cavity to engage and withdraw the thoracic portion of the liver. *6,* Liver entirely withdrawn and hernial opening completely exposed. *K,* Kidney. Withdrawal of the liver should be left until the last part of the reduction. Diaphragmatic defect is repaired as illustrated in Fig. 198.

22

that there is insufficient room to pull the liver down without damaging it. In these cases it is essential to withdraw the intestines first, then the colon, and finally the liver.

Suture of Hernial Opening.—The next step in the operation consists of denuding the edge of the hernial ring of serous membrane, and approximat-

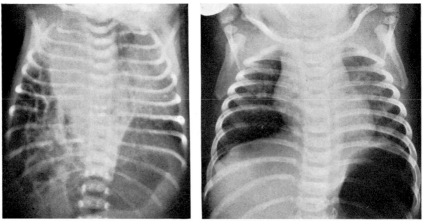

Fig. 202.—Roentgenograms of eleven-day-old infant with right-sided hernia (Case 6, Table 34). *Left,* Preoperative film. *Right,* Film taken three weeks after operation.

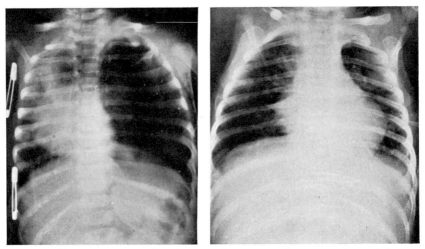

Fig. 203.—Roentgenograms showing rapid postoperative expansion of lung when patient is placed in a tent with 90 to 95 per cent oxygen. *Left,* Film taken at completion of operation for left diaphragmatic hernia. There is an extensive left pneumothorax. *Right,* Film taken five days later, showing complete expansion of lung.

ing the muscle edges with a row of mattress sutures of silk. A second row of interrupted sutures closes the peritoneal layer.

Replacement of Abdominal Viscera and Closure of Wound.—The abdominal viscera—which had been kept out on the abdominal wall during the herniorrhaphy—are now replaced into the peritoneal cavity and the abdominal wound is closed *in layers* if there is not too much tension. Oftentimes the abdomen is poorly developed because it has never contained all of its viscera and, hence, the operator has great difficulty in finding room for the intestines and others organs. This might seem to be an insuperable problem, but it can be met by undercutting the skin to allow it to slide and then closing only the subcutaneous fascia and skin (Fig. 205). This, of course, leaves an *incisional hernia,* but this can be repaired five or six days

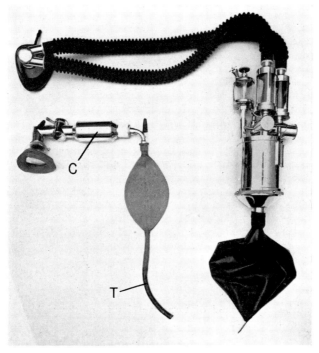

Fig. 204.—Above and to the right is a typical connecting system and canister which is used for adults. Below is a smaller system which has been found satisfactory for administration of cyclopropane to babies. The container (*C*) is filled with soda lime. The tube (*T*) brings oxygen and cyclopropane from the gas-mixing machine.

later when the abdominal wall has been sufficiently stretched and before the cutaneous stitches have cut through. This plan is superior to prolonged efforts at closing the abdominal wall in the usual layers if this latter must be done under great tension, because: (1) it is far less shocking; (2) it avoids placing undue strain on the diaphragmatic suture line; and (3) it avoids pressure embarrassment of the respiratory, alimentary, and circulatory systems.

Satisfactory closure of the abdominal wall is the most perplexing step in treatment of a congenital diaphragmatic hernia. In the first part of our operative series, the abdominal wound was always closed in layers in spite of the resulting high intraperitoneal tension. With this policy, deaths were frequent because upward pressure on the diaphragm led to respiratory distress or else compression of the inferior vena cava interfered with the proper circulation of blood. The conclusion is obvious, that it is wrong to approximate the peritoneum, rectus muscles, and rectus fasciae unless these layers can be brought together without tension. With these considerations in mind we now close the abdominal wall in the difficult cases *by only approximating the subcutaneous fascia and skin.* In five or six days this wound is reopened

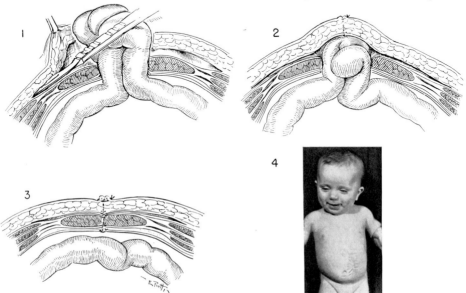

Fig. 205.—Satisfactory method of two-stage closure of the abdominal wound when there is such tension that the muscles and peritoneum cannot be approximated. *1,* Wide undermining of the skin flaps. *2,* Closure of the subcutaneous fascia and skin, with the muscles and peritoneum left separated. This produces a slightly bulging hernia which must be adequately supported with a sterile dressing and adhesive tape. *3,* At secondary operation five or six days later the abdominal wall has stretched so that all layers can now be closed. *4,* Postoperative photograph of a baby (Case 8) showing satisfactory condition of the abdominal wall after a two-stage repair.

and a careful suture of all layers is done. During this interval, the infant has largely recovered from the first operation, the abdominal wall has sufficiently stretched to allow adequate closure and the dangers of evisceration have not yet appeared. In every case, this delayed, two-stage closure of the abdomen has been satisfactory.

Treatment of Patients with True Hernial Sacs.—Patients with a true hernial sac can also be treated satisfactorily by a *transabdominal approach.* After the sac has been emptied of its contents a small incision is made in it to allow air to enter the pleural cavity. After this has been done the sac can be delivered into the abdomen and the margin of the diaphragm muscle defined. The sac is then completely excised, so that denuded muscle shows all the way around the edge of the hernial ring. The defect is now closed with two rows of silk sutures, as already described for cases having no sac. (See Fig. 198.)

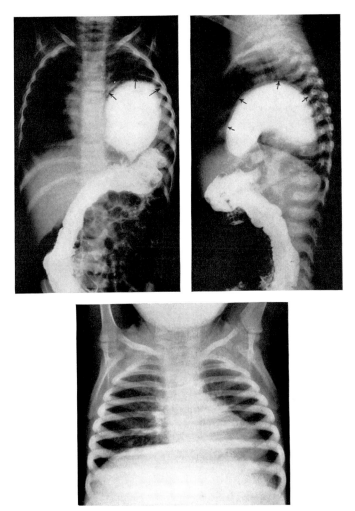

Fig. 206.—Roentgenograms from a two-year-old girl with left-sided hernia which had a sac (outlined by arrows). *Above,* Barium meal outlines the inverted stomach within the sac, and a barium enema shows relation of the colon to this. *Below,* Film after diaphragmatic herniorrhaphy

Treatment of Esophageal Hiatal Hernias.—Individuals with esophageal hiatal hernias (Fig. 207) should be operated upon only if there are important symptoms, such as recurrent lower thoracic or epigastric pain, gastric or intestinal obstruction at the hernial ring, or sufficient constriction of the stomach by the hernial ring to cause mucosal ulceration and severe bleeding. It is frequently difficult or even impossible to repair esophageal hiatal hernias if the esophagus is congenitally short and will not permit replacement of the entire stomach into the abdomen. If there is a short esophagus and a part of the stomach lies above the level of the diaphragm, a row of sutures can be placed to anchor the hernial ring to the adjacent gastric serosa. These will prevent other abdominal viscera from prolapsing upward into the hernial sac. Hiatal hernias may be approached through an *abdominal* or a *thoracic transpleural incision.* The latter gives an admirable exposure and is preferable if much dissection and freeing of the esophagus is anticipated.

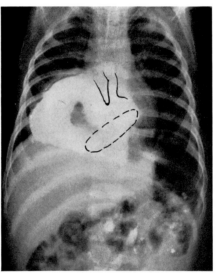

Fig. 207.—Roentgenogram from a nine-month-old boy with hernia at the esophageal hiatus. Lower portion of the short esophagus and adjacent fundus are indicated with ink lines. Circle indicates position of the diaphragmatic opening. Patient subsequently operated upon with a transthoracic approach; the major portion of the stomach was replaced in the abdomen and the hernial sac was plicated.

Postoperative Care.—The postoperative care of these patients is important. A *blood transfusion* should be given at the end of the operation. This should be large enough to replace any blood which has been lost, and to control any bleeding tendency which might exist. It should be small enough to avoid any risk of embarrassing the right side of the heart, which is a very real danger in these individuals. For four or five days the infant is placed in an *oxygen tent* with 90 to 95 per cent oxygen, for three reasons: (1) to make breathing less labored; (2) to keep the intestine deflated; (3) to remove quickly any room air which might have been trapped in the pleural cavity. *Feedings* are regulated so that a proper water balance is maintained, but little attempt should be made to fulfill the caloric requirements for the first few days. If sufficient fluids cannot be given by mouth, they are supplemented by parenteral routes.

RESULTS OF TREATMENT

In 1936 Orr and Neff[16] collected seventeen cases of diaphragmatic hernia from the literature, including one of their own which had been operated on in the first year of life, with nine successful results. A partial review of the literature now reveals fourteen additional operative cases with eight satisfactory results.[2, 12, 13, 17, 19]

TABLE 34

DATA FROM CHILDREN'S HOSPITAL CASES OF SUCCESSFULLY TREATED DIAPHRAGMATIC HERNIA

No.	Age and Sex	Major Symptoms	Site of Hernia	Operations*	Result	Anesthesia
1	4 weeks, F.	Vomiting, cyanosis	Esophageal hiatus	Diaphragm repair	Slight recurrence. Symptomatic cure.	Ether
2	2 years, F.	Vomiting, cyanosis	Left posterolateral†	Phrenic crush; diaphragm repair	Cured	Ether
3	3 weeks, M.	Cyanosis	Left posterolateral	Diaphragm repair	Cured	Ether
4	9 months, M.	Vomiting	Esophageal hiatus	Diaphragm repair	Symptomatic cure	Cyclopropane
5	6 weeks, F.	Cyanosis	Left posterolateral	Phrenic crush; diaphragm repair	Cured	Ether
6	11 days, M.	Cyanosis requiring constant oxygen	Right posterolateral	Phrenic crush; diaphragm repair; 4 months later abdominal wall repair	Cured	1st: Cyclopropane 2nd: Cyclopropane
7	18 months, M.	Vomiting, dyspnea	Right posterolateral	Phrenic crush; diaphragm repair	Cured	Cyclopropane
8	40 hours, M.	Cyanosis requiring oxygen	Left posterolateral	Phrenic crush; diaphragm repair; 8 days later abdominal wall repair	Cured	1st: Cyclopropane 2nd: Ether
9	48 hours, M.	Cyanosis requiring oxygen	Left posterolateral	Phrenic crush; diaphragm repair; 4 days later abdominal wall repair	Cured	1st: Cyclopropane 2nd: Ether
10	3 months, F.	Recurrent vomiting, dyspnea	Left posterolateral	Phrenic crush; diaphragm repair	Cured	Cyclopropane
11	10 years, F.		Left anterolateral	Phrenic crush; diaphragm repair	Cured	Cyclopropane
12	2 years, M.	Recurrent vomiting	Left posterolateral	Phrenic crush; diaphragm repair	Cured	Cyclopropane

* A transthoracic approach was employed in Case 4. An abdominal approach was used in all the other cases.
† This child also had absence of the pericardium.

At the Children's Hospital there have been twenty-eight patients with diaphragmatic hernia in infancy or early childhood, nineteen of whom have been operated on and nine of whom had no operation. Of the nine subjects without operation, five have died, three cannot be traced, and one is alive. This last child has a hernia at the esophageal hiatus, she apparently has a short esophagus, and a portion of her stomach is above the level of the diaphragm. Her only symptoms are recurring bleeding from the gastro-intestinal tract (positive benzidine tests on the stools) and a consequent anemia which requires continued administration of iron to maintain the red blood count at a normal level. Of the nineteen patients who have been operated on, twelve have recovered. Improvement in handling of these cases is shown by the fact that there have been eleven recoveries in the last thirteen patients operated upon—a survival of 85 per cent.

It should be again strongly emphasized that in the last ten years a change from a 75 per cent mortality in infants with congenital hernias, as estimated by Hedblom,[4] to an 85 per cent recovery has taken place. The main factors bringing about this change are: resorting to operation in the first few days of life, the two-stage closure of the abdominal wall, improved surgical technic, and better preoperative and postoperative care.

BIBLIOGRAPHY

1. Barrett, N. R., and Wheaton, C. E. W.: Pathology, Diagnosis and Treatment of Congenital Diaphragmatic Hernia in Infants. Brit. J. Surg., *21:* 420, 1934.
2. Donovan, E. J.: Congenital Diaphragmatic Hernia. Ann. Surg., *108:* 374, 1938.
3. Dunhill, T.: Diaphragmatic Hernia. Brit. J. Surg., 22: 475, 1935.
4. Hedblom, C. A.: Diaphragmatic Hernia. J. A. M. A., *85:* 947, 1925.
5. Johnson, H. and Bower, A. G.: Strangulated Diaphragmatic Hernia in an Infant. California and West. Med., *36:* 48, 1932.
6. Keith, A.: Remarks on Diaphragmatic Herniae. Brit. M. J., *2:* 1297, 1910.
7. Kerr, H. D., and Steinberg, S. S.: Right Sided Diaphragmatic Hernia, with Report of Three Cases. Am. J. Roentgenol., *34:* 735, 1935.
8. Ladd, W. E.: Congenital Absence of the Pericardium. New England J. Med., *214:* 183, 1936.
9. Ladd, W. E., and Gross, R. E.: Congenital Diaphragmatic Hernia. New England J. Med., *223:* 917, 1940.
10. Lauenstein, H.: Zur Symptomatologie und Diagnostik der Zwerchfellhernien im Säuglings- und Kindesalter. Ztschr. f. Kinderh., *54:* 117, 1932.
11. Lepoutre, L. de: Sur un cas de hernie diaphragmatique congenital chez un enfant de trois mois. Bull. et Mem. Soc. der Chir. de Paris, *48:* 170, 1922.
12. Meyer, K. A., Hoffman, S. J., and Amtman, J. K.: Diaphragmatic Hernia in the Newborn. Review of the Literature and Report of a Case. Am. J. Dis. Child., *56:* 600, 1938.
13. Miller, E. M., Parmelee, A. H., and Sanford, H. N.: Diaphragmatic Hernia in Infants: Report of Two Cases. Arch. Surg., *38:* 979, 1939.
14. Morton, J. J.: Herniation through the Diaphragm. Surg., Gynec. and Obst., *68:* 257, 1939.
15. Ochsner, A., deBakey, M., and Murray, S.: Absence of the Anterior Mediastinum with Report of Case Associated with Congenital Diaphragmatic Hernia. Surgery, *6:* 915, 1939.
16. Orr, T. G., and Neff, F. C.: Diaphragmatic Hernia in Infants under One Year of Age Treated by Operation. J. Thoracic Surg., *5:* 434, 1935–36.
17. Schönbauer, L., and Warkany, J.: Zur Frage der Behandlung Angeborener Diaphragmalhernien. Ztschr. f. Kinderh., *50:* 125, 1930.
18. Truesdale, P. E.: Diaphragmatic Hernia in Children with a Report of Thirteen Operative Cases. New England J. Med., *213:* 1159, 1935.
19. Weinberg, J.: Diaphragmatic Hernia in Infants; Surgical Treatment with Use of Renal Fascia. Surgery, *3:* 78, 1938.

CHAPTER XXVIII

INTRA-ABDOMINAL HERNIA

Sites.—Concealed, or intra-abdominal, hernia is one of the rarer causes of acute intestinal obstruction. The sites at which these are likely to occur are indicated in Fig. 208. Herniation through the *foramen of Winslow* or through preformed openings in the *broad ligament* and *omentum* deserves only passing mention. Congenital rents may appear in any part of the *mesentery,* particularly in that of the *terminal ileum,* and through such holes loops of small intestine can pass and become incarcerated. Indeed, this is the most common intra-abdominal hernia in the childhood period. A similar but much rarer opening is found in the *ascending mesocolon,* which leads in behind the cecum or ascending colon. Finally, there are *paraduodenal hernias,* the orifices of which are situated just below the ligament of Treitz.

Paraduodenal (Mesentericoparietal) Hernia.—*Pathology.*—A considerable literature has accumulated regarding paraduodenal or "mesentericoparietal" hernia—an escape of intestines through a small posterior wall opening, to gain access to the space behind the mesentery or behind the descending mesocolon. As the midgut rotates in fetal life, the mesentery becomes fused to the posterior abdominal structures from the ligament of Treitz downward and outward toward the right iliac fossa. This process of attachment may be complete except for a small zone just below the junction of duodenum and jejunum where the former emerges from its retroperitoneal position. The pocket thus formed may extend to the right behind the mesentery, behind the ascending colon, or up behind the transverse mesocolon. Conversely, the pocket may extend to the left behind the descending mesocolon and descending colon. When intestines enter these two spaces the resulting lesions are called, respectively, *right* and *left* mesentericoparietal (paraduodenal) hernia. Only a loop or two may be caught in these hernias or the major part of the small intestine may be confined within them.

Etiology.—It was formerly thought that these lesions were *acquired* and that the sacs were produced by intestines forcing their way into some small recess or indentation below the ligament of Treitz. Such a theory is scarcely plausible because there is insufficient differential pressure within the confines of the abdominal walls to allow such a dissection to take place. The more recent studies rather conclusively support the view that these pouches are always *congenital* in origin and that they result from an incomplete posterior fixation of the mesentery and mesocolon. This "congenital" theory is not vitiated by the fact that when intestines once enter such a sac they can accumulate increasing amounts of fluid and gas and can thereby distend a small preexisting sac into one of considerable proportions.

Anatomic Considerations.—Mesentericoparietal hernia on the left is about three times as common as that on the right. The left-sided hernia has

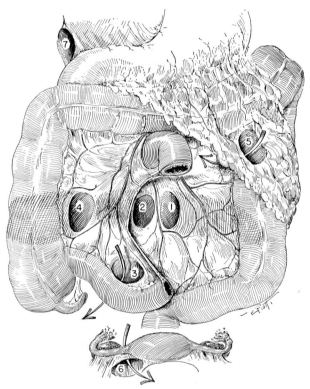

Fig. 208.—Sites of intra-abdominal hernias. 1, *Left mesentericoparietal (paraduodenal) hernia.* Opening below and to left of duodenojejunal junction leads behind descending mesocolon and descending colon. 2, *Right mesentericoparietal (paraduodenal) hernia.* Opening below and to right of duodenojejunal junction leads behind mesentery and possibly behind ascending colon. 3, *Defect in mesentery,* which is most common in mesentery of terminal ileum. 4, *Hernia into ascending mesocolon.* Intestines can get in behind the ascending colon. 5, *Defect in omentum.* 6, *Defect in broad ligament.* 7, *Herniation through the foramen of Winslow* into the lesser peritoneal cavity.

Nos. 5, 6, and 7 are surgical curiosities. Nos. 1, 2, 3, and 4 are uncommon, but yet important enough for the surgeon to be familiar with, because they may be unexpectedly met at the operating table. No. 3 is the most common type of internal hernia (except for diaphragmatic hernia) in childhood.

a mass lying largely to the left of the vertebral column and an orifice facing toward the right. Around the inferior and anterior border of this opening are the *inferior mesenteric artery and vein,* an anatomic fact which precludes slitting of the constricting ring in the surgical reduction of the hernia.

The right mesentericoparietal hernia has a mass lying largely to the right of the vertebral column and an orifice facing to the left. In or near the anterior border of the constricting ring are the *superior mesenteric artery and vein*, structures which must be carefully protected during reduction of the hernia. The locations of these arteries and veins are important for two

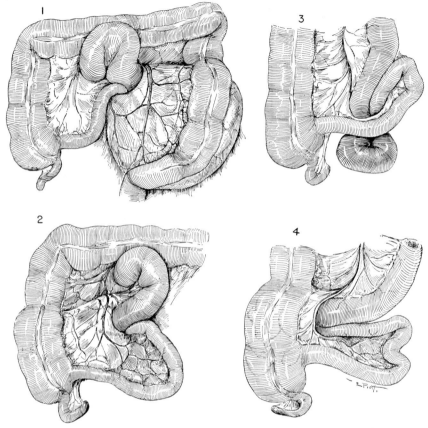

Fig. 209.—Forms of the more common intra-abdominal hernias. 1, *Left mesentericoparietal hernia*. The inferior mesenteric artery and the inferior mesenteric vein course along the neck of the sac; hence the neck cannot be cut when the hernia is being reduced. 2, *Right mesentericoparietal hernia*. The superior mesenteric artery and vein course near the orifice of the sac, so the neck cannot be slit to reduce the hernia. 3, *Mesenteric hernia* with intestine prolapsing through the defect. 4, *Hernia into ascending mesocolon* with intestines prolapsed in behind colon.

reasons: First, stretching of the hernial ring by entrapped viscera may compress the blood vessels and bring about extensive infarction of intestine or colon. Second, although it is permissible for the surgeon to open the presenting, less vascular dome of a hernial sac to release tension before pulling intestines out of the hernial orifice, in no case should he continue the incision close enough to the orifice to endanger these vessels.

Symptoms of Intra-abdominal Hernia.—The symptoms of all forms of intra-abdominal hernia are primarily those of intestinal obstruction. *Nausea* and *vomiting* combined with diminishing passage of flatus and stools are the rule; severe *abdominal pain* is observed in most cases. Pain may be intermittent and referred to the umbilicus, or it may be more continuous and maximal in other regions. If the intestine or colon has been infarcted below the obstructed segment, variable amounts of *blood* appear in the stool. In one of our patients this was the outstanding symptom. The history may include previous minor episodes of vomiting or pain, presumably related to temporary bouts of incarceration which were spontaneously relieved.

Physical Findings.—The physical findings are those of an acutely and seriously ill patient. *Vomiting, dehydration,* and abdominal *tenderness* are usually observed. A *localized mass* can often be felt, corresponding to the entrapped group of intestines, though dilatation of intestine above the point of obstruction may be sufficient to make abdominal palpation unsatisfactory. Increased peristalsis and borborygmi may be heard. The pulse is elevated. The white blood count is apt to be raised, particularly if infarction is present.

Roentgenologic examination of the abdomen in some cases gives valuable aid in suggesting the diagnosis. Dilated intestine appears above the obstructed point, or (in the mesentericoparietal type of hernia) a group of intestines may appear to be crowded into and encapsulated in one section of the abdomen, while the remainder of the abdomen is more or less empty.

Treatment.—It is almost impossible to establish the correct diagnosis in these patients before operation. Indeed, it is not necessary to do more than make a diagnosis of acute intestinal obstruction and to explore the abdomen on this basis. It is important, however, to be familiar with the types of hernia which have been discussed, because this knowledge will enable the operator to recognize more quickly the pathology at hand and to institute the proper therapeutic measures without delay. Reduction can be effected in most cases with little difficulty; but resection will be necessary when the delivered intestine is not viable.

Results of Treatment.—Our familiarity with these lesions in children is limited to seven cases which were of the following types: mesenteric defect hernia, three (with one death); ascending mesocolic hernia, one; right mesentericoparietal hernia, two; left mesentericoparietal hernia, one (died). Both of the fatalities were in children with extensive intestinal gangrene, who died in shock.

BIBLIOGRAPHY

1. Alexander, F. K.: Roentgen Diagnosis of Intraabdominal Hernia. Am. J. Roentgenol., *38:* 92, 1937.
2. Baty, J. A.: Internal Strangulation through Aperture in Mesentery. Brit. M. J., *1:* 671, 1938.

3. Callander, C. L., Rusk, G. Y., and Nemir, A.: Mechanism, Symptoms, and Treatment of Hernia into the Descending Mesocolon (Left Duodenal Hernia). Surg., Gynec. and Obst., *60:* 1052, 1935.

4. Chamberlain, J. W.: Acute Intestinal Obstruction Following Hernia into Ascending Mesocolon; Case Report. New England J. Med., *216:* 299, 1937.

5. Cutler, G. D.: Mesenteric Defects as a Cause of Intestinal Obstruction. Boston M. and S. J., *192:* 305, 1925.

6. Dowdle, E.: Right Paraduodenal Hernia. Surg., Gynec. and Obst., *54:* 246, 1932.

7. Halpert, B.: Right Retromesocolic Hernia. Surgery, *3:* 579, 1938.

8. Halpert, B.: Left Retromesocolic Hernia. Surgery, *5:* 379, 1939.

9. Hansmann, G. H. and Morton, S. A.: Intra-abdominal Hernia; Report of Case and Review of Literature. Arch. Surg., *39:* 973, 1939.

10. Longacre, J. J.: Mesentericoparietal Hernia. Surg., Gynec. and Obst., *59:* 165, 1934.

11. Martzloff, K. H.: Prolapse of the Intestine through a Preformed Opening in the Great Omentum. Surg., Gynec. and Obst., *50:* 899, 1930.

12. Masson, J. C., and Atkinson, W.: Hernias Into Broad Ligament and Remarks on Other Intraabdominal Hernias. Am. J. Obst. and Gynec., *28:* 731, 1934.

13. Mitchell, G. F.: Acute Intestinal Obstruction in Baby 15 Months Old; Hernia through Foramen of Winslow. Brit. J. Surg., *26:* 648, 1939.

14. Moynihan, B. G. A.: On Retroperitoneal Hernia. New York: William Wood & Co., 1906.

15. Paul, M., and Hill, W. C. O.: Right "Duodenal" Hernia. Brit. J. Surg., *25:* 496, 1938.

16. Short, A. R.: On Retroperitoneal Hernia; With a Report of the Literature. Brit. J. Surg., *12:* 456, 1925.

17. Snyder, J. W.: Paraduodenal Hernia. Surgery, *5:* 389, 1939.

18. Watson, J. R.: Acute Intestinal Obstruction Due to Mesenteric Defect. Ann. Surg., *106:* 1097, 1937.

CHAPTER XXIX

INGUINAL HERNIA

Inguinal hernia in the child is almost invariably of the indirect type and represents a persistence of the fetal condition in which the peritoneum has an outpocketing along the inguinal canal. In embryonic life the testis develops high on the posterior wall of the abdomen, whence it gradually descends to its final resting place in the scrotum. This migration is apparently initiated and facilitated in some poorly understood way by the *gubernaculum,* a mass of tissue containing smooth muscle which is attached to the lower pole of the testicle.

Before the testis enters the inguinal canal, the *processus vaginalis* projects down from the peritoneum through the various muscle and fascial planes but still retains a communication with the general peritoneal cavity. The fully descended testicle comes to rest alongside of this sac, the lowermost bit of which is pinched off to form the ensheathing tunica vaginalis. The upper part of the processus vaginalis normally atrophies, but if it does not do so the sac remains as a congenital indirect inguinal hernia. If the entire processus vaginalis remains patent, then the resulting hernia extends downward as far as the lower tip of the testicle.

The right testicle descends at a somewhat later date than does the left, and accordingly the right processus vaginalis is closed off at a later time than is the left one. This delayed series of events—when accentuated—probably accounts for the greater frequency of congenital indirect inguinal hernia on the right.

In the female, the processus vaginalis develops in a similar manner and can persist into postnatal life. The hernial sac is contiguous with the round ligament of the uterus.

SYMPTOMS

A hernia is frequently discovered at or shortly after birth, and indeed some of the largest scrotal variety are found during the neonatal period. The majority, however, are first noticed during the second or third month when the child becomes stronger and straining or crying forces intestines down into the persisting sac.

Size and Contents of Inguinal Hernias.—The bulge may be small and appear at the internal ring, or it may be elongated and extend through the entire canal. Less often, the mass fills the scrotum on the involved side. The size of the swelling depends upon the dimensions of the sac and the degree to which it is distended. In a neglected case, the hernia has a tendency to become progressively larger and permit more and more viscera to enter it. Most hernias contain only loops of small intestine. In babies the omentum is usually quite short and cannot reach this far, but in older children it occasionally projects out through the internal ring. A fallopian tube or ovary, and rarely the appendix, may prolapse into the sac.

Subjective Symptoms.—Varying degrees of *discomfort* are observed, according to the tenseness with which structures are crowded into the constricted space. Some children show little concern and have surprisingly little disturbance. Others are quite fretful, have a loss of appetite, and gain weight poorly. In the majority of cases the existence of the swelling is the only complaint. The hernial sac is usually large enough to permit easy ingress and egress of intestinal loops; the mass therefore appears frequently and is easily reduced by local pressure or by assuming a recumbent position. About 60 per cent of inguinal hernias are right-sided, 20 per cent bilateral, and 20 per cent left-sided. Ninety per cent of all hernias appear in males.

Incarcerated Hernia.—Incarceration occurs with considerable frequency in childhood. Thorndike and Ferguson[5] made a recent study of these cases at the Children's Hospital. In one decade 106 patients with incarcerated or strangulated hernias were treated, and during the same period 1740 individuals were operated upon for inguinal hernia, making an incidence of 6 per cent for this complication. In approximately 30 per cent of these children an inguinal hernia had not been recognized prior to the time of incarceration.

When incarceration occurs, the local swelling is quite painful, and the baby or child shows evidence of intense discomfort or agony. *Reflex vomiting* is common, and indeed all the major symptoms of obstruction may appear if intestine is caught for several hours. Incarceration is most frequent in the first six months of life (Fig. 212); it becomes less common after the second year and is relatively rare after the fifth or sixth year. About 80 per cent of incarcerated hernias are on the right, and 95 per cent are in males.

PHYSICAL FINDINGS

The examination for an inguinal hernia must be quite different from that which is routinely employed in the adult. It is useless to invert the scrotum with a finger in the hope of feeling the hernial sac or to poke a finger tip up through the external ring. Such manipulations are very disturbing to a child and important information is seldom gained in this way. If the confidence and cooperation of the child are not first obtained, the ensuing palpation on a squirming or kicking subject may be worthless.

Inspection.—Everything possible should be learned from inspection before the patient is touched. The appearance and regression of an inguinal swelling during coughing or straining may be all that is required to make the diagnosis. The child should be permitted to stand up, if he so desires, for the erect position may produce sufficient intra-abdominal pressure to bring on the inguinal bulge. When a hernial mass is found, gentle pressure should be exerted on it from below upward to see if it can be reduced. When the lump is reducible, other local lesions such as inguinal adenitis, suppurative iliac adenitis, and hydrocele of the cord are at once ruled out.

Light Touch Palpation.—Often there is a good history of recurrent swelling but an inguinal mass is not apparent during the examination. In such cases a great deal can be learned by laying a single finger (preferably the middle one) over the inguinal structures (Fig. 210) and then lightly

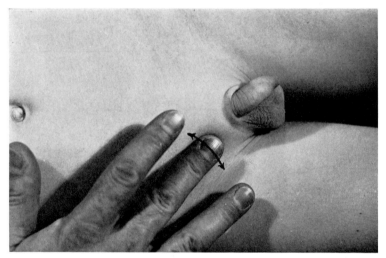

Fig. 210.—Method of examining a child with a suspected inguinal hernia. The middle finger rests lightly over the canal and is rubbed gently from side to side in the direction of and within the limits of the arrows. If the canal contains a hernial sac, an increased thickness can be felt.

rubbing from side to side. This will not disturb the child and yet a good estimate can be gained of the thickness of the tissue within the canal. When compared to the normal, the side with a hernia is found to be slightly thicker even though the hernial sac is empty. There is often imparted to the finger a sensation similar to that obtained by rustling together two surfaces of silk. With a little experience this simple examination will be found to be very valuable.

Incarcerated Hernia.—When a hernia is incarcerated, a flattened or elongated mass can be felt along the inguinal canal which usually does not extend beyond the external ring, though in some cases it may fill the scrotum on the same side. This is quite tender; the subcutaneous tissues are edematous; the child is very fretful. If the incarceration has been of some standing, vomiting, abdominal distention, borborygmi, and intestinal patterning may give evidence of intestinal obstruction.

TREATMENT

Spontaneous Cure.—Parents often inquire about the possibility of a spontaneous cure if no therapy is instituted. There can be little argument about the fact that obliteration of the processus vaginalis (which should have been completed in late fetal life) can continue into the first months of postnatal existence, but a natural closure is a rare exception and not the rule. This process of atrophy has been observed as late as five or six months. It can be encouraged by avoiding constipation, crying, coughing, or other conditions which raise the intra-abdominal pressure and thereby tend to dilate the sac. It can also be aided by applying some form of external support which will constantly give light pressure over the inguinal region. For this purpose a *yarn truss* serves admirably, and is the only satisfactory form of truss for infants. The essential aim of these measures is to keep the sac collapsed so that its walls can coalesce. If a hernia is found after six months of age, almost no hope for a natural cure should be entertained.

Injection Treatment.—During recent years the injection treatment of hernias has been enthusiastically supported in some clinics. To this form of therapy in childhood we are unalterably opposed. Without doubt, sclerosing fluid can cause a reaction which induces fibrosis and obliteration of the sac, but it is difficult to accomplish this without extensive and possibly permanent injury to the delicate spermatic vessels and vas deferens. There is no question that some hernias have been closed without deleterious effects on the surrounding structures, but it is impossible to repeat these results uniformly in a large number of cases. The percentage of cures certainly cannot compare with those obtained by the operative exposure and removal of the sac. Furthermore, the repeated regional injections of irritating substances are more upsetting to a child than is a properly executed herniorrhaphy.

Use of Trusses.—Treatment of an inguinal hernia in infancy and childhood therefore resolves itself into a choice between two methods: the conservative application of a truss or the more radical yet safe method of herniorrhaphy. Operation can be performed at any time, and, indeed, many of our patients have been so treated a few weeks after birth. However, there is some disadvantage in operating before a year and a half or two years of age, because prior to this time the cord and the hernial sac are so delicate that the dissection requires a considerable amount of skill, patience, and care. With proper surgical technic and with adequate facilities in a well organized children's hospital, where contamination of the wound by urine can be avoided, the results of an early operation are quite as good as those

23

at a later age. It is usually more satisfactory for both doctor and parent
to postpone the operation beyond the first year. For these reasons it has
been our practice to apply a yarn truss for hernias in babies, and to continue this until herniorrhaphy can be more easily done. In some infants
the hernia is so large that it is difficult to keep it reduced with a truss, and
it is wiser to operate early, regardless of age.

Concerning the use of trusses, it is our opinion that *rubber, spring,* or
leather appliances should be completely dispensed with. They are usually

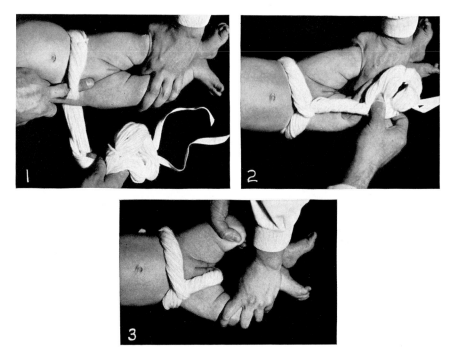

Fig. 211.—Method of applying a yarn truss for an inguinal hernia. *1,* The hernia
has been reduced and is held back with the finger, as shown. *2,* The wool has been
threaded through the first loop. This makes a lump which is brought to rest over the
internal ring. *3,* The yarn presses down over the inguinal canal and is passed up over
the buttock to be tied posteriorly. It must be tied in the *midline* posteriorly to prevent
slipping of the truss when the thigh is flexed.

irksome to a child and may do harm by placing too much pressure on the
spermatic cord.

The Yarn Truss.—A most satisfactory support can be quickly and
cheaply fashioned from ordinary soft, white knitting yarn. A loop is prepared so that it is about 24 inches long and contains about fifteen strands
of yarn. For older babies and young children the loop may be longer and
thicker; its dimensions depend, of course, on the size of the patient. To
apply this truss the child is placed in a recumbent position and the hernia

is reduced. A finger is passed through one end of the yarn loop and the tip of the finger is then placed over the internal inguinal ring (Fig. 211). The free loop of yarn is then passed medially and completely around the trunk so that it can be threaded through the end where the finger is. This will make a knot or lump directly over the internal ring. The free end of the yarn is now turned downward along the inguinal canal and then between the legs so that it can be tied up posteriorly to that portion which runs across the back. Such a truss can be easily and quickly applied. It gives firm but yielding pressure over the canal, and prevents intestines from entering the hernial sac. If the skin is powdered, there is practically no chafing. This form of truss is cheap; it can be washed; and when badly soiled it can be discarded.

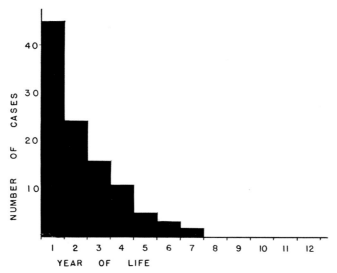

Fig. 212.—Age incidence of 106 children with incarcerated inguinal hernia.

Operative Treatment.—The operative treatment of inguinal hernia may be of two forms. English and Scottish surgeons commonly use the *Mitchell Bankes operation,* by which a ½- or ¾-inch incision is made over the upper end of the canal, the sac is pulled out and ligated at the internal ring, and no attempt is made to repair the canal. This simple operation is reported to be followed by a very low incidence of recurrences. Instead of resorting to this incomplete procedure we prefer a thorough removal of the sac and careful closure of the inguinal canal.

Modified Ferguson Operation.—The operation which is best suited to children is some modification of the Ferguson technic. The Bassini type of operation, with transposition of the cord, is not to be recommended because of the danger of compressing the delicate spermatic vessels and bringing about atrophy of the testicle. The type of operation (Fig. 215) which we have used for many years with satisfactory results begins with the usual incision over the inguinal canal down to the aponeurosis of the external

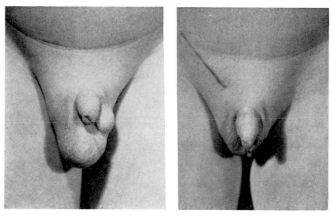

Fig. 213.—Photographs before and after right inguinal herniorrhaphy.

oblique muscle. The canal is then opened by splitting the aponeurosis fibers from the external to the internal ring. The sac is next freed from the cord and surrounding structures up to the internal ring. It is opened, transfixed,

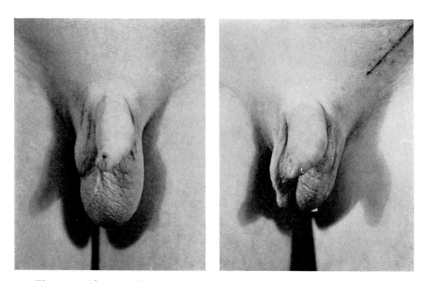

Fig. 214.—Photographs before and after left inguinal herniorrhaphy.

tied, and cut off. The stump is then anchored away from the internal ring by suturing it up inside of the abdominal wall. The spermatic cord is placed in its normal position. It should be emphasized that the vessels of the spermatic cord should not be injured, because this will often lead to atrophy of the testicle. While the veins may appear numerous and large they should not be considered as a varicocele and should never be excised.

With care not to include the ilio-inguinal nerve in the sutures, the canal is closed by bringing the external oblique fascia and the internal oblique muscle to Poupart's ligament with one row of stitches. The lower flap of the external oblique is then overlapped from below upward and sutured with a second row of stitches. The subcutaneous fascia and skin are likewise closed with interrupted stitches and a small collodion dressing is applied. The same operation is performed in the female, except that the external ring is tightly closed and the round ligament is anchored to Poupart's ligament to prevent displacement of the uterus. There is little question about the superior qualities of *fine silk,* as compared to catgut, for routine use in herniorrhaphies.

Treatment of Incarcerated Inguinal Hernia.—*Conservative Measures.*—An incarcerated hernia should always have a sufficient trial of conservative therapy before operative measures are resorted to. If light pressure will not reduce the mass, no forceful efforts should be made to accomplish this. The child should be given an adequate dose of *morphine* to abolish pain, to induce sleep, and to relax the abdominal wall. The patient should then be placed on his back in a bed the foot of which is elevated so that the mattress is inclined at an angle of about 20 degrees with the horizontal. An ice bag placed over the scrotum and inguinal region will help to reduce local edema. When this position has been maintained for an hour or two the intestines may spontaneously return to the abdomen, or they will do so when the fingers gently press upon the mass. With this management, 80 per cent of incarcerated inguinal hernias can be reduced without operation.

Conservative treatment should always be tried for three or four hours, but not longer than this because of the danger of strangulating the entrapped intestine. Surgical reduction of an incarcerated hernia is a difficult undertaking in babies or young children. Edema obscures the various landmarks and once the hernia has been reduced it is difficult to repair the inguinal canal satisfactorily. It is better, therefore, to reduce the hernia by conservative means, if this is at all possible, and then wait for two or three days until the edema and vascular engorgement subside before proceeding with the herniorrhaphy.

Operation.—If operation is necessary for an irreducible, incarcerated hernia, general anesthesia should always be employed and an adequate exposure provided for. The external oblique fascia and internal oblique muscle should be slit upward and outward from the internal ring, in order to approach the constricted gut from above downward. The intestine must

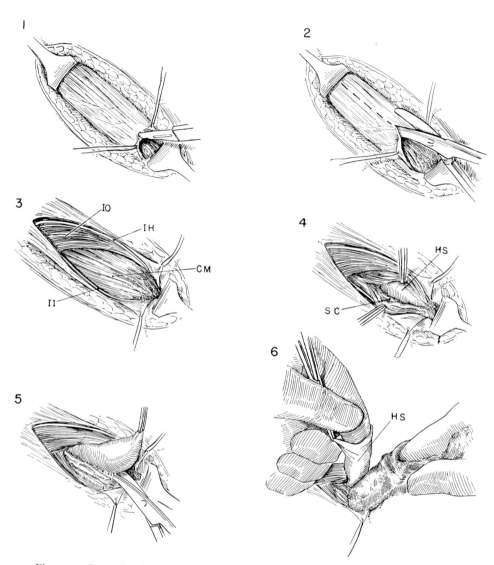

Fig. 215.—Steps for inguinal herniorrhaphy; modified Ferguson repair. *1*, External oblique fascia and external ring exposed. Cutting external ring. *2*, Slitting external oblique fascia along direction of its fibers. *3*, Internal oblique muscle (*IO*) bared. Ilio-hypogastric (*IH*) and ilio-inguinal (*II*) nerves identified. Cremaster muscle (*CM*) exposed. *4*, Blunt separation of cremaster fibers with smooth forceps to bare hernial sac (*HS*) and spermatic cord (*SC*). *5*, Tip of sac picked up. Sharp dissection of it from surrounding structures. *6*, Hernial sac (*HS*) opened and left forefinger inserted into it. A hemostat catches its end so that it will not slip off the finger. Gauze-covered right forefinger continues dissection bluntly.

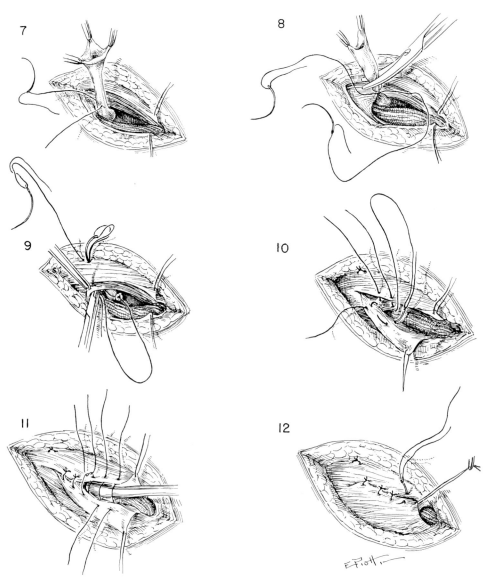

Fig. 215 (*Continued*).—*7*, Freed sac held up. Its neck is transfixed with a silk suture. *8*, Neck of sac tied. Cutting away excess sac. *9*, Ligature (of hernial sac) fitted with double needles, which are passed (backwards) out through internal oblique muscle and external oblique fascia. When tied externally they will draw the hernial neck up and away from the internal ring. *10*, Spermatic cord in normal bed. Silk sutures through edge of external oblique fascia and internal oblique muscle and finally through inguinal ligament. *11*, Blunt periosteal elevator holding cord out of way while sutures are tied. *12*, Imbricating lower flap of external oblique fascia upward with interrupted stitches. Reconstructed external ring shown.

not be allowed to slip back into the abdominal cavity until it can be thoroughly examined, because a necrotic loop may thus disappear and evade all efforts to locate it again through the small peritoneal opening. In occasional cases of incarceration the pressure against the adjacent spermatic vessels is sufficient to induce infarction of the testicle (Fig. 216) and orchidectomy may be required.

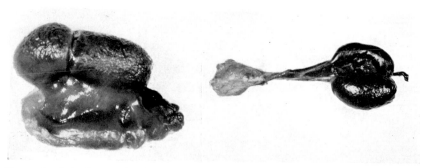

Fig. 216.—*Left*, Hemorrhagic ovary which had been caught in an incarcerated hernia of a nine-month-old baby. *Right*, Infarcted testicle, removed from one-month-old boy with incarcerated hernia.

Strangulation of intestine is relatively rare. In the 106 cases of incarcerated hernia studied by Thorndike and Ferguson, there was strangulation with gangrene in only four instances. When it is necessary to resect a portion of dying or perforated intestine, an adequate peritoneal opening is essential. This can be obtained by enlarging the internal ring laterally along the direction of the external oblique fibers.

POSTOPERATIVE CARE

A most important consideration in the postoperative care of these cases is that of keeping the wound dry and clean. This is best accomplished with a *Stiles dressing*, consisting of a cradle from which a diaper is hung down between the patient's thighs (Fig. 217). When the child voids, the urine will be directed against this diaper, which absorbs it (Fig. 218). Only a small covering is placed over the incision, and a collodion-sealed dry dressing is sufficient. The child should be restrained and kept on his back. Oddly enough, the most active boy submits to this restriction and sedatives are seldom required.

The healing process is rapid and it is not necessary to keep such patients in bed in the hospital for more than seven or eight days. During the second week they are allowed to go home where they must stay in bed, but may turn, sit up, or play as desired. After the second week, standing and walking are permitted and graded physical exercise is begun.

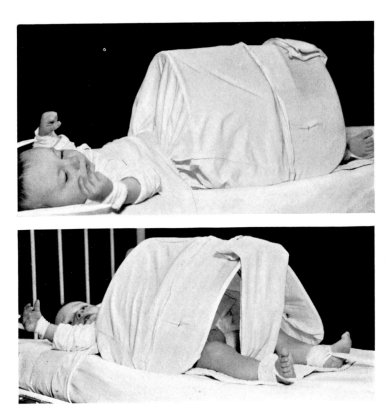

Fig. 217.—Stiles dressing for postoperative herniorrhaphy in an infant or child. The cradle keeps bed clothing off the body. A diaper is suspended from lower end of the cradle to catch any urine which is passed. The wound is thereby kept dry. The arms and legs are restrained.

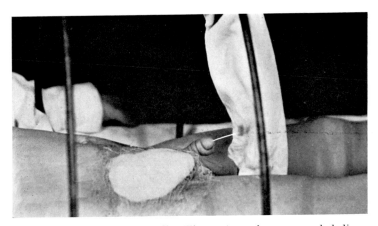

Fig. 218.—Side cover removed from cradle (Fig. 217) to show suspended diaper and how it catches voided urine. The wound area is never soiled.

RESULTS OF TREATMENT

During the twenty-five-year period of 1915 through 1939, 4133 inguinal herniorrhaphies were performed on the public and private ward services of the Children's Hospital. This figure does not include herniorrhaphies which were done during operations for undescended testes (which would add more than 400 other cases). There have not been long-time follow-up observations on all of these patients for an evaluation of the final results of operation. However, the majority of these children have been seen for at least a year, and most of them have returned to the hospital at later times for other medical or surgical treatment. While accurate statistics are not yet available, the impressions of the staff and the perusal of the hospital records give a fairly good idea of the condition of these subjects. There have come to our attention only ten instances of *recurrence*. Slightly greater in frequency than recurrence of the hernia is *postoperative atrophy of the testicle*. This complication is fortunately rare, but it again stresses the importance of carefully preserving the testicular blood supply and also reconstructing an inguinal canal so that it is large enough to accommodate the spermatic cord without undue constriction.

BIBLIOGRAPHY

1. Anson, B. J., and McVay, C. B.: Inguinal Hernia; Anatomy of Region. Surg., Gynec. and Obst., *66:* 186, 1938.
2. Herzfeld, G.: Hernia in Infancy. Am. J. Surg., *39:* 422, 1938.
3. MacLennan, A.: The Radical Cure of Inguinal Hernia in Children. Brit. J. Surg., *9:* 445, 1922.
4. Rea, C. E.: Sterility Following Injection Treatment of Hernia; Determination of Its Incidence. Ann. Surg., *105:* 351, 1937.
5. Thorndike, A., Jr., and Ferguson, C. F.: Incarcerated Inguinal Hernia in Infancy and Childhood. Am. J. Surg., *39:* 429, 1938.

CHAPTER XXX

HYDROCELE

In fetal life the peritoneum has a downward, fingerlike projection—the *processus vaginalis*—which reaches into the scrotum. The inferior tip of this sac precedes the descending testicle and then becomes pinched off and surrounds the testis to form the *tunica vaginalis*. Accumulation of fluid within this forms a hydrocele of the tunica. The upper part of the processus vaginalis lies alongside of the spermatic cord (or the round ligament in the female) and normally atrophies. If it persists, and still maintains a communication with the peritoneal cavity, the individual has an indirect inguinal hernia. If it persists and is closed off from the peritoneum, the individual has a hydrocele of the *spermatic cord* (or hydrocele of the *canal of Nuck* in the female).

SYMPTOMS AND DIAGNOSIS

Hydroceles are frequently encountered in infants and young children. They are rounded or oblong, cystic, and rather soft. In order of decreasing

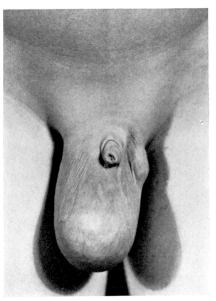 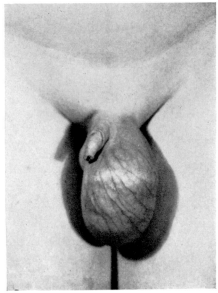

Fig. 219.—Right hydrocele in a nine-year-old boy.

Fig. 220.—Left hydrocele in a six-year-old boy.

frequency they are found around the testicle, along the spermatic cord, and in the canal of Nuck. Hydroceles usually give rise to few symptoms other than those of mild local *discomfort*. Even this may be very slight in proportion to the large dimensions which some of them attain. A hydrocele of the spermatic cord or of the canal of Nuck, constricted as each is by the inguinal canal, is seldom more than 1 cm. in diameter and possibly 2 cm. in length. In contrast, hydroceles of the tunica vaginalis may be much larger, and can greatly distend the scrotum on the affected side (Figs. 219 and 220).

A hydrocele of the canal of Nuck or of the spermatic cord may be confused with an *incarcerated inguinal hernia*. However, the persistence of the mass over a long period of time and the absence of local pain are more suggestive of a hydrocele. These lesions of the cord do not transmit light readily, since they are small and are covered by the external oblique fascia.

A hydrocele of the tunica vaginalis seldom causes any difficulty in diagnosis. The mass is soft, nontender, and envelops the testicle. The upper end of the sac can be palpated at or just below the external inguinal ring. The structure transmits light quite readily, and in some instances the shadow of the encased testicle can be faintly outlined by *transillumination*. A hydrocele of the tunica vaginalis is occasionally accompanied by an indirect hernia; hence the inspection and palpation should always be extended to include the inguinal canal.

TREATMENT

Spontaneous Cure.—A hydrocele of the *tunica vaginalis* seldom requires operation within the first year of life. Small accumulations of fluid will often disappear without treatment, and infants need not be operated upon unless the mass is large enough or tense enough to cause discomfort. Hydroceles of the tunica which persist after the first year of life or which appear after this age usually require treatment, since they have little tendency to regress spontaneously.

It is seldom necessary to treat a hydrocele of the *canal of Nuck* or of the *spermatic cord* in the first year of life. These lesions result from a pinching off of the upper end of a small, unsuspected hernia, and if left alone they usually obliterate spontaneously in several months' time. In contrast, hydroceles of the canal of Nuck or of the spermatic cord appearing after the first year usually persist, and will require operative removal.

Aspiration; Injection Treatment.—Aspiration of hydroceles in children should always be avoided. Recurrence almost invariably takes place and the dangers of sepsis are small but real. The injection of sclerosing fluids is valueless and even harmful. The local accumulation of fluid may be increased and the testis or spermatic cord is apt to be permanently injured. The reaction which follows such injections is certainly more troublesome and painful than that which follows surgical excision.

Operative Treatment.—In the operative removal of a hydrocele from the *canal of Nuck* or from the *spermatic cord*, an oblique incision in the direc-

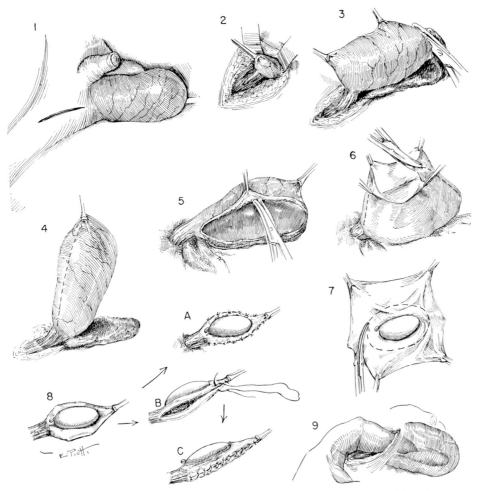

Fig. 221.—Operative treatment of a hydrocele of the tunica. *1*, Incision down to, but not into scrotum. *2*, Pulling hydrocele up into wound. *3*, Entire hydrocele delivered. Lower end being severed from inverted scrotum. *4*, Hydrocele freed from inferior and posterior attachments. Starting at dotted line, superficial coats will be peeled back. *5*, Peeling superficial layers back and exposing the thin serous membrane. *6*, Serous membrane being opened along the dotted line. *7*, Sac opened. Testicle exposed. Excess membrane will be trimmed away along the dotted line. *8*, Excess membrane discarded. *A*, Bleeding points ligated around cut serosal edge, which will not be sewed back behind epididymis. *B, C*, Alternate method of turning serosal edge backward behind epididymis. *9*, Pushing testicle down into its scrotal bed.

tion of the inguinal canal is made over the mass. The various superficial layers are teased apart, the hydrocele is freed, and the inner sac is severed from its attachments.

A hydrocele of the *tunica vaginalis* should be exposed through an incision over the external inguinal ring which does not run down onto the scrotum (Fig. 221). It is preferable to keep the wound above the wrinkled skin of the scrotum, which is difficult to sterilize and to approximate accurately. Any hydrocele can be grasped and drawn up through the high cutaneous opening—a process which is aided by inversion of the scrotum with a finger pressing upward through the draping sheet. It is not always necessary to dissect the hydrocele entirely away from the inverted scrotum, but if this is done the subsequent procedures are facilitated. The cremasteric fibers and fasciae are pushed posteriorly by sharp and blunt dissection, to lay bare the thin, innermost serous layer of the sac. This delicate membrane is now opened and the major portion of it is trimmed away.

Some operators prefer to leave two narrow edges and reflect these behind the epididymis—the so-called *bottle operation*. Reflection of the tunica vaginalis in this manner is not routinely necessary. It is simpler and also satisfactory to trim away the membrane close to the testicle, provided care is taken in ligating all of the small bleeding points. Any oozing should be fully stopped by applying warm, wet saline sponges before replacing the testicle in its scrotal bed. The subcutaneous fascia and skin can now be closed without drainage.

From 1915 through 1939, 507 patients with hydrocele have been operated upon at the Children's Hospital. There was no mortality from operation and in no case has there been a recurrence.

BIBLIOGRAPHY

1. Greene, L. B.: Hydrocele and Varicocele: Operative and Injection Treatment. Am. J. Surg., *36:* 204, 1937.
2. Langer, M.: Über die Hernie und Hydrokele des Kindesalter. Arch. f. klin. Chir., *181:* 418, 1934.
3. Rolnick, H. C.: Hydrocele, Spermatocele, Varicocele. S. Clin. North America, *15:* 757, 1935.
4. Young, H. H.: Radical Cure of Hydrocele by Excision of Serous Layer of Sac. Surg., Gynec. and Obst., *70:* 807, 1940.

CHAPTER XXXI

UNDESCENDED TESTICLE (CRYPTORCHIDISM)

The testicle develops in a rather high position in the posterior abdomen, from which it normally descends along the retroperitoneal tissues to pass along the inguinal canal into its final resting place within the scrotum. This process may be interrupted at any point, so that the testicle stops within the inguinal canal or even within the abdomen itself. Whether or not the testicle enters the inguinal canal, the fingerlike processus vaginalis extends from the peritoneum out through the structures of the inguinal canal. Therefore, the undescended testicle is almost always associated with an *indirect inguinal hernia*.

The truly undescended testis (in contrast to one which is held up by a strong cremasteric reflex) always has *adhesions* which anchor it to near-by structures. The origin of these adhesions is not clear, but doubtless they are an important factor in arresting the descent of the organ. Since the testicle has never resided in the scrotum, the dartos muscle and the scrotal skin on the involved side are small and shrunken.

Differential Diagnosis.—True cryptorchidism must be clearly distinguished from *ectopic testis* and from *retracted testis*. In the former condition the testicle and its spermatic cord have normally progressed along the inguinal canal, but after escaping from the external ring the testicle assumes an abnormal position. It may pass upward outside of the external oblique fascia and lie in the subcutaneous tissues of the lower abdominal wall, or it may go downward and end its migration in the upper thigh or even within the perineum. By the term "retracted testis," attention is directed to the strong cremasteric reflex, so frequently observed in infants and young children, which may hold the testicle in the upper part of the scrotum or indeed within the canal itself. This is not a true undescended testicle, because as the child matures the testicle enlarges, the cremaster muscle is less active, and the testicle normally drops into the scrotum.

Complications.—When the testicle does not normally complete its descent several complications may arise. First of all, and not the least important, is the *cosmetic* deformity. In some individuals this may be a source of considerable anxiety because of the feeling of physical or sexual inferiority. Second, a testicle which lies within the canal is somewhat exposed to the *dangers of trauma*, because the more or less rigid posterior wall of the canal does not afford the cushioning which is provided by the soft and elastic scrotum. Third, a testicle which resides within the canal, and particularly the one within the abdomen, has a *diminished spermatogenic activity* which may advance to complete deterioration of the germinal epithelium. These retrogressive changes are presumably related to the higher temperature of the abdominal cavity. Finally, an undescended testicle is said to be subject to *malignant degeneration* in a slightly higher percentage of cases than is a normally placed one.

CLINICAL FINDINGS

These patients are usually brought to the physician because a small scrotum has been noticed and the parent is concerned about the future development of the sexual apparatus. An undescended testicle is rarely the cause of discomfort.

Inspection.—Inspection shows that the entire scrotum, or one side of it, is smaller than normal and has an incompletely developed appearance. Before palpating the genitalia, careful inspection in a proper light may show a slight bulge along some part of the canal, indicating the position of the testicular mass.

Palpation.—By gentle palpation the testicle may be felt just outside the external ring or along the canal. If it cannot be felt at all, it is presumably atrophied, or else it resides within the abdomen. The finger tips should be placed at the upper lateral edge of the mass and attempts made to push it obliquely downward toward the scrotum. With this maneuver some idea may be gained about the mobility of the testicle. If it is fixed by adhesions it can be displaced but little. If it is merely held in a high position by an overactive cremasteric reflex it can be pushed downward along the canal and made to appear in the scrotum.

In some boys the cremasteric reflex is so active that the testicle is drawn up as high as the internal ring and cannot be palpated at all. It is common experience to find that a testicle entirely eludes detection on one or two examinations but that it can be readily palpated at a subsequent time— presumably when the cremasteric reflex is less active. Mere exposure of the child for examination is often sufficient to make the testicle retreat completely within the abdomen. The cold hands of an examiner have been responsible for many erroneous diagnoses of imperfectly descended testis.

Repeated examination may be necessary because it is not always easy to decide whether an individual has a retracted testis or an imperfectly descended one. Hence, there should be no rush about the institution of therapy because the testis may spontaneously descend into the scrotum if the individual is only kept under observation until the prepubertal years.

About 50 per cent of undescended testes are right-sided, 20 per cent are bilateral, and 30 per cent are left-sided. Most of these individuals have an *indirect inguinal hernia*. The lower tip of this sac usually reaches down into the scrotum. The hernial sac is often large, and the recurring swelling may be quite troublesome.

TREATMENT

Spontaneous Descent.—In all of these cases sufficient time should be allowed to make sure that the testicle will not ultimately assume its proper position without the clinician's aid. In most individuals the normal processes of descent are completed before birth, but they can be delayed and can continue during childhood years. Oftentimes an undescended testicle does not enter the scrotum until or just before puberty. Without question a large number of testicles have been operated upon which would have normally descended if left untouched for a few years. Likewise, many of the so-called cures under hormone therapy recorded in the literature in the last decade actually represent testicles that would have descended whether treated or not. One cannot deny that in a certain number of cases the testicle will enter the scrotum under hormone therapy, but this is undoubtedly the type of testicle which would descend anyway when the boy reached pubertal years and produced his own hormones in sufficient quantity.

Hormone Treatment.—In recent years the treatment of undescended testicles has raised the question of therapy by injection of various hormones. The physiologic mechanism, which is accelerated by gonadotropic hormones, is poorly understood. It is difficult to believe that the testicle plummets downward solely because it is larger and heavier. It is possible that the hormones have some effect on contracting smooth musculature within the gubernaculum, thus aiding in pulling the testicle downward. A third factor is possibly related to the increased size and length of vessels of the spermatic cord; when the structures of the cord are thus lengthened, the testicle can possibly descend more easily.

The literature is filled with reports of so-called triumphs for the treatment of undescended testicles by injection of *gonadotropic substances.* Anyone who carefully evaluates the results must entertain considerable skepticism. First of all, it is well known that many testicles will spontaneously descend in the prepubertal years. This process can be brought on at an earlier age by injection treatments; but there is no advantage in doing this. Furthermore, the surgeon who has had any breadth of experience with these patients knows that fibrous adhesions often hold the testicle or the cord to various parts of the inguinal canal and to the posterior abdominal wall. It is almost inconceivable that injected hormones could produce any downward movement of the testicle in this type of case.

The hormone treatment of undescended testicles has several *disadvantages:* (1) The injections, which must be repeated once or twice a week over a period of some months, are disturbing to the child and the accumu-

24

lative discomfort is far worse than that experienced for a few days after properly performed surgical orchidopexy. (2) The cost is considerable at the present market values of such materials. This expense usually approximates that of surgical therapy and in many cases exceeds it. The problem of expense is doubly important in those individuals who, after a long course of injections without results, must submit to a surgical procedure. (3) Hormone treatment accomplishes little or nothing of permanent value. It precipitates the descent of only those testicles which would spontaneously descend if left alone for a few more years. (4) Excessive stimulation of the testicle by gonadotropic hormones is not without danger, because a compensatory atrophy has at times followed the cessation of injections.

Several staff members of the Children's Hospital have accumulated a considerable amount of unpublished data from cases which have been treated with various preparations of hormones. An objective study of the results has led us to abandon the use of hormone treatment for undescended testicles. The only exception to this rule would be the boy who is fat and has generalized underdevelopment of the genitalia. Injections of gonadotropic substance for this *Fröhlich type* of individual have considerable value when combined with properly performed orchidopexy.

Orchidopexy.—Under no circumstances should any form of *truss* ever be worn, for while it will adequately support the hernia, the pressure will almost certainly damage the testicle. Most of these individuals can be tided over until the optimum age for operation at nine or ten years by the avoidance of increased intra-abdominal pressure such as is caused by constipation, chronic cough, or strenuous exercise. If a hernia is troublesome despite these precautions, early operation can be performed—while this is difficult and less sure of a perfect result, it is far preferable to the use of a temporary truss.

Optimal Age for Operation.—Consideration of operative treatment introduces the question of the proper age at which the operation should be undertaken. One of the prime reasons for placing the testicle in the scrotum where the temperature is lower is to maintain the spermatogenic function of the organ. It has been shown that the intra-abdominal testicle will continue to produce small numbers of spermatozoa for some years, but that, if both testicles are thus retarded, sterility will occur in 90 per cent of the individuals. Therefore, it is not necessary to treat these cases in early childhood, but the testicle should be given its optimum conditions for function prior to the onset of puberty. We have found that the optimal age for therapeutic placement of the testicle in the scrotum is *between the ninth and twelfth years.* If the associated hernia is troublesome and demands earlier treatment, herniorrhaphy may be required in the first few years of life, but the operator must be prepared to perform orchidopexy at the same time. If dissection is exacting and delicate, this combination has fairly good promise of success, but the results of the orchidopexy are not as favorable as those following operation at an older age.

The results of orchidopexy have made some individuals rather skeptical about this procedure, but there should be little foundation for this pessimistic view. Without question there are surgical failures, but with experience and attention to detail, the careful operator can reduce these unfortunate results to an acceptable minimum. Properly performed orchidopexy requires an adequate exposure, a complete separation of the testicle and cord from the surrounding structures, a severance of adhesions about the internal ring, and possibly extensive dissection of fibrous bands in the retroperitoneal spaces.

Exposure and Separation of Testicle and Cord from Surrounding Structures.—A long cutaneous incision is made over the inguinal canal (Fig. 222). The external oblique fascia is opened and under the edge of the internal oblique muscle the testis will usually be found lying alongside of a patent processus vaginalis. This entire mass is lifted up and the gubernaculum is completely separated from its inferior attachments. The hernial sac is opened and is carefully dissected away from the cord. This peritoneal sac often forms a thin invisible layer over one side of the testicle so that the inexperienced operator gets the erroneous impression that the testicle lies within the sac itself. It is often very difficult to find a plane of cleavage and the filmlike sac is easily torn. Just below the internal ring the peritoneal layer can be more easily separated from the cord, which lies posterolaterally. After the hernial sac is freed the peritoneal orifice is closed.

The testicle may be found folded upward on the cord and bound there by fibrous adhesions, the severance of which will allow it to turn downward into a lower position. The testicle and cord are now raised from their bed in the inguinal canal; all filmy and fibrous adhesions holding them to surrounding structures are divided by sharp dissection. The spermatic cord is thus lengthened as much as possible.

Severance of Adhesions about Internal Ring.—Attention is now turned to the internal inguinal ring. The peritoneum is held upward and medially by a narrow malleable retractor. By blunt dissection the peritoneum is pushed forward from the posterior pelvic wall. When this is accomplished the spermatic artery and vein can be seen coursing upward and disappearing in the depths of the wound. Likewise the vas deferens will be found running over the internal ring and disappearing downward toward the seminal vesicle. By very gentle traction on the spermatic vessels fine adhesions are discovered between them and the posterior abdominal musculature. As these strands are divided the testicle will be found to have a longer pedicle. This intra-abdominal dissection may have to be carried 4 or 5 inches or more above the internal ring, because it is this extensive freeing which gives sufficient length to the cord and allows the testicle to move into a scrotal position without tension. The vas deferens is rarely shorter than

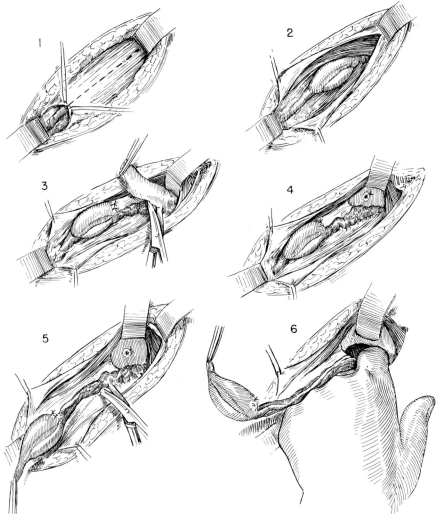

Fig. 222.—Operative treatment of a left undescended testis. *1*, External oblique fascia will be opened along the dotted line. *2*, Canal opened. Testicle lies just below internal ring. *3*, Internal oblique muscle retracted. Hernial sac has been bisected; its lower portion is left as a tunica vaginalis and the upper part is being dissected free. *4*, Hernial sac removed and peritoneal neck sutured. *5*, Testicle held up by gubernaculum. Spermatic cord being freed up and straightened. *6*, Cord entirely liberated and unkinked. Peritoneum held forward with retractor; finger dissecting along posterior abdominal wall behind the peritoneum.

normal, but when this is so, additional freedom can be obtained by cutting the transversalis fascia of the internal ring and allowing the vas to assume a more medial position.

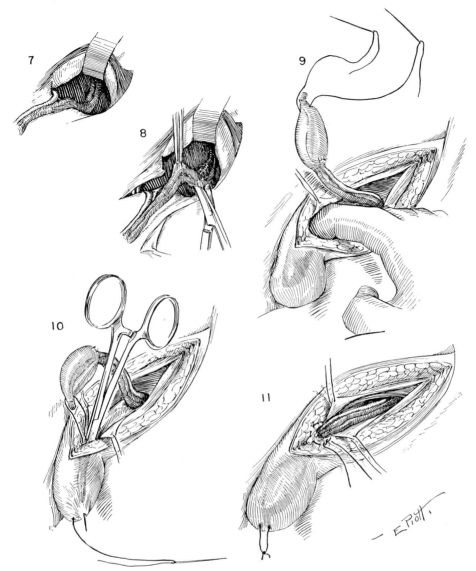

Fig. 222 (*Continued*).—*7*, Peritoneum stripped free and held forward. The spermatic vessels disappear up along the retroperitoneal tissues. *8*, Cutting adhesions and liberating spermatic vessels. The internal ring has been slit to allow the vas deferens to slip medially toward the inferior epigastric vessels. *9*, Double-headed silk or silkworm gut suture through lower tip of testicle. Scrotum being forcibly stretched with the finger. *10*, Sutures being passed outward through lower tip of scrotum. *11*, Traction suture loosely tied (see Fig. 223). Silk purse-string suture around cord—but not constricting it —to prevent upward movement of testicle. (The canal will be repaired by a modified Ferguson technic.)

Preparation of Scrotum for Receiving Testicle.—After sufficient mobility and lengthening of the cord have been obtained, the scrotum must be prepared for receiving the testicle. Inasmuch as this sac is always under-developed, it must be stretched; this is best done by passing two fingers down through the operative wound, and then forcibly distending the dartos and scrotal skin. If the dartos is unusually small it is well to pierce it at its lower extent and then pass the finger into the subcutaneous tissues of the scrotum to form an adequate bed there for the testicle. A single stitch of silkworm gut or silk is now taken through the lower pole of the testis to be subsequently used as a *traction suture*. If the stitch is passed through the gubernaculum this may subsequently stretch or give way; it is therefore better to take the suture through the lower 2 or 3 mm. of the testicle itself. Two straight needles are threaded on the ends of this suture and are passed downward through the prepared bed and out through the very bottom of the scrotal skin. Tension on these sutures will pull the testicle down into the scrotum.

Anchoring of Testicle and Closure of Wound.—As the testicle is pulled into its bed the cord must not be twisted. The inguinal canal is closed by

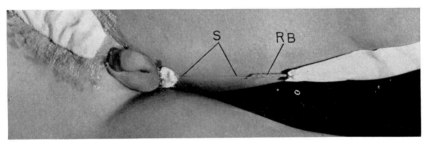

Fig. 223.—Postoperative traction apparatus. The suture (S) is attached to the lower pole of the testicle and is connected by the rubber band (RB) to the leg adhesive strap.

the type of repair described in the chapter on Inguinal Hernia. After the cutaneous wound has been approximated and dressed, the tension suture (piercing the scrotum) is lightly tied and is attached to a thin, slightly taut rubber band, the lower end of which is anchored to the lower thigh by adhesive tape (Fig. 223). This tension apparatus is left in place for about one week, and is then removed.

After operation an unattached testicle may retract by cremasteric action into a high position and become adherent there. Hence, a traction suture should always be used to hold the testicle in its scrotal position until it becomes adherent to the scrotum. This appliance is not used with the idea of stretching the cord, because pulling unduly on the cord may squeeze its blood vessels and induce testicular atrophy. *The success of an orchidopexy depends on adequate freeing of various structures so that the testicle can lie in the scrotum without tension on the cord.*

In occasional instances it is possible to perform *bilateral* orchidopexy, but either this is a very long procedure, or else the surgeon feels hurried while operating on the second side. It is probably better judgment to treat bilateral cases with two separate operations, which, however, may be completed during one hospitalization.

In no case have we employed the *Torek operation,* or any modification of it, which anchors the testicle through the scrotum to the inner aspect of the thigh. These procedures have been designed with the idea of stretching the structures of the cord for several months before cutting the testicle free from the thigh and allowing it to reside finally in the scrotum. We

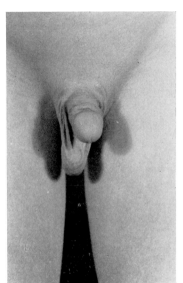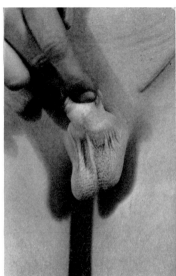

Fig. 224.—Left undescended testicle in an eight-year-old boy before operation and six months after orchidopexy. The testicle resides in a satisfactory position in the scrotum.

believe that such operations are entirely unnecessary and to use them is an admission that sufficient freedom of the cord structures has not been obtained.

RESULTS OF TREATMENT

During the twenty-five-year period, 1915 through 1939, 457 boys have been operated upon at the Children's Hospital for undescended testes. The results of operation have been judged primarily by postoperative observations on the size of the testicle, consistency of the testicle, and the final position of this organ.

Handicaps and Complications.—In any such series a certain number of disappointing results are bound to occur. In some cases the testicle is found to be *small and underdeveloped* at the time of operation and it always remains so thereafter. In other cases a testicle which appears normal at the time it is brought down into the scrotum subsequently *atrophies* because of interference with its blood supply. Ischemia can be produced by actual severance of the spermatic blood vessels or it can result when too

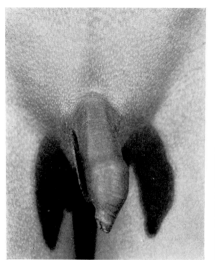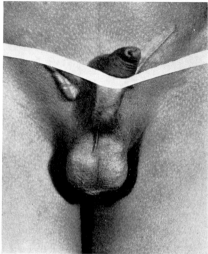

Fig. 225.—*Left,* Bilateral undescended testes in a twelve-year-old boy. *Right,* Photograph seven months after bilateral orchidopexy, showing normal position of the testicles.

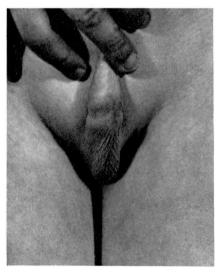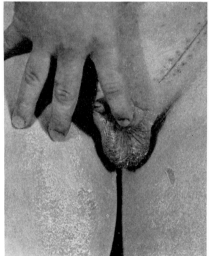

Fig. 226.—*Left,* Bilateral undescended testicles in a ten-year-old boy. The scrotum is underdeveloped. *Right,* Postoperative photograph. The testes lie within the scrotum.

great a tension is applied with the traction mechanism. In a few cases the structures of the cord are so short that the testicle cannot be brought into the scrotum by any means. In occasional patients the testicle does not become firmly anchored in the scrotum and will *retract* up to the external ring or even higher. These are the most common handicaps and complications, but in spite of them good results can be obtained in more than 80 per cent of the cases. By this is meant that the scrotum can be made to contain a testicle (or testicles) of normal size and consistency.

Functional Capacity of Testicle after Operation.—It is difficult and almost impossible to estimate what power the unilateral surgically treated testicle has for producing spermatozoa and testicular hormones, because the opposite normal organ simultaneously carries on these functions. However, in cases of bilateral cryptorchidism the postoperative functional results are more susceptible to analysis. MacCollum[7] studied twenty-two adults who had previously had bilateral orchidopexy and found definite fertility in fifteen and potential fertility in three others who had reduced counts but who had more than 25,000,000 actively motile spermatozoa per cc. of ejaculate. The percentage of probable fertility could then be computed as 82 per cent. This is in distinct contrast to the estimated 10 per cent fertility in persons with bilateral cryptorchidism who have not been treated. These studies conclusively showed that not only can good cosmetic results be obtained by operation, but that the functional results are likewise satisfactory.

BIBLIOGRAPHY

1. Bigler, J. A., Hardy, L. M., and Scott, H. V.: Cryptorchidism Treated with Gonadotropic Preparations; Surgical Repair of Cryptorchidism with and without Gonadotropic Therapy. Am. J. Dis. Child., *56:* 989, 1938.
2. Christofferson, W. G., and Owen, S. E.: Neoplasms in Cryptorchids. Am. J. Cancer, *26:* 259, 1936.
3. Eisenstaedt, J. S., Appel, M., and Fraenkel, M.: The Effect of Hormones on the Undescended Testis: An Experimental and Clinical Study. J. A. M. A., *115:* 200, 1940.
4. Gilbert, J. B., and Hamilton, J. B.: Studies in Malignant Testis Tumors. III.—Incidence and Nature of Tumors in Ectopic Testes. Surg., Gynec. and Obst., *71:* 731, 1940.
5. Hinman, F., and Benteen, F. H.: Relationship of Cryptorchidism to Tumor of Testis. J. Urol., *35:* 378, 1936.
6. Jones, A. E., and Lieberthal, F.: Perineal Testicle. J. Urol., *40:* 658, 1938.
7. MacCollum, D. W.: Clinical Study of the Spermatogenesis of Undescended Testicles. Arch. Surg., *31:* 290, 1935.
8. Mason, W. R., Jr., and Lehman, E. P.: Undescended Perineal Testis; Report of Case. Surgery, *5:* 932, 1939.
9. Rea, C. E.: Treatment of Undescended Testis; with Special Reference to Therapy with Hormones. Surgery, *4:* 552, 1938.
10. Rea, C. E.: Functional Capacity of Undescended Testis. Arch. Surg., *38:* 1054, 1939.
11. Smith, R. E.: Observations on Descent of Testicle with Special Reference to Spontaneous Descent at Puberty. Arch. Dis. Childhood, *14:* 1, 1939.
12. Thompson, W. O., and Heckel, N. J.: Undescended Testes; Present Status of Glandular Treatment. J. A. M. A., *112:* 397, 1939.
13. Wangensteen, O. H.: The Undescended Testis. Arch. Surg., *14:* 663, 1927.
14. Zelson, C., and Steinitz, E.: Treatment of Cryptorchidism with Male Sex Hormone. J. Pediat., *15:* 522, 1939.

CHAPTER XXXII

TORSION OF THE TESTIS AND THE APPENDIX TESTIS

TORSION OF THE TESTIS

Etiology.—Torsion of the testis is less frequent in childhood than in adult life. It may be produced by a sharp blow to the scrotum or by the individual's being jounced in a roughly riding vehicle. Torsion may spontaneously occur without history of trauma.

Symptoms.—There is sudden onset of excruciating local *pain* and *tenderness*. *Nausea* and *vomiting* are frequent. The testicle rapidly becomes swollen and *edema* may extend up along the cord. As infarction of the testicle proceeds, the local symptoms become more severe and low-grade *fever* appears.

Differential Diagnosis.—Diagnosis of the condition rarely offers any difficulty. The absence of urethral discharge and seminal vesicle tenderness, as well as the rarity of gonorrheal infection in young boys, should rule out *epididymitis* in most cases.

Treatment.—The treatment of testicular torsion consists of *immediate exploration* of the organ as soon as the diagnosis is made. The longer that operation is delayed the greater are the chances of irreparable infarction. Exploration should be done through a low, oblique incision, and the inguinal canal should be laid open if necessary. Inspection of the spermatic cord will quickly indicate in which direction the twist has taken place. The surrounding structures are edematous and the tissues distal to the twist are hemorrhagic or dusky in color. *Reduction* of the torsion may permit a return of circulation if the injury has been of short standing. Slitting open the tunica vaginalis and directly viewing the testicle allows a better estimate of its viability. When the state of the circulation is in doubt, five or ten minutes' observation, to find out how much the color will improve, is preferable to undertaking a too hasty *orchidectomy*. If the testicle is extensively damaged and its viability is lost, it must be removed. Seven cases have been treated at the Children's Hospital; the torsion could be reduced and the testicle saved in one, while excision was necessary in the other six. Three of these torsions occurred in undescended testes.

TORSION OF THE APPENDIX TESTIS

The appendix testis, or hydatid of Morgagni, is a small, pedunculated structure several millimeters in diameter arising from the superior portion of the testis and lying within the tunica vaginalis. It represents a remnant of the degenerated Müllerian system.

Symptoms.—The appendix testis occasionally becomes twisted upon its pedicle (Figs. 227 and 228) and the resulting infarction produces symptoms somewhat the same but not as severe as those of torsion of the testicle. While torsion of the appendix testis has been reported in infancy, it is chiefly a condition of boys and young adults. Eighty per cent of the patients are between five and fifteen years of age. The disorder is marked by sudden onset of sharp *pain*. At first this is of moderate severity, but later it tends to subside—a fact possibly related to the gradual killing of the nerve which passes through the twisted pedicle. *Local swelling* and *tenderness* follow within a few hours and are sharply confined to the affected side of the scrotum. *Redness* of the overlying skin may appear in thirty-six to forty-

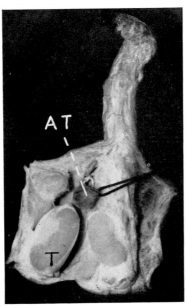

Fig. 227.—Torsion and infarction of an appendix testis. The darkly discolored appendix testis (*AT*) is seen in the upper pole of the normal testis (*T*).

eight hours. If the condition is not relieved by surgical means the swelling may persist for many days. Particularly striking is the *absence of systemic reaction;* nausea and vomiting are rarely observed. The temperature is normal, or only slightly elevated. In some instances the swollen and tender hydatid can be felt at the upper pole of the testicle, but in most cases there is early accumulation of fluid within the tunica vaginalis which prohibits accurate palpation of the structures within it.

Differential Diagnosis.—Torsion of the appendix testis may be confused with *torsion of the testicle* itself. The mildness or the absence of general reaction and the less striking local changes suggest that the process is limited to the appendix. In some instances the past history will indicate that there have been similar episodes of minor pain or swelling which probably represented slight twists of the appendix testis which were spontaneously reduced.

Treatment.—The treatment in all cases should be *operative removal* of the appendix testis. It is important to know that this condition can exist, for all too often orchidectomy is performed in the belief that the patient has had a torsion of the testicle. In the exploration of one of these cases edema and vascular engorgement along the cord without a frank twist of the cord should always arouse one's suspicions regarding torsion of the appendix testis. *When there is any question about the pathology concerned it is best to open the tunica vaginalis and inspect the hydatid.* If this is

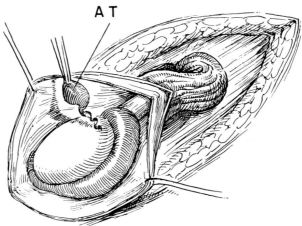

A T

Fig. 228.—Operating table sketch from an eight-year-old boy with torsion and infarction of the appendix testis (*AT*). This gangrenous structure was excised and the testicle was returned to its bed in the scrotum.

twisted and infarcted it can be rapidly excised and the testicle can be spared. In the first patient we encountered with this lesion (a sixteen-month-old boy), regional vascular engorgement was believed to indicate infarction of the testicle. Hence, this organ was removed. However, postoperative examination of the surgical specimen (Fig. 227) showed that the important pathology was confined to the twisted appendix. Accordingly, in five subsequent cases (ages twenty-eight months to twelve years) precaution was always taken to open the tunica at operation so that the gangrenous appendix testis could be removed and the testis saved.

BIBLIOGRAPHY

1. Foshee, C. H.: Torsion of the Appendix Testis; Report of Two Cases. J. A. M. A., *99:* 289, 1932.
2. McFadden, G. D. F.: Torsion of Appendix of Testis. Lancet, *1:* 320, 1939.
3. Randall, A. J.: Torsion of Appendix Testis (Hydatid of Morgagni). J. Urol., *41:* 715, 1939.
4. Rolnick, H. C.: Torsion of Hydatid of Morgagni. J. Urol., *42:* 458, 1939.

CHAPTER XXXIII

DISEASES OF THE FEMALE GENITAL TRACT

HYDROMETROCOLPOS

Etiology.—Enormous distention of part of the genital tract sometimes appears in female babies during the first month or two of life. This results from a complete obstruction of the vagina either at an *imperforate hymen* or just above it, where there is an *atresia*. Since obstruction alone does not produce symptoms in girls until puberty when bloody material accumulates and gives rise to a hematocolpos, one must find an additional factor for the development of hydrometrocolpos in the period shortly after birth. The explanation presumably lies in the fact that a sufficient amount of estrogenic substance is absorbed from the maternal circulation to stimulate the baby's cervical and endocervical glands into abnormal secretory activity before birth and for a few weeks thereafter. In short, it is believed that hydrometrocolpos depends upon: (1) *mechanical obstruction* of the vagina, and (2) an *unusual secretion* by glands of the uterine cervix.

Pathology.—In hydrometrocolpos the vagina (which is normally but 1 or 2 cm. in length and 5 or 6 mm. in width at this age) reaches the proportion of a golf ball or a tennis ball, or may even be larger. The accumulated fluid may so stretch the uterine body and the cervical canal that their contours are greatly distorted. The ballooned genital tract may assume a dumbbell shape and rise from the pelvic floor into the abdominal cavity with the constricted portion representing the junction of the uterus and the vagina. It may be impossible to recognize the true nature of the lesion until the more or less normal uterine tubes and ovaries are identified at the upper pole. When such a specimen is opened, the vagina is obstructed by a thin diaphragm across its lower third, or by an imperforate hymen. The lumen is filled with clear or brownish mucoid fluid. The cervix is widely patulous, and the uterine body is also greatly distended. Microscopic examination shows an overproduction of mucus by the cervical glands, which have been presumably stimulated by estrogens. Keratinization of the vaginal epithelium likewise gives evidence of an increased hormone activity.

Clinical Findings.—Clinically, this condition appears as a pelvic or lower abdominal swelling which may produce: (1) Anterior pressure and *urethral* obstruction; (2) posterior pressure and *rectal* obstruction; or (3) upward displacement of intestines and *respiratory* embarrassment. The *enlarged uterus* may be palpable, and indeed can reach up to or beyond the navel.

It is apt to be tensely filled and give the impression of a smoothly rounded, solid tumor. Not infrequently it is mistaken for a distended bladder, until drainage of the bladder with a urethral catheter fails to diminish the size of the abdominal swelling.

By *rectal examination* the pelvis is found to be filled by a mass projecting backward against the hollow of the sacrum. Gentle separation of the labia and inspection of the vaginal orifice or canal shows a bulging membrane either at the hymen itself or at a slightly higher level.

Treatment.—It is important to recognize this condition, because the unwary operator may open the abdomen, excise the presenting mass, and

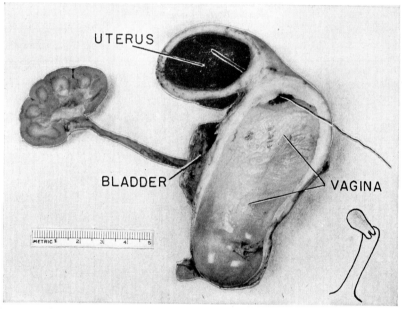

Fig. 229.—Photograph of hydrometrocolpos removed at autopsy in a week-old baby. The specimen had contained mucoid fluid. The vagina and uterus are greatly distended. (The outline at the right indicates the relative size of a uterus and vagina from a normal baby of this age.)

not realize until it collapses that he has removed the uterus and a large part of the vagina. In most instances treatment is possible by the simple measure of *nicking the membrane* which presents at or near the vaginal orifice. The operator should insert a small needle and aspirate some of the fluid to make certain of the diagnosis, before plunging a knife into the structure. If mucoid fluid (which may be slightly hemorrhagic) is obtained, the occluding diaphragm can be slit and the opening dilated with a hemostat. There will be an immediate discharge of the entrapped fluid and the pelvic or abdominal mass will disappear.

In one of their cases, Mahoney and Chamberlain[2] injected Diodrast through a needle which had been passed through the vaginal membrane. Subsequent films (Fig. 230) confirmed the impression of a dilated genital tract and this baby was successfully treated by mere incision of the membrane.

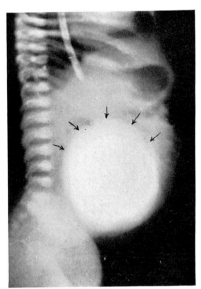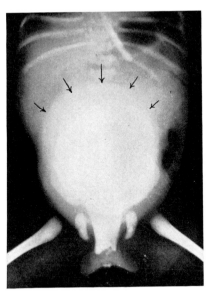

Fig. 230.—Roentgenograms of a hydrometrocolpos in a two-day-old baby made by injection of iodide into it through the vaginal membrane. (Case of P. J. Mahoney and J. W. Chamberlain.)

HEMATOCOLPOS

In girls with an *imperforate hymen* the uterine discharge of blood at puberty leads to a collection of hemorrhagic material within the vagina.

Clinical Findings.—These patients, eleven to thirteen years of age, have *abdominal* or *pelvic pain* which may be constant or crampy. Constitutional symptoms are absent or minimal; nausea and vomiting are rarely observed. *Tenderness* is found by rectal examination or by suprapubic midline pressure.

Diagnosis.—Intraperitoneal pathology, such as appendicitis, may be suspected and it is well to remember that lower abdominal pain in a female of this age can be caused by a distended vagina. This possibility is to be especially considered if the individual has not yet menstruated but has other signs of beginning sexual maturation, such as appearance of pubic hair and enlargement of the breasts. Satisfactory examination of the vaginal outlet should immediately establish the correct diagnosis. The occluding vaginal membrane will be bulging and will have a dark color because of the blood which is dammed up behind it.

Treatment.—A simple incision of the imperforate hymen permits escape of the entrapped fluid and brings immediate relief to the girl.

OVARIAN CYSTS

Cysts of the ovary are not uncommon in girls prior to puberty. They have been found at birth, shortly afterward, or at any period of childhood.

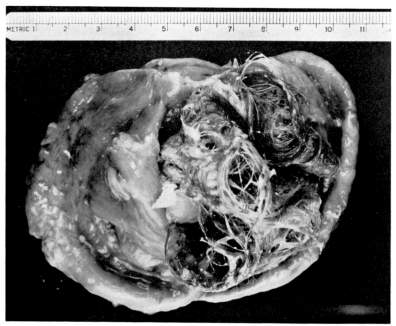

Fig. 231.—Dermoid of the ovary removed from eight-year-old girl.

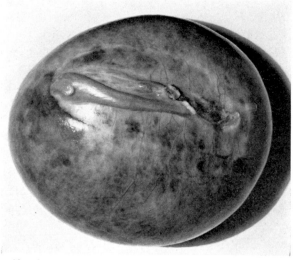

Fig. 232.—Simple cyst of the ovary removed from a six-month-old baby.

They attract attention by intermittent *lower abdominal discomfort,* by progressive *enlargement of the abdomen,* or by acute episodes of severe *abdom-*

inal pain resulting from torsion of the pedicle. Abdominal or rectal examination reveals a cystic mass, which is usually nontender but which may be quite tender if it is twisted and infarcted. In some cases the cyst rides up out of the pelvis and is thought to originate from some other organ, such as the mesentery or omentum. When dermoid cysts contain teeth, they can be detected by roentgenologic studies.

Simple cysts (Fig. 232) and *dermoids* (Fig. 231) occur with about equal frequency. The former are filled with a clear serous fluid and the latter contain hair, sebaceous material, teeth, or other structures which can develop from the ectoderm. Some data from seven cases of ovarian cyst in childhood surgically treated at the Children's Hospital are summarized in Table 35.

TABLE 35

OVARIAN CYSTS IN CHILDREN

Age	Type of Cyst	Size
6 months	Simple (with torsion)	16 by 13 by 11 cm. 1100 cc. of fluid
6 years	Dermoid	7 by 3 by 3 cm.
6 years	Multilocular (with torsion)	6.5 by 4 by 3 cm.
8 years	Dermoid	6.5 by 7 by 4 cm.
10 years	Dermoid	12 by 10 by 9 cm.
11 years	Dermoid (with torsion)	10 by 7.5 by 6.5 cm.
13 years	Simple	4 cm.

NEOPLASMS OF THE OVARY

Well over 100 examples of ovarian neoplasms in girls have been recorded in the literature. Of all the tumors and cysts of ovarian origin which have been described, approximately 60 per cent are malignant neoplasms, about 20 per cent are dermoids, and about 20 per cent are simple cysts.

Sarcoma.—Sarcoma of the ovary is one of the rarest of malignant tumors in this age group. It proliferates rapidly and tends to metastasize early. In fortunate cases the incidental discovery of the mass during an abdominal examination, or the torsion and infarction of the growth, has led to early excision and permanent cure.

Teratomas.—Teratomas are a little more common, and of course have a better prognosis regarding local extension, metastases, and recurrence. They may be largely composed of sebaceous material, but microscopic study of the solid portions shows other forms of tissue which indicate a derivation from ectoderm, mesoderm, and entoderm. Portions of teeth or bone can be frequently identified by roentgenologic examination of the abdomen. These lesions vary considerably in size; they may become extremely large and still

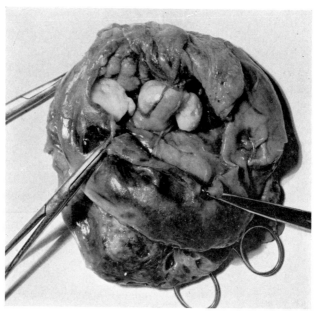

Fig. 233.—A granulosa cell carcinoma of the ovary from a thirteen-month-old child, showing cystic portions and the internal pedunculated solid tissue. This baby entered the hospital because of uterine bleeding.

TABLE 36

Ovarian Neoplasms in Children, Occurring in the Children's Hospital

Age	Type of Growth	Size	Postoperative Result
13 months	Granulosa cell carcinoma	15 by 11.5 by 12 cm.	No recurrence 4 years later
19 months	Fibrosarcoma	7 by 5 by 5 cm.	No recurrence 4 years later
5 years	Fibrosarcoma (with torsion)	11 by 6 by 4 cm.	No recurrence 10 years later
5 years	Adenocarcinoma	12 by 9 by 6 gm.	No recurrence 11 years later
6 years	Teratoma	5 by 4 by 4 cm.	No recurrence 14 years later
10 years	Embryoma	1500+ gm.	Recurrence and metastases in 3 months
11 years	Teratoma	2055 gm.	No recurrence in 7 years
11 years	Adenocarcinoma	700 gm.	Metastases. Death in 6 months

retain rather benign features. Surgical excision is almost always followed by an excellent chance of permanent cure.

Carcinoma.—Carcinoma of the ovary is a rare condition which has most of the characteristics found in this type of neoplasm in women. The lesion is usually unilateral. It is apt to be solid, though portions may be cystic or necrotic. While growth is rapid, encapsulation may exist for a considerable period of time, a fact which enhances the possibility of cure if early removal can be performed. These tumors may be an embryonal type of *epithelioma,* a more slowly growing *adenocarcinoma,* or even the more highly differentiated *granulosa cell* neoplasm (Fig. 233). With the latter lesion so much estrogenic substance may be produced that menstrual periods appear, breast tissue develops, and the bone growth exceeds the normal.

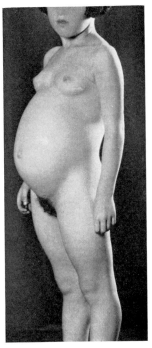

Fig. 234.—Photograph of a seven-year-old girl with a granulosa cell carcinoma of the ovary, showing pubic hair, enlargement of the breasts, and advanced physical development. (From Bland and Goldstein in Surgery, Gynecology and Obstetrics.)

Clinical Findings in Ovarian Tumor.—The clinical features of ovarian tumors are those of an enlarging lower abdominal or pelvic mass which may or may not be fixed. *Pain* is rare unless torsion has occurred or peritoneal implantations have taken place. *Sexual precocity* (Fig. 234) and *uterine bleeding* appear if the neoplasm produces sufficient amounts of estrin.

Treatment.—If physical examination and roentgenologic study do not demonstrate metastases, *exploration* should be performed, because the neoplasm may be a comparatively benign teratoma or else a more malignant growth with an unbroken capsule. In either case the chances of a complete cure are better than has been generally supposed.

When a malignant ovarian neoplasm has been found at operation and has been apparently completely removed, the question naturally arises of whether *x-ray irradiation* should be given postoperatively over the abdomen and pelvis as a precautionary measure. We customarily withhold postoperative irradiation because it will permanently sterilize and will prevent the full maturation of the individual. If malignant cells have been left in the operative field, x-rays will probably not destroy all of them; if neoplasm has not been left, x-ray treatment is superfluous and will bring on the detrimental effects of destruction of the remaining ovary.

VAGINITIS

Vaginitis is occasionally found in young girls and has been described in epidemic form in foundling homes where there are inferior toilet facilities and poor hygienic care. Gonococcal vaginitis and purulent discharge is uncommon but yet is a well recognized entity. Foreign bodies of various sorts may be introduced into the vagina by the child and their presence is often unsuspected until persistent discharge leads to an adequate vaginal examination.

Most cases of vaginitis in children will permanently subside with proper attention to local *cleanliness,* occasional vaginal *irrigations* with a catheter and syringe, and possibly instillation of mild *antiseptics* (which can be introduced on a throat swab). If local irritation has been produced by a foreign body, the removal of this object is the principal therapeutic measure which is necessary.

Treatment of Gonococcal Vaginitis.—Gonococcal vaginitis often responds to repeated douches and application of mild antiseptics, but a more rigorous treatment is sometimes required. Injection of *estrogenic substances* in sufficient amounts will change the vaginal epithelium to a squamous form which is more resistant to bacterial growth, but this treatment is expensive and deserves little more than theoretical consideration. Chemotherapy is cheaper and is easier to administer. *Sulfathiazole* has been described as giving very satisfactory results when the drug is employed for ten days to two weeks in moderate doses, according to the age and size of the individual.

BIBLIOGRAPHY

Hydrometrocolpos

1. Cranwell, D. J.: Congenital Hydrocolpos. Rev. de gynec. et de chir. abd., *9:* 635, 1905.
2. Mahoney, P. J., and Chamberlain, J. W.: Hydrometrocolpos in Infancy. Congenital Atresia of the Vagina with Abnormally Abundant Cervical Secretions. J. Pediat., *17:* 772, 1940.
3. Spencer, H. F.: Imperforate Hymen in a Baby. Lancet, *1:* 823, 1916.

Hematocolpos

4. Calvin, J. K., and Nichamin, S. J.: Hematocolpos Due to Imperforate Hymen. Am. J. Dis. Child., *51:* 832, 1936.

5. Tompkins, P.: Treatment of Imperforate Hymen with Hematocolpos; Review of 113 Cases in Literature with Report of 5 Additional Cases. J. A. M. A., *113:* 913, 1939.

Ovarian Cysts and Neoplasms

6. Bland, P. B., and Goldstein, L.: Granulosa Cell and Brenner Tumors of the Ovary. Surg., Gynec. and Obst., *61:* 250, 1935.

7. Gross, R. E.: Neoplasms Producing Endocrine Disturbances in Childhood. Am. J. Dis. Child., *59:* 579, 1940.

8. Mayo, C. W., and Butsch, W. L.: Ovarian Tumors among Young Girls. Minnesota Med., *21:* 256, 1938.

9. Mazzola, V. P., and Ryan, L. M.: Dermoid Cyst of Ovary in Child 5 Years Old, with Comments on Value of X-ray in Diagnosis. Am. J. Obst. and Gynec., *35:* 696, 1938.

10. Schaeffer, M. H., and Cancelmo, J. J.: Cavernous Hemangioma of Ovary in Girl 12 Years of Age. Am. J. Obst. and Gynec., *38:* 722, 1939.

11. Trout. H. F., and Marchetti, A. A.: A Consideration of So-Called "Granulosa" and "Theca" Cell Tumors of the Ovary. Surg., Gynec. and Obst., *70:* 632, 1940.

Vaginitis

12. Burpee, C. M., Robinow, M., and Leslie, J. T.: Gonorrhoeal Vaginitis in Girls Treated with Estrone (Theelin), Fever, and Sulfanilamide. Am. J. Dis. Child., *57:* 1, 1939.

13. Hoffman, S. J., Schneider, M., Blatt, M. L., and Herrold, R. D.: Sulfanilamide in Treatment of Gonorrheal Vulvovaginitis. J. A. M. A., *110:* 1541, 1938.

14. Jacoby, A., Madonia, D. E., Till, S. M., and Wood, T. H.: Treatment of Gonococcal Vaginitis by Estrogenic Hormone. Am. J. Obst. and Gynec., *38:* 140, 1939.

15. Schauffler, G. C., Kanzler, R., and Schauffler, C.: Management of 256 Cases of Infection of Immature Vagina; Practical Deductions, with Study of Use of Sulfanilamide in Treatment. J. A. M. A., *112:* 411, 1939.

CHAPTER XXXIV

EXSTROPHY OF THE BLADDER

Exstrophy of the bladder is one of the most distressing congenital malformations which the surgeon must treat. In this condition, the bladder, opening as it does on the anterior abdominal wall, allows a continual escape of urine which produces malodor and disagreeable wetting of the clothing. The everted and exposed mucous membrane is very sensitive and is easily irritated by any overlying pad or dressing. The deformity is always associated with a *wide separation of the pubic bones,* so that there is a *waddling and unstable gait.* These individuals rapidly become socially ostracized because of the uriniferous odor which always attends them; furthermore, they are quite apt to become introspective and retiring because of the physical deformity which bothers them.

The therapeutic problems are threefold: (1) to provide an adequate receptacle which can receive and discharge urine at suitable intervals; (2) to remove the discomfort caused by the exposed mucous membranes; (3) to stabilize the pelvis and thereby improve the manner of walking.

CLINICAL FINDINGS

Exstrophy of the bladder in males or females is a deformity in which the entire lower urinary tract from the apex of the bladder to the external

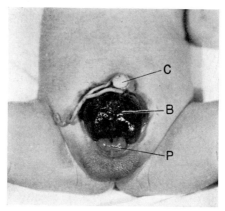

Fig. 235.—Exstrophy of bladder in a day-old boy. *C,* Cord stump. *B,* Bladder. *P,* Penis.

urethral meatus is opened (as if by an anterior midline cut) and lies exposed and everted on the abdominal wall. The trigone and its ureteral orifices can be viewed in the center of this mass. Below this is the verumontanum (in the male) and a complete *epispadias.* The exposed bladder mucosa is thrown into folds and has a bright *cherry-red color,* in contrast

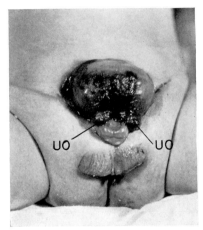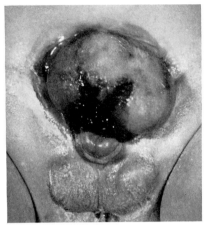

Fig. 236.—Exstrophy of bladder. *Left,* At seven months of age. *UO* indicates the ureteral orifices. *Right,* At four years of age. Note how squamous epithelium has now covered about three fourths of the bladder.

to the surrounding skin (Figs. 235, 236, and 238). The ureteral orifices intermittently dilate and discharge droplets of urine. The mucous membrane of the urethra is smooth, red, and moist. Touching any portion of

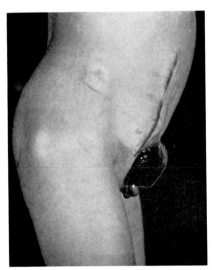

Fig. 237.—Lateral view of a four-year-old boy showing the bulging exstrophied bladder.

these various membranes will make the child wince and cry out with discomfort and pain. This *sensitivity* diminishes with advancing years because squamous epithelium replaces a portion but not all of the bladder mucosa

(Fig. 236). As much as a half or two thirds of the bladder may be thus spontaneously covered and rendered less irritable.

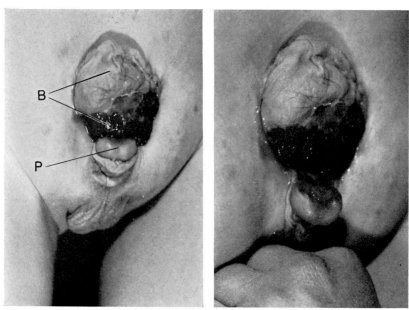

Fig. 238.—Exstrophied bladder in an eight-year-old boy. B, Bladder, the upper half of which is covered by squamous epithelium. P, Penis, which has a complete epispadias.

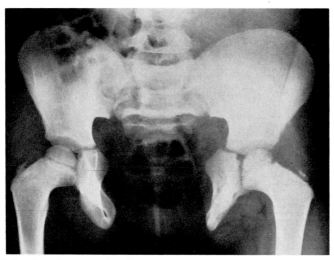

Fig. 239.—Pelvis of a six-year-old boy with exstrophy of the bladder, showing the wide separation of the pubic bones.

As stated previously, such a forward dislocation of the bladder and urethra is always accompanied by a complete separation of the pubic bones, which is associated with a wide *diastasis recti* below the umbilicus. By palpating either lower abdominal wall lateral to the bulging bladder the rounded ends of the pubic bones can be felt. The two sides may be separated from each other by as much as 2 or 3 inches. Many of these individuals have bilateral indirect *inguinal hernias,* and *undescended testicles* are not infrequently found in the males.

The external opening of the ureters would naturally lead one to believe that ascending staphylococcal or streptococcal infections would be common, yet it is quite unusual to find an important ureteritis or pyelitis. Numerous observations on untreated children have shown little or no microscopic changes in the urine and no dilatation of the pelves or ureters by retrograde or intravenous pyelograms.

TREATMENT

Historical.—The earliest efforts to treat this malformation were directed toward anatomic restoration of the bladder and urethra. The bladder was turned in, closed, and was given an intra-abdominal position, but these operations were never successful, because it was impossible to reconstruct a suitable vesical outlet and sphincter muscle.

Subsequent surgical attempts were confined to excision of the bladder and transplantation of the ureters into the loin, groin, or onto the penis itself. With the ureters in such positions, various types of rubber apparatus could be strapped to the body or thigh to collect the urinary discharges. Such attachments were very cumbersome and this form of treatment has fallen into disuse.

Ureterocolonic Anastomoses.—For a long time the rectum has been employed as a urinary reservoir, but the methods for anastomosing the ureters to this structure have passed through many modifications. In 1894 *Maydl* accomplished this task by excising and discarding most of the bladder, and then implanting the trigone (with the ureters attached) into the colon. In this way he hoped to save the valvelike action of the ureterovesical junctions. Unfortunately, the implanted trigone frequently sloughed because its blood supply had been impaired. In 1901 *Peters* improved upon this technic by implanting the ureters separately and carrying along only a narrow rim of trigonal tissue with each ureter. This procedure was followed by quite a few successes and some individuals are still alive and in good health twenty to thirty years after the operations. The first child treated by this means at the Children's Hospital (by Ladd), in 1918, was in excellent health during the sixteen years that he could be followed until 1934. Since that time the patient has been lost track of.

In 1909 Coffey[1] suggested that a valvelike structure could be obtained if ureters were run along for a sufficient distance between the coats of the colonic wall. The first operations employing this principle were done in the next few years at the Mayo Clinic. During the following two decades Coffey made numerous studies of the methods for best performing a ureterocolonic anastomosis. The *Coffey No. 1 technic* was quite elaborate; it involved an extensive preparation of the bowel, then implantation of the ureters into the sigmoid, and use of inlying ureteral catheters which were led down through the rectum and anus for external drainage during the week or ten days following operation. In this way a continuous flow of urine could be maintained, because the postoperative edema and swelling at the anastomotic site could not close off the ureters.

The *Coffey technic No. 2* was similar, but in addition a sleeve of rubber tubing was placed over that segment of the catheter which passed through the implanted part of the ureter. This was done to insure making a sufficiently large tunnel through the bowel wall, and thus avoid a constriction of the ureter after the catheters were removed. In the *Coffey No. 3 technic* no ureteral catheters were used. Only one ureter was transplanted at a time and the lower end of it was temporarily closed by a constricting suture which sloughed through in a few days and established a communication between the ureteral and colonic lumina. In all three of his modifications Coffey used the oblique submuscular position of the ureter to obtain a valvelike action, and this is his important contribution to this field of surgery.

Since Coffey's publications there have been numerous reports on experimental studies of modifications for ureteral transplantations. In many of these the ureter has been purposely obstructed by a catgut suture, silk suture, a dress snap, or other contrivance which spontaneously sloughs through in a few days' time. This is done in the hope of avoiding early bacterial contamination along the ureteral lumen or the periureteral lymphatics. We are absolutely opposed to all these *occlusive types* of anastomosis because they are unnecessary, they are unduly complicated, and there are adequate clinical observations to show that the simpler anastomotic methods are more certainly productive of uniform and satisfactory results.

Bilateral Ureterosigmoidostomy (Children's Hospital Technic).—During the decade prior to 1930 the operative results in the Children's Hospital cases were not good. Most of the patients had been treated by the elaborate Coffey No. 1 technic, and in some an extraperitoneal approach had been used. The operative mortality from peritonitis was high. Postoperative kidney function was often impaired by a considerable degree of urinary tract infection. The methods employed were poorly suited to children, because they were too time-consuming and complicated. The inlying catheter often set up a severe traumatic ureteritis which paved the way for a superimposed and chronic secondary infection. Because of these unsatisfactory results, animal experimentation was performed by Lanman and Colby,[9] and it is largely from this work that the Children's Hospital methods of ureterosigmoidostomy (since 1930) have been evolved.

Principles of the Operation.—The principles which are regarded as of fundamental importance are: (1) simplification of technic; (2) a transabdominal exposure; (3) establishment of a long, intramural, submuscular implantation of the ureter; (4) careful walling off of the operating field and avoidance of contamination so that the dangers of peritonitis are minimal; (5) omission of inlying ureteral catheters (after operation) so that the dangers of ureteritis are lessened; (6) noninterruption of the urinary flow during operation or in the early postoperative period; (7) transplantation of the ureters in separate stages.

The steps in the operative procedure (Fig. 240) may be described as follows.

Stage 1. Transplantation of the Right Ureter.—The child should have a low-residue diet and daily saline enema for several days prior to operation. In this way fecal material in the rectum can be kept at a minimum during and shortly after operation. Avertin, 80 mg. per kg. of body weight, supplemented by ether, is a very satisfactory anesthesia. The tube by which the avertin is administered is left in the rectum but is clamped. The exstrophied bladder is suitably walled off with sterile guttapercha or oiled silk and adhesive tape.

Since it is technically easier to transplant the right ureter first, a low right rectus incision is made, and the muscle is retracted laterally. The ureter is identified at the pelvic brim and from this point downward the posterior parietal peritoneum is opened so that the ureter can be dissected from its bed. It is freed almost to the bladder, where it is divided with the actual cautery or endothermy knife. The lower end is ligated and allowed to retract down behind the peritoneum.

A small No. 10 or 12 soft-rubber catheter is now inserted into the upper end of the ureter and maintained here only during the course of the operation, so that urine can be collected and suitably carried away from the field. Furthermore, this catheter keeps the ureter slightly distended while being planted into the bowel, and thus insures that a large enough tunnel will be made in the colonic wall. The sigmoid is then brought over to a proper position so that the ureter may be directed into it without angulation. A portion of the sigmoid must be selected which will allow the intramural portion of the ureter to be in a straight line with the superior retroperitoneal segment of the ureter. Furthermore, there must be no tension or kinking of the colon itself.

The rectal tube (which had been used for administration of the avertin) is now unclamped and the sigmoid is milked downward to express its

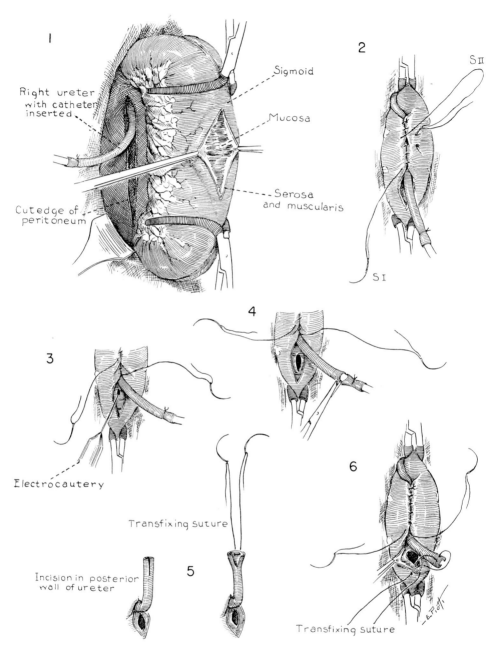

Fig. 240.—Method of establishing a ureterosigmoidostomy. *1*, Portion of sigmoid isolated by right angle clamps. Bowel wall opened down to mucosa. Small catheter tied into mobilized and severed ureter. *2*, Ureter laid into bowel wall. *S-I* and *S-II*, First and second layers of sutures closing sigmoid. *3*, Piercing mucosa with electrocautery. *4*, Ureter cut off to suitable length and catheter removed. *5*, Slitting ureter and placement of double-headed silk suture. *6*, Ureter sutures run into lumen of sigmoid and then passed out through sigmoid wall to anchor ureter.

gas and liquid contents. Two right-angle rubber clamps are placed so that no further gas or fluid can enter the sigmoid. A longitudinal incision 2½ or 3 inches in length is made by sharp dissection through the serosa and muscularis; a small flap is freed up on either side from the underlying submucosa. The ureter is now laid directly on this bared submucosa and the divided muscularis and serosa are brought together over it from above

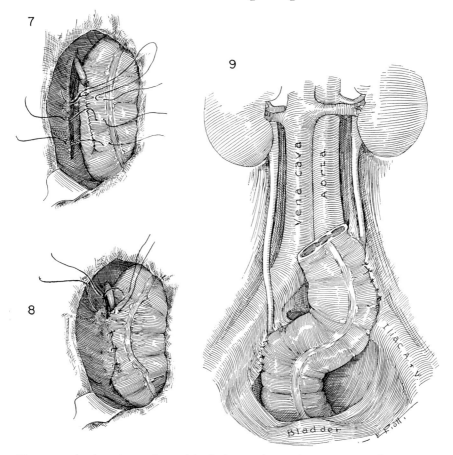

Fig. 240 (*Continued*).—*7,* Lateral leaf of posterior peritoneum sutured to bowel with interrupted silk sutures. *8,* Tightening of sutures to anchor bowel to posterior peritoneum. *9,* Position of viscera after completion of bilateral ureteral transplantation.

downward with a continuous suture. A second continuous suture is then placed, which folds in and supports the first line of sutures.

The rubber catheter is now withdrawn and any excess of ureter is cut off. A longitudinal slit is made in the posterior border of the ureter so that the small opening at its end is transformed into a long oblique one. A double-headed fine silk suture is passed through this free end of the ureter; the needles are threaded from within outward. The mucosa of the bowel is opened with an endothermy knife and the ureter is carried into the lumen by the double-headed suture, the needles of which are passed through the bowel wall from within outward. When this suture is tied externally the ureter will be anchored to the internal aspect of the sigmoidal wall, its orifice will be directed into the lumen of the gut, and the ureteral opening will be large enough so that it will never become scarred and constricted. During this step there is, of course, the possibility of soiling the operative field, but if care is taken and the instruments employed are discarded, important contamination is rare.

The two previous layers of sigmoidal wall suture are now continued downward to close the gut and also to cover over the ureteral anchor suture. The posterior peritoneum (which had been opened to isolate the ureter)

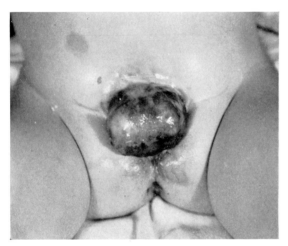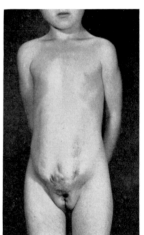

Fig. 241.—*Left,* Exstrophy of bladder in a three-year-old girl. *Right,* Photograph at five years, after completion of ureteral transplants and cystectomy in three stages.

is now closed. With great care the sigmoid loop must be suitably anchored to the posterior abdominal wall so that the ureter is kept in a straight line and is not angulated at the point at which it enters the bowel. Silk sutures are always used for this stabilizing of the sigmoid in order to insure permanency. The abdomen is closed in layers without drainage.

Following operation a high fluid intake should be urged for several days, in order to maintain an adequate flow of urine. If the child does not drink well, fluid should be given by parenteral routes. The time when urine appears in the rectum is variable and probably depends upon the amount of edema at the operative site and the resulting temporary constriction of the implanted ureter. Urinary discharge into the rectum usually begins in twenty-four to forty-eight hours, but it may be delayed as long as three or four days.

Stage 2. Transplantation of the Left Ureter.—The left ureteral transplantation is done through a left rectus incision at a subsequent time. It is usually possible to carry this out in two or three weeks, according to how much reaction the individual has had to the first procedure.

Stage 3. Removal of Bladder and Repair of Abdominal-Wall Hernia and Epispadias.—After both ureters have been transplanted, the next surgical problem is concerned with removal of the bladder and repair of the abdominal-wall hernia and epispadias. If the child is in good condition this may be undertaken during the same hospitalization. Inasmuch as the third-stage procedure is a lengthy one, it is preferable in most cases to defer it for several weeks until the child has fully recuperated from his first two operations. The best method we have found for repair of the epispadias is the one described by Ladd and Lanman.[8] The general principle of this is to save a strip of bladder mucosa to form an anterior wall for the urethra while the superior surface of the penis is covered with skin which is brought backward from a flap of the foreskin. In this way a canal representing the full length of the urethra is maintained, so that the reproductive tract of the individual is established. The steps in this procedure are indicated in Fig. 242.

The bladder mucous membrane and the exposed urethra and penis must be cleansed thoroughly with soap solution and alcohol or other mild antiseptic. The skin of the surrounding abdomen and scrotum is prepared with ether and half-strength tincture of iodine. An incision is made around the entire bladder, except inferiorly. At the upper pole of the bladder the marginal incisions are carried upward in an apex above the umbilicus. The bladder mucous membrane is now dissected free from the underlying structures and is turned forward and downward, as a flap, still maintaining its attachment with the base of the penis. It is sometimes extremely difficult to accomplish this without opening the peritoneum, but every effort should be made to avoid doing so. If the peritoneum is accidentally nicked it should be immediately closed. The hernia between the widely separated rectus muscles is repaired by turning over a flap from one anterior rectus fascia and suturing it to the fascia of the opposite side.

Attention is now returned to the freed bladder mucosa; the lateral portions of the bladder are cut off and discarded, while a midline strip (about ¼ to ½ inch wide) is saved and reflected forward onto the superior surface of the penis, to form the roof of the urethral gutter of the epispadias. This raw surface is now covered over with a pedicle flap of skin which is obtained from the foreskin in the manner shown in the drawing. If this skin has been sewed into place as indicated, there remain small lateral tabs or "ears" of tissue, at the points *B* in Fig. 242. These have a tendency to shrink and become less objectionable following operation,

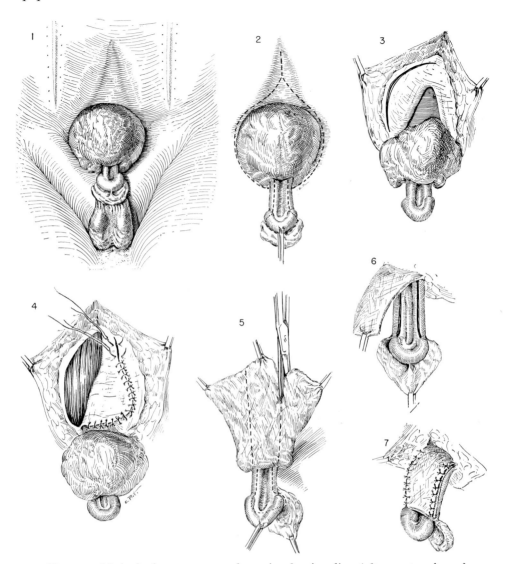

Fig. 242.—Method of cystectomy and repair of epispadias (after ureters have been transplanted to the colon). *1*, View of exstrophied bladder and penis. The two abdominal scars are from the ureteral transplantation operations. *2*, Outline of incision for excising bladder. *3*, Entire bladder freed up and reflected downward, exposing rectus fascia and peritoneum. Lateral cut made in rectus fascia. *4*, Flap of rectus fascia turned to close the diastasis recti. *5*, Bladder flap trimmed along dotted lines; lateral portions to be discarded. *6*, Lateral cuts made on either side of the urethral membrane to receive the bladder flap. *7*, Bladder flap sutured into place, its membrane forming the anterior wall of the urethra.

and they should not be trimmed down at this time for fear of interfering with the blood supply of the foreskin flap.

The postoperative appearance of one of these patients is shown in

Fig. 243. While an anatomic repair is by no means obtained, all of the previously exposed mucous membrane is either removed or covered, the genital canal of the penis is completed, and the local region is considerably improved from the cosmetic standpoint.

Stabilization of Bony Pelvis.—To date no one has attempted to restore the anterior continuity of the bony pelvis. It would be technically possible to inlay a graft of bone to stabilize the two sides of the pubic structures, but since three operations are necessary for rearrangement and repair of the genito-urinary tract, further extensive operations would be seldom

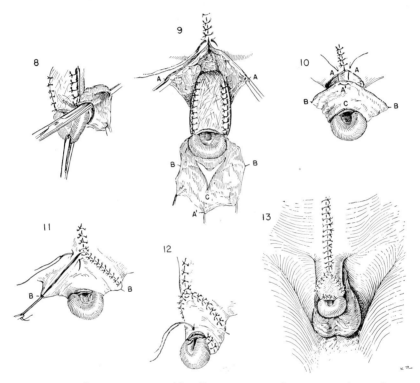

Fig. 242 *(Continued)*.—*8*, Foreskin slit open around corona and two layers of its skin being separated by blunt dissection. *9*, Foreskin flap is unfolded and will be threaded over the glans. *10*, Foreskin over the glans and being anchored to skin of abdominal wall. *11*, Continuation of suture of foreskin to abdominal wall skin. *12*, Anchoring of foreskin to the tip of the bladder flap. *13*, Completed repair.

justified. While these individuals tend to have a waddling gait in childhood, the pelvis becomes more stabilized in later years. Walking improves as the child grows older and, indeed, one of our patients has indulged in athletics, including football. If the pelvis is quite unsteady a considerable amount of support can be given by a longshoreman's type of belt which is placed below the crests of the ilia so that the sides or the pelvis are com-

26

pressed. An adaptation of this is shown in Fig. 244; this wide canvas strap can be tightened by the suitably placed buckles.

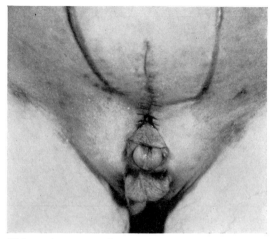

Fig. 243.—Five-year-old boy after ureteral transplants, cystectomy, and repair of epispadias outlined in Fig. 242.

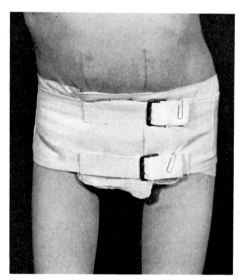

Fig. 244.—Type of belt employed to stabilize the pelvis and thereby improve the gait.

RESULTS OF OPERATION

Safety of Bilateral Ureterosigmoidostomy.—Since 1930, twenty-six chil dren at the Children's Hospital have been subjected to bilateral ure-terosigmoidostomy, according to the principles above described. There have been no deaths either during the postoperative period or subsequent thereto. Two patients developed abdominal abscesses and peritonitis following a ureteral transplant, but both of these recovered after suitable drainage of the peritoneal cavity. These infections obviously resulted from contamination of the peritoneum at the time of operation, or from a temporary leak at the site of anastomosis. The comparative rarity of peritonitis (two instances in fifty-two ureterosigmoidostomies) makes it evident that the transperitoneal approach is a relatively safe one. For this reason *we do not believe that an extraperitoneal operation for implantation of the ureters into the bowel is necessary.* There is considerable objection to this latter procedure because it is impossible to determine the exact intra-abdominal positions of the sigmoid and attached ureters. Hence,

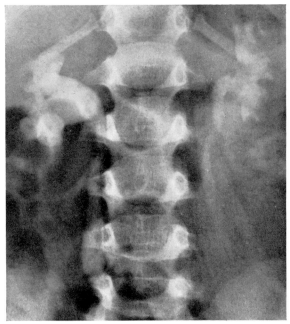

Fig. 245.—Intravenous pyelograms from a four-year-old girl, three months after transplantation of ureters. There is only a slight dilatation of the ureters and renal pelves.

there is considerable danger of unknowingly angulating the bowel or ureters at the site of anastomosis.

Obstructive Symptoms after Operation.—If for any reason a stricture develops at the anastomotic site or if too short a segment of ureter has been led into the sigmoid (so that the luminal pressure of the bowel is transmitted up the urinary tract) dilatation of the ureters and pelves will result. A slight degree of *hydronephrosis* is found in most cases (Figs. 245 and 247), but minimal dilatation will not impair the individual's health if there is no superimposed infection. In an occasional patient the urinary tract is quite dilated for several months after operation, but then is smaller in size when visualized a few years later (Fig. 247). Presumably, edema or low-grade infection at the anastomosis partially obstructs these ureters for weeks or months, but when this reaction subsides the ureter obtains a free drainage and shrinks to more normal proportions.

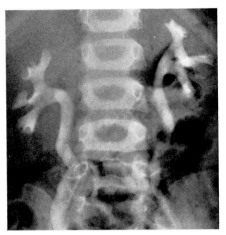

Fig. 246.—Intravenous pyelograms from a four-year-old boy, eight months after the right ureteral transplantation and four months after the left ureteral transplantation. The ureters are only slightly dilated. The calices are quite sharp and have only minimal blunting.

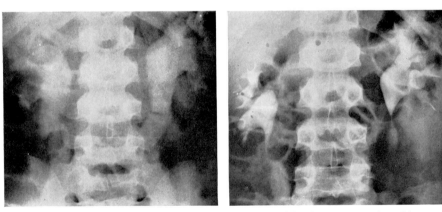

Fig. 247.—Films from a boy who was eight years old when ureterosigmoidostomies were established. The ureters and pelves became dilated after operation, but they subsequently diminished in size. *Left,* Two months after ureteral transplants. *Right,* Two and a half years after operations.

In one girl a very large ureter (which had been previously obstructed by another congenital anomaly) was unwisely implanted into the colon, and subsequently this kidney and ureter had to be removed because of poor function and infection. In two other children, recurrent flank pain and evidence of nonfunctioning kidney by pyelographic studies led to reexploration of the abdomen and inspection of the ureteral anastomoses; in one there was a ureteral angulation and in the other there was a stricture. The correction of each obstruction was followed by relief of symptoms and return of kidney function.

Postoperative Pyelitis.—While the Coffey technic of establishing a valve at the junction of ureter and sigmoid has undoubtedly been one of the greatest advances in the treatment of these cases, there is little question that bacteria from the colon occasionally get into the ureters and give rise to an ascending infection. Prior to the days of chemotherapy this complication resulted in bouts of pyelitis which were at times very difficult to control. Since most of these infections are caused by the colon bacillus, a potent agent is now available in the form of *sulfanilamide* for treating those individuals who develop pyelitis. *Sulfathiazole* is more effective

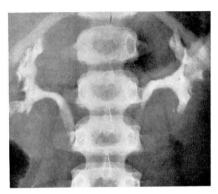

Fig. 248.—Intravenous pyelograms from a boy six years after establishment of ureterosigmoidostomies. Note the excellent preservation of calices, pelves, and upper portions of the ureters.

against the enterococcus and some other organisms which may be present, but experience has shown that sulfanilamide alone is usually sufficient (and less dangerous) for controlling the infection, provided there is no concurrent ureteral obstruction.

Sphincter Control after Operation.—Individuals with discharge of urine into the rectum can gain an adequate control of the anal sphincter, if cooperation is good and adequate training is provided. During the day these children can go as long as two, three, or four hours without emptying the rectum, and without soiling themselves between times. They may have to get up once at night, but some can sleep through the entire night without defecation or soiling. These considerations raise the question of the *best age* for performing ureteral transplantation, and the period from three to five years has been arbitrarily selected as the optimum time. In infancy it is technically possible to transplant the ureters, but there is some question of whether a baby would acquire adequate bowel habits, and we have deferred operation until the child is already trained.

Summary and Conclusions.—The results of surgical treatment of exstrophy of the bladder have been very encouraging. These individuals who were previously ostracized are now able to play with other children, to attend school, and to have an improved cosmetic appearance. While the functional reproductive state of males must remain in doubt, cases have been reported in which females have borne children. While the life expectancy of patients with ureteral transplants will be undoubtedly diminished below normal because of recurring kidney infections, it is important to note that there are published accounts of individuals who are in satisfactory health twenty-five to thirty years after ureteral transplantation.

BIBLIOGRAPHY

1. Coffey, R. C.: Pancreato-enterostomy and Pancreatectomy. Ann. Surg., *50:* 1238, 1909.
2. Coffey, R. C.: Transplantation of the Ureters into the Large Intestine in the Absence of a Functioning Urinary Bladder. Surg., Gynec. and Obst., *32:* 383, 1921.
3. Coffey, R. C.: Transplantation of the Ureters into the Large Intestine. Surg., Gynec. and Obst., *47:* 593, 1928.
4. Coffey, R. C.: Further Studies and Experiences with Transfixion Suture Technic (Technic 3) for Transplantation of Ureters into Large Intestine. Northwest Med., *32:* 31, 1933.
5. Estes, W. L.: Exstrophy of the Urinary Bladder; Implantation of Both Ureters into Rectum; Prolongation of Life Twenty-four Years. Ann. Surg., *99:* 223, 1934.
6. Higgins, C. C.: Transplantation of Ureters in Infants. J. Urol., *41:* 464, 1939.
7. Ladd, W. E., and Lanman, T. H.: Exstrophy of the Bladder. New England J. Med., *216:* 637, 1937.
8. Ladd, W. E., and Lanman, T. H.: Exstrophy of the Bladder and Epispadias. New England J. Med., *222:* 130, 1940.
9. Lanman, T. H., and Colby, F. H.: Report of the Society of Clinical Surgery. Nov., 1931.
10. Peters, G. A.: Transplantation of Ureters into Rectum by an Extraperitoneal Method for Exstrophy of Bladder. Brit. M. J., *1:* 1538, 1901.
11. Randall, L. M., and Hardwick, R. S.: Pregnancy and Parturition Following Bilateral Ureteral Transplantation for Congenital Exstrophy of the Bladder. Surg., Gynec. and Obst., *58:* 1018, 1934.
12. Turner, G. G.: The Treatment of Congenital Defects of the Bladder and Urethra by Implantation of the Ureters into the Bowel: With a Record of 17 Personal Cases. Brit. J. Surg., *17:* 114, 1929–30.
13. Von Geldern, Charles E.: The Etiology of Exstrophy of the Bladder. Arch. Surg., *8:* 61, 1924.
14. Walters, W., and Braasch, W. F.: Ureteral Transplantation to Rectosigmoid for Exstrophy of Bladder, Complete Epispadias, and Other Urethral Abnormalities with Total Urinary Incontinence: Study of 85 Operative Cases. Am. J. Surg., *23:* 255, 1934.

CHAPTER XXXV

EMBRYOMA OF THE KIDNEY (WILMS' TUMOR)

Embryoma of the kidney is one of the most common tumors of the abdomen in childhood. The neoplasm is a highly malignant one and has been variously called "renal carcinoma," "sarcoma," "rhabdomyosarcoma," "angiosarcoma," and so on, depending upon the predominating type of tissue. While any given tumor may be largely comprised of one histologic substance, an adequate microscopic examination of blocks from different parts of the specimen always shows a mixed structure. Hence, it is preferable to designate these lesions as *embryomas,* or *mixed tumors,* of the kidney.

Considerable pessimism has sprung up regarding the prognosis for children with this neoplasm, and while it is still true that the mortality is high, the outlook is not as hopeless as many textbooks and reports would suggest. A review of the Children's Hospital material indicates that about 25 per cent of patients can be permanently cured by the methods which will be subsequently presented.

PATHOLOGY

For many years the Children's Hospital pathological material on Wilms' tumor of the kidney has been carefully preserved and studied by Dr. Sidney Farber. His records have been used liberally in summarizing data for previous reports[8, 9] and for the following section.

Gross Pathology.—An embryoma always arises within the renal substance and as it grows the kidney capsule is expanded and surrounds the neoplasm for a considerable period of time before rupturing. Embryomas vary greatly in size; a few are as small as a fist; many are as large as a grapefruit; some have the proportions of a football. The growth tends to be spherical or oblong. The external surface is smoothly rounded or only slightly lobulated. For the most part the neoplasms are solid, though cystic spaces and areas of degeneration are common. The color is gray to grayish white, but some zones may have a pinkish or yellowish tint. The tissue may be quite firm, or else highly cellular and rather soft. On the whole, the vascularity is poor, but the surface vessels can be quite large. The neoplasm tends to be sharply demarcated from the compressed kidney substance by a narrow band of connective tissue, but it is impossible to dissect the neoplasm away at such a septum. The kidney may retain a more or less normal contour, but it is more apt to be squeezed into a distorted shape. Likewise, the kidney pelvis may be narrowed, elongated, or otherwise deformed.

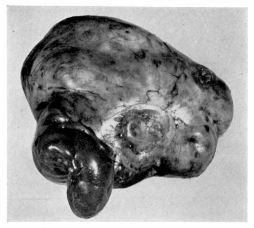

Fig. 249.—Surgically removed embryoma of the kidney. Kidney in lower left corner. The tumor is encapsulated and has a smooth surface.

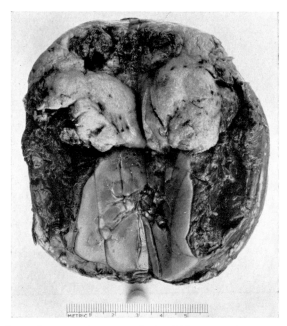

Fig. 250.—Opened specimen, embryoma of the kidney. Variegated appearance of cut surface. Kidney in lower center.

Tumor tissue may project into the renal pelvis, but in the great majority of cases it does not do so. The tumor metastasizes either by invasion of the renal vein or of the retroperitoneal regional lymphatics.

Histologic Features.—Microscopic examination shows tissues of many types. Epithelial cells predominate and vary from sheets of rapidly growing embryomatous elements to more or less well-differentiated, epithelial-lined spaces which are often reminiscent of renal tubules. Connective-tissue structures are always found to some extent, and indeed they dominate

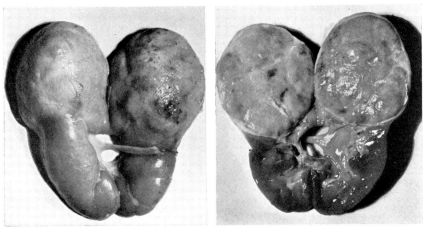

Fig. 251.—Embryoma of kidney removed from a thirteen-month-old boy who is alive and well two years later (Case 13, Table 38).

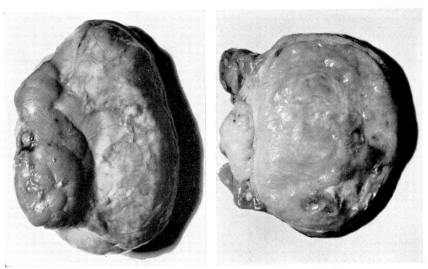

Fig. 252.—Embryoma of kidney from a one-year-old boy.

the picture in some specimens. Smooth muscle and immature or even fully developed striated muscle are commonly observed. Small bits of bone and cartilage may be found. The preservation may be good, but hemorrhage and degenerative changes are common. Careful microscopic examination may show nests of cells within blood vessels.

Prognosis on Basis of Pathologic Findings.—A great deal of time has been spent in the Children's Hospital Department of Pathology in the effort to

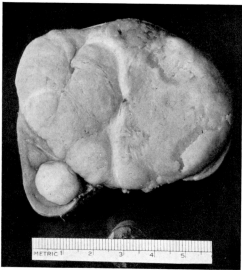

Fig. 253.—Embryoma of kidney removed from a ten-month-old female. Patient alive and well five years later (Case 9, Table 38).

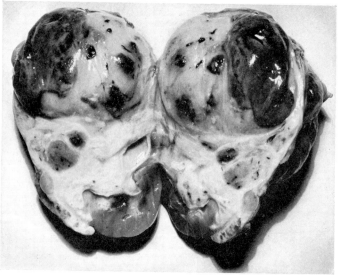

Fig. 254.—Renal embryoma from a three-year-old girl who died eight months later with pulmonary and intracranial metastases. Tip of kidney shows at bottom of photograph.

classify our fifty-six embryomas into subdivisions, with the hope of establishing the prognosis in a given case from the histologic findings of the specimen which has been surgically removed. The studies to date have been fruitless, and we are convinced that nothing is to be gained from subclassifying the embryomas. However, a thorough examination of the specimen gives some important information to the surgeon, because extensive hemorrhage and necrosis, rupture of the capsule, extension of tumor through the capsule, or invasion of renal veins are all findings of almost certain fatal import. The absence of all of these changes does not necessarily mean that the outlook will be excellent, because cells may have broken into the blood stream before or during the operation and no evidence of this propagation can be detected by the pathologist. The size of a tumor is no measure of its capability for setting up metastases. A large growth which completely fills the flank may be followed by a permanent cure, whereas two of our smallest tumors had renal veins blocked with tumor cells at the time of operation.

Summary of Observations.—The tumor can then be characterized by: (1) occurrence in the early years of life; (2) a variegated histology; (3) complete encapsulation for an undetermined length of time before its membrane is broken; (4) a very high degree of malignancy; (5) common occurrence of hemorrhage and necrosis; (6) a tendency to reach a large size before metastases occur; (7) dissemination by way of the regional lymphatics or by blood stream invasion.

CLINICAL DATA

Symptoms and Physical Findings.—Unfortunately, this lesion is silent for a long time and the primary complaint is usually related to a firm *swelling* in one flank which is discovered by the mother while dressing or bathing the child. It is extraordinary to see how large it can become before being noticed. The mass is characteristically quite painless until it reaches enormous proportions and even then there is seldom more than a dull ache or discomfort. Careful questioning will sometimes disclose that the child has been pale or below par for several months, but this is the exception rather than the rule. Urinary complaints are quite rare, but *hematuria* is observed in a few instances.

Inspection and *palpation* discloses a nontender mass (Figs. 255 and 256) which fills the renal fossa and possibly projects down into the pelvis and forward into the peritoneal cavity. It is rounded or ovoid and has a smooth surface or a gently lobulated one. The larger growths fill a third or even half of the abdomen. The superior margin disappears beneath the costal edge; the lower border can extend below the crest of the ilium; the anteromedial border can project well into the abdominal cavity as far as the midline of the body. The mass is quite fixed; it cannot be moved in relation to the posterior abdominal structures; it does not move during respiration. The diaphragm on the affected side may be somewhat elevated, but there is no respiratory embarrassment. When an embryoma of the kidney appears on the right, its upper anterior border may be hard to define from the adjacent liver, except for a shallow groove between these two structures.

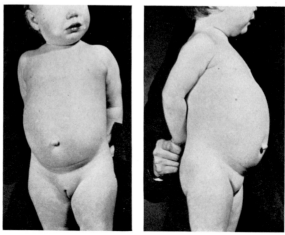

Fig. 255.—Twenty-six-month-old girl with large embryoma of right kidney.

Low-grade concomitant *fever* can be explained on the basis of hemorrhage and tumor decomposition; it does not necessarily imply that there is infection in this or another part of the body.

The urine is normal in most cases; occasionally a few red or white blood cells are found; rarely there is gross hematuria. The nonprotein nitrogen level of the blood is within normal limits.

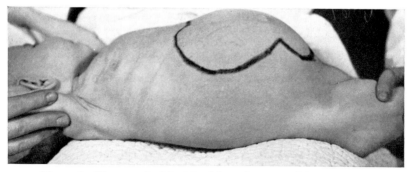

Fig. 256.—Five-month-old girl with embryoma of left kidney.

Diagnosis.—The *age incidence* of embryoma of the kidney is of considerable help in establishing the diagnosis. The neoplasms are most frequently discovered between two and three years of age, though the youngest in our series was two months and the oldest child was seven years old. Females and males are affected in about equal numbers. Embryoma appears with about equal frequency on the two sides, while in rare individuals both kidneys are the sites of separate neoplasms. In the present series twenty-five were on the left, twenty-eight were on the right, and three were bilateral.

It is important to have as little trauma as possible in the handling of these patients, because repeated palpation of the mass, squeezing of the tumor, or disturbing it with a puncture biopsy instrument, may discharge malignant cells into the blood stream and give rise to distant metastases which vitiate any possibility of a permanent cure. *Aspiration biopsy* has been recommended by some writers for confirming the diagnosis by microscopic study. This procedure is a thoroughly unsound one, since puncture

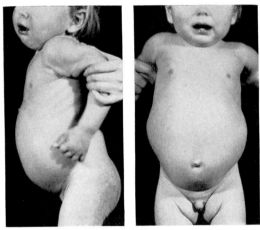

Fig. 257.—One-year-old boy with embryomas of both kidneys. Each kidney tumor was apparently a separate, primary growth.

of the mass may seed the peritoneal cavity or the surrounding tissues with neoplasm and spoil the surgeon's opportunity for complete removal of a lesion the prognosis of which is favorable. We abandoned this procedure more than twenty years ago.

ROENTGENOLOGIC EXAMINATION

Films of the abdomen without contrast media almost always show a slightly opaque mass with displacement of intestines to the middle or opposite side of the abdomen. *Pyelograms* by intravenous or retrograde routes give additional information but need not be considered necessary for establishing the diagnosis. The pelvis of the kidney may be compressed, greatly elongated, or completely normal. It can remain in its customary position, but it often rides at the upper or lower pole of the tumor shadow. Hence, the dye-filled pelvis can be found well up toward the diaphragm or quite low in the iliac fossa. The kidney pelvis and ureter are almost never displaced laterally, but they are frequently pushed medially to a considerable degree. Lateral films may show the kidney pelvis displaced forward or backward in relation to the shadow of the neoplasm. It has been our practice to obtain an *intravenous* pyelogram in all cases when the diagnosis is in doubt. *Retrograde* studies have usually been omitted because they require an additional anesthesia and seldom give more information than can be obtained by the simpler intravenous method.

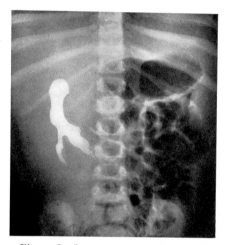 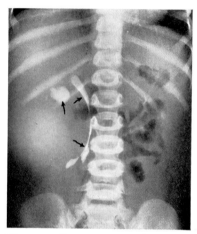

Fig. 258.—Intravenous pyelogram from a child with an embryoma. Opaque shadow fills the right half of the abdomen. The right renal pelvis is enlarged and distorted.

Fig. 259.—Intravenous pyelogram from a girl with an embryoma of the kidney. Note the opaque shadow on patient's right and the distorted pelvis (arrows).

An embryoma of the kidney can almost always be recognized without roentgenologic studies, but x-ray findings aid the surgeon because it is desirable to have preoperative knowledge of the position of the renal pedicle and blood vessels.

DIFFERENTIAL DIAGNOSIS

In infancy and childhood, embryoma of the kidney must be differentiated from several other solid tumors which may occur in this region.

Neuroblastoma Sympatheticum.—This tumor (see Chapter XXXVI), which arises from the adrenal gland medulla, or from other neural tissue in the retroperitoneal spaces, is the most common neoplasm which is apt to be confused with embryoma of the kidney. It is a highly malignant lesion and is found in the same age groups. In general, it is not as large as most of the embryomas. It metastasizes early and even when the primary tumor is small there may be widespread secondary growths in the liver and particularly the skeleton. The primary neoplasm is firm or hard and generally has a pebbly or finely nodular surface, in contrast to the more smoothly rounded or gently lobulated contour of an embryoma. The neuroblastoma usually has an irregular outline, poorly defined borders, and possibly an extension across the midline of the abdomen, whereas an embryoma has a spherical or oblong shape, well delineated borders, and no extension beyond the vertebral column.

The metastases of these two growths are quite different. Embryomas spread to regional lymph nodes and to the lungs where the nodules are large and fuzzy in outline. Neuroblastoma metastases are more widely scattered to the liver, kidneys, brain, orbits, lungs, and particularly the skeleton which is peppered with small destructive lesions. The roentgenologic characteristics of the metastases (when they exist) will often differentiate between the two forms of neoplasm.

Since a neuroblastoma can invade the adjacent kidney and distort its pelvis, pyelographic study is of little aid in differentiating the two conditions.

Hypernephroma of the Kidney.—Hypernephroma, or the *Grawitz tumor*, is a solid neoplasm arising within the kidney and composed of cells with clear, foamy cytoplasms resembling those of an adrenal cortex. It is believed that such growths arise from rests of adrenal cortical tissue which are not infrequently found in otherwise normal kidneys. The Grawitz tumor is one which appears in middle, or even late, adult life. It is exceedingly rare in childhood and we have not encountered a single specimen during the last twenty-five years at the Children's Hospital. It is important to recognize the difference between these two entirely different neoplasms of the kidney, and we would scarcely need to mention the hypernephroma in this section on differential diagnosis, except to clarify the hazy impressions which some physicians still hold concerning the two conditions. The practical absence of hypernephroma in childhood makes it unnecessary to consider this lesion further.

Unattached Retroperitoneal Embryoma.—This term has been employed[4] to describe a solid or partially cystic mixed tumor which may appear anywhere along the posterior abdominal (or thoracic) wall. The adjective "unattached" is meant to imply that it is not connected with the kidney in spite of the fact that histologic resemblance to renal embryoma may be close. This neoplasm is believed to arise from remnants of the primitive pronephros or mesonephros and hence may be found on either side of the vertebral column from the fourth cervical segment downward as far as the internal genitalia. It often attains a very large size before attracting attention. The prognosis is somewhat dependent upon the degree of malignancy and upon the promptness with which the lesion is recognized and removed. If a massive, unattached retroperitoneal embryoma has a high position, it is usually impossible to distinguish it before operation from an embryoma of the kidney. If it should arise in the lower abdomen, embryoma of the kidney can be excluded because the mass does not extend into the renal fossa. Retroperitoneal embryomas are rare; most of them are found in adult life. During a period of years in which we have encountered fifty-six embryomas of the kidney, only five retroperitoneal embryomas have been seen.

Hydronephrosis.—Hydronephrosis is not rare in this age group; it usually results from some congenital obstruction either at the ureteropelvic junction or at the ureterovesicle valve. While a kidney pelvis can attain enormous proportions and even fill half of the abdomen, it may be unaccompanied by pain in its dilated state. However, the history will usually indicate that there have been previous bouts of pain in the flank or loin of the involved side. By palpation the fluid nature of a hydronephrosis is usually evident, but a tensely distended hydronephrotic sac has not infrequently been mistaken for a solid tumor. If physical findings leave the physician in doubt, intravenous or retrograde pyelograms will quickly settle the differential diagnosis.

TREATMENT

When the diagnosis of embryoma of the kidney has been made, the course of therapy must be decided upon. If left untreated, these individuals rapidly develop metastases in the retroperitoneal lymph nodes or lungs, and possibly in the liver or brain. If no metastases are demonstrable the primary growth should be removed in all cases no matter how large it might be. While the size of the abdominal swelling may make the prognosis appear dubious, *surgical excision* holds the only hope of cure.

Preoperative Irradiation.—Some clinicians, notably Kerr,[5] Kretschmer,[6] Wharton,[12] Priestley and Broders,[11] and Prather and Friedman,[10] have advocated the use of preoperative irradiation over the growth with two thoughts in mind: (1) to reduce the size of the local mass so that it will be technically easier to remove it; (2) to kill off the more malignant cells and possibly prevent their escape into the blood stream during the manipulations of operation. Some surgeons have employed x-ray irradiation to shrink the tumor so that it can be removed through an oblique flank incision (which gives a totally inadequate exposure in a child). However, if a transperitoneal approach is used, sufficient room can be obtained to remove even the largest embryoma, so that preoperative irradiation can be dispensed with.

Preoperative irradiation implies that there must be a deferment of operation for several weeks to gain the optimum effects of the x-rays. During this time the tumor may begin to seed the blood stream and set up metastases, and the one chance for a permanent cure has been lost. Preoperative irradiation refutes one of the cardinal principles for treatment of these cases—namely, *removal of the mass as soon as it is discovered.* We are convinced that x-ray therapy has been too widely employed without due consideration of the end results obtained in patients so treated.

A fairly extensive, but not entirely complete, review of the English literature shows sixteen cases which may be listed as probable cures following nephrectomy. To these may be added fourteen more from our own service. Of these thirty cases (Table 37), ten had preoperative irradiation and twenty did not. While the total number of cases treated with and without preoperative irradiation is obviously too small to warrant any sweeping conclusions, the figures certainly suggest that recourse to immediate surgery gives the highest possibility of permanent cure.

Immediate Excision of the Tumor.—In recent years at the Children's Hospital the large size of a tumor has in no instance been considered a contraindication to immediate operation. Furthermore, the operative mor-

TABLE 37

WILMS' TUMOR CURED MORE THAN EIGHTEEN MONTHS

	No. of Cases
With Preoperative Irradiation and Nephrectomy:	
From literature	9
From Children's Hospital	1
Nephrectomy without Preoperative Irradiation:	
From literature	7
From Children's Hospital	13
Total	30

tality has not been high, even though the tumors have been removed without preoperative x-ray shrinkage. During the last thirteen years thirty-seven patients have been subjected to excision of an embryoma with two operative deaths. One of these had intra-abdominal metastases and probably should not have been operated upon. The other died of shock. In the last eight years twenty-two embryomas have been removed, and with no operative mortality. These figures refute the statements that preoperative irradiation is necessary to obtain a low operative mortality.

Preoperative Preparations.—If anemia is present, preoperative *transfusion* is indicated. Preparation must be made to administer blood during or immediately after operation, because the extent of the dissection often produces considerable shock which can be adequately combated only by transfusion. While it is not absolutely necessary, it is a good precautionary measure to place an inlying cannula in one of the ankle veins before starting the laparotomy so that intravenous fluids and blood can be given at a moment's notice if the need arises.

27

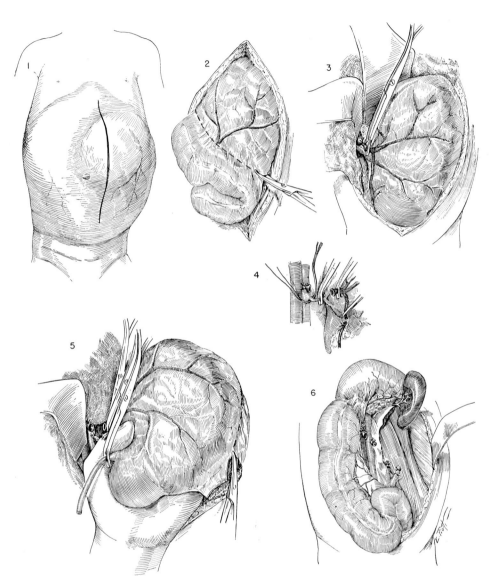

Fig. 260.—Operative excision of an embryoma of the left kidney. *1,* Position of the bulging mass and the long left rectus incision. *2,* Colon displaced downward and medially by tumor. Peritoneum will be cut along the dotted line to mobilize colon and expose the neoplasm. *3,* Colon pulled medially. Renal pedicle treated before the tumor is disturbed. Vein being tied and clamped. *4,* Renal vein divided. Spermatic (or ovarian) vein divided. Renal artery clamped; ligature being passed around it. *5,* Renal vein, artery and ureter all divided. Inferior and posterior dissection of mass being carried out. *6,* Tumor removed from renal fossa. The colon will be dropped back into this raw space.

Transabdominal Exposure.—There can be no question about the best method for removal of an embryoma of the kidney. It is unwise to attack one of these lesions through an oblique posterolateral incision in the flank, because this gives too small an opening between the closely approximated ribs and iliac crest of a child, whereas an anterior abdominal wound can be more liberal and gives a better view of the mass. Furthermore, the postero-lateral approach implies that the neoplasm will be handled a great deal before it is circumvented and the renal pedicle reached, whereas the trans-abdominal exposure allows the renal vessels to be ligated and divided before the tumor is disturbed. It is highly important to close the renal vein early in the operation to diminish the dangers of liberating tumor cells into the blood stream.

The *incision* should run from the costal margin downward as far as the circumstances of the case dictate (Fig. 260); not infrequently it must be carried almost to the pubis. The rectus muscle can be split, but it is preferable to retract it laterally and thus gain a stronger postoperative wound. The ascending or descending colon, according to whether the tumor is right- or left-sided, is freed from its lateral peritoneal reflection and is turned toward the midline of the body, to expose the renal mass and pedicle.

Liberation of the Tumor Mass and Closure of Wound.—The renal artery and vein are divided. It may be necessary to remove a portion or all of the adrenal gland, but in most cases the adrenal can be saved. The ureter is next divided as low down as it can be freed. Dissection is now begun to free the tumor from its extensive posterior bed. All of the fat which clings to its capsule or pedicle should be left attached to the tumor and removed with it. Branches of the lumbar veins course over the surface of the tumor and must be severed. When the mass is completely liberated and lifted out of the belly, there is a large raw area in the posterolateral abdominal wall. This must be carefully inspected and all bleeding points ligated. The colon is allowed to drop back in place to cover over the raw zone. The abdominal wound is quite long, but if it is carefully closed no disturbance in healing is encountered in the postoperative period.

There is always a tendency to worry about the general condition of the child, and whether he will stand continuation of the operation. Because of this the operator is apt to feel hurried; thus a necrotic tumor may be roughly pressed or pulled upon, and its capsule thereby ruptured. Every effort should be made to handle it carefully to avoid this catastrophe. If an inlying venous cannula has been previously placed in one of the extremities so that blood can be continually administered during operation, the surgeon will be considerably reassured and will be able to undertake a slower and better type of operation.

RESULTS OF TREATMENT

In our series of fifty-six patients with embryoma of the kidney, fifty-four were operated upon, and two died without operation. Almost all those who died after operation had evidence of recurrence (by physical examination or roentgenogram of the chest) within six months. In all but one of the fatal cases, death occurred within one year of operation. These observations have led us to believe that if a patient survives operation for a year and a half without evidence of recurrence, he can probably be regarded as a permanent cure. The high degree of malignancy in this tumor does not make it necessary to set up minimal limits of five or seven years as criteria for claiming a permanent cure. In no instance have we seen a late recurrence some years after operation, such as is occasionally found with cancers of the breast, colon, and uterus in adults.

TABLE 38

CHILDREN'S HOSPITAL CASES WITH PROBABLE CURE OF RENAL EMBRYOMA
(Preoperative irradiation used only for Patient 13. Only Patient 12 had postoperative irradiation)

Case	Sex	Age at Operation	Nephrectomy	Well after Operation for:
1	M.	5 months	Left	$21\frac{1}{2}$ years
2	F.	31 months	Right	15 years
3	F.	12 months	Right	12+ years
4	M.	10 months	Left	12 years
5	F.	5 months	Left	9+ years
6	F.	5 years	Right	9 years
7	M.	22 months	Right	$7\frac{1}{2}$ years
8	F.	7 months	Right	$6\frac{1}{2}$ years
9	F.	10 months	Left	5 years
10	F.	5 months	Left	$3\frac{1}{2}$ years
11	F.	8 months	Right	$3\frac{1}{2}$ years
12	M.	5 months	Left	$2\frac{1}{2}$ years
13	M.	13 months	Right	2 years
14	M.	$4\frac{1}{2}$ years	Right	20 months

Of the fifty-four patients operated upon, thirty-five are known to be dead, three are alive but are regarded as hopeless because of demonstrable metastases, and two others are alive and have a hopeful prognosis. These two individuals have been recently operated upon, are in good health, and show no evidence of recurrence; they cannot be regarded as cures because one and one-half years have not yet fully elapsed. Fourteen children are regarded as probable cures, since they are alive and well for periods ranging from one and one-half to twenty-one and one-half years after excision of an embryoma of the kidney. Some data regarding these successful cases are listed in Table 38. It is interesting to note that whereas the average age of all patients (cured and uncured) was twenty-nine months at the time of operation, the fourteen individuals who are cured had an average age of seventeen months at the time of operation. Furthermore, of these fourteen cured children ten were thirteen months or less of age at the time of operation. One can speculate that the younger the individual at the time of operation, the better is the prognosis. This point is all the more striking when a review of all patients operated on in the first year of life shows that 50 per cent of them have permanent cures.

Symptoms of Recurrence.—If recurrence is found after operation, a firm irregular mass is eventually felt in the renal fossa, in the liver, or in some other portion of the abdomen. The first evidence of recurrence is sometimes detected by respiratory distress or roentgenologic examination of the chest. Development of pulmonary metastases heralds the onset of a rapidly downhill course. Extreme emaciation, intestinal obstruction, or superimposed pulmonary infection usually precedes exitus. Heavy x-ray irradiation will greatly shrink recurrent tumors in the abdomen or metastases in the chest, but this treatment has a limited usefulness and will only temporarily check the advance of the neoplasm. While the child is made more comfortable, life is seldom prolonged for more than a few months beyond that expected without such x-ray treatment.

Postoperative Irradiation.—Whether postoperative irradiation should be employed as a routine measure for all surgically treated cases is a moot question. Theoretically, a few viable cells might be left, in the renal fossa or scattered in the lungs, which could be killed by x-rays reaching these areas in high enough concentration soon after operation. For this reason it has been our recent policy to employ postoperative irradiation over the operative field and over the lungs. There has been an insufficient experience with this adjunct to make any statement regarding its effectiveness in producing a higher number of permanent cures. Certainly postoperative irradiation deserves a continued and more extensive trial.

BIBLIOGRAPHY

1. Bradley, J. E., and Pincoffs, M. C.: Association of Adeno-myo-sarcoma of Kidney (Wilms' Tumor) with Arterial Hypertension. Ann. Int. Med., *11:* 1613, 1938.
2. Campbell, M. F.: Primary Malignant Tumors of the Urogenital Tract in Infants and Children. J. A. M. A., *109:* 1606, 1937.
3. Dean, A. L., Jr., and Pack, G. T.: Embryonal Adenosarcoma of the Kidney. J. A. M. A., *98:* 10, 1932.
4. Hansmann, G. H., and Budd, J. W.: Massive Unattached Retroperitoneal Tumors; Explanation of Unattached Retroperitoneal Tumors Based on Remnants of Embryonic Urogenital Apparatus. J. A. M. A., *98:* 6, 1932.
5. Kerr, H. D.: Treatment of Malignant Tumors of Kidney in Children. J. A. M. A., *112:* 408, 1939.
6. Kretschmer, H. L.: Malignant Tumors of Kidney in Children. J. Urol., *39:* 250, 1938.
7. Kretschmer, H. L., and Hibbs, W. G.: Mixed Tumors of the Kidney in Infancy and Childhood. Surg., Gynec. and Obst., *52:* 1, 1931.
8. Ladd, W. E.: Embryoma of the Kidney (Wilms' Tumor). Ann. Surg., *108:* 885, 1938.
9. Mixter, C. G.: Malignant Tumors of the Kidney in Infancy and Childhood. Ann. Surg., *96:* 1017, 1932.

10. Prather, G. C., and Friedman, H. F.: The Immediate Effect of Preoperative Radiation in Cortical Tumors of the Kidney. New England J. Med., *215:* 655, 1936.
11. Priestley, J. T., and Broders, A. C.: Wilms' Tumor; Clinical and Pathological Study. J. Urol., *33:* 544, 1935.
12. Wharton, L. R.: Preoperative Irradiation of Massive Tumors of the Kidney. Arch. Surg., *30:* 35, 1935.
13. Wharton, L. R.: Transperitoneal Nephrectomy for Malignant Tumors of the Kidney. Surg., Gynec. and Obst., *60:* 689, 1935.

CHAPTER XXXVI

NEUROBLASTOMA SYMPATHETICUM

Neuroblastoma is the most common neoplasm of the abdominal cavity in childhood; embryoma of the kidney is a close second. During the ten-year period ending September 1, 1939, a series of 301 malignant tumors from all parts of the body in childhood were reviewed by Farber.[5, 6] In this group were forty neuroblastomas, of which thirty-two originated in the abdomen. During the same period there were thirty embryomas of the kidney. The neuroblastoma should be classified with the neurologic tumors, for it is now known to originate from tissue which gives rise to the adrenal medulla or other portions of the sympathetic system. This tumor is a highly malignant one, it metastasizes early and widely, and it has a serious but by no means always fatal prognosis. The curability of neuroblastoma has been pointed out by Farber[5, 17] who has reviewed and followed up the Children's Hospital cases. Neuroblastoma has been described under various names, including "sympathicoblastoma," "sarcoma of the adrenal gland," and "neuroblastoma sympatheticum."

PATHOLOGY

The sympathogonia are the formative cells from which the sympathetic nervous system develops. They can differentiate into the sympathoblast and the sympathetic ganglion cell on one hand or the chromaffin cells of the adrenal medulla on the other. From these various types of cells may originate four different types of tumors: (1) the more embryonic and extremely malignant *sympathogonioma;* (2) the malignant *neuroblastoma sympatheticum,* with which the present chapter is concerned; (3) the benign *ganglioneuroma;* and finally (4) the *chromaffinoma* or adrenalin-secreting tumor of adrenal medullary tissue. Of these four types of tumors the neuroblastoma is by far the most common.

Gross Pathology.—The neuroblastoma grows with considerable rapidity and while it may remain encapsulated for a short period of time it has a marked tendency to break out, spread along tissue planes, and invade surrounding organs, including blood vessels. Specimens vary greatly in size. Some of them are so small that they cannot be felt and yet they give rise to widespread metastases; others form a large mass which is readily palpable or which may even distend one side of the abdomen. The tumors, if small and encapsulated, are smooth and rounded (Fig. 261), but the great ma-

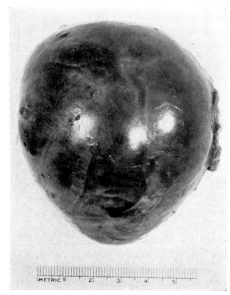

Fig. 261.—Encapsulated neuroblastoma of the adrenal, removed from an infant.

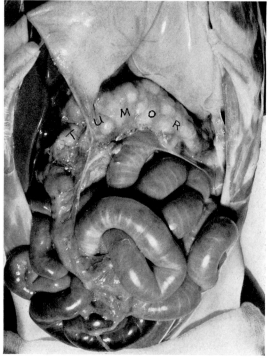

Fig. 262.—Two-and-one-half-year-old child with a neuroblastoma, arising from the retroperitoneal sympathetics (extra-adrenal origin). Note the nodular character of the tumor.

jority of them are larger and attain a finely lobulated or nubby surface (Fig. 262). This nodularity frequently enables the physician to distinguish the lesion from the smoother and possibly larger embryoma of the kidney.

Neuroblastomas may arise on either side of the vertebral column, but they not infrequently extend across the midline and indeed give rise to a secondary growth of lesser size in the opposite paravertebral gutter. This tendency to spread across the midline is again in contrast to the findings with embryomas of the kidney which only occasionally are bilateral. The tumor surface is extremely vascular; the vessels are rather small and appear as a fine network. The external surface therefore has a distinct reddish or

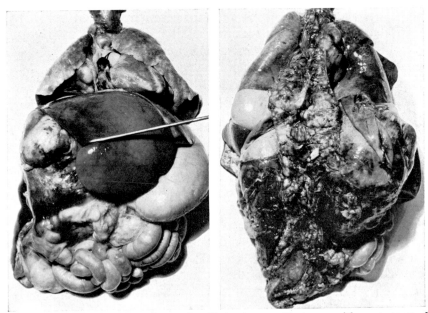

Fig. 263.—Viscera from patient who died of neuroblastoma with metastases. *Left,* Liver pulled away to show the primary tumor which arose from the right adrenal gland. *Right,* Posterior view of the viscera, showing the widespread extension of neoplasm behind the abdominal and mediastinal organs.

grayish-red color when viewed during life. While some of the growths can be dissected away clearly from surrounding organs, the more advanced lesions infiltrate and directly invade the adjacent kidney, renal pelvis, regional veins, root of the mesentery, body of the pancreas, lymph nodes, etc. There is a tendency to spread up and down along the retroperitoneal and even along the retropleural tissues (Fig. 263). It may be extremely difficult to delineate the pancreas, lymph nodes, retroperitoneal vessels, and other structures, when these are permeated by neoplasm. The growth may extend into the vertebral bodies and on occasions has pressed into the spinal canal.

The cut surface of the tumor is spongy, soft, grayish or yellowish gray, highly cellular, and possesses little supporting stroma. Some of the tumors have a mushy consistency, and bits of substance will extrude or ooze out when the specimen is cut open. The blood vessels are numerous but small; necrosis and hemorrhage are common.

Metastases.—Metastases take place by way of both lymphatic and blood stream invasion. In isolated cases the metastases are more or less limited to regional lymph nodes or massive invasion of the liver. More frequently the metastases are widely disseminated and are seeded through the lungs, kidneys, orbits, brain, and other organs, with a special predilection for the skeletal system. Pepper (in 1901) called attention to "sarcoma of the adrenal" and involvement of the liver, and for many years this combination was spoken of as the *Pepper syndrome*. In 1907 Hutchinson described primary adrenal tumors with metastases to the skull and orbits, producing unilateral or bilateral exophthalmos. This group of findings was referred to as the *Hutchinson syndrome*. There is no need for perpetuation of these designations, since the pathology in either instance is the same and the clinical manifestations are merely dependent upon what part of the body is invaded by the tumor.

Histologic Features.—Microscopic examination shows a highly cellular, rapidly growing neoplasm with great invasive qualities. The supporting stroma is quite scanty. Blood vessels are usually of rather small caliber. The tumor cells occur in broad sheets and clusters. They have somewhat the appearance of lymphocytes but are a little larger than such cells. Because of this feature, the tumors were often described in the past as sarcomas or lymphoblastomas. The cell nuclei are polygonal but in general have a spherical contour. There is a moderate amount of chromatin which has either a fairly even distribution or a peripheral arrangement. One to several nucleoli are often seen. The cystoplasms are amphophilic. Since these stain poorly in improperly preserved specimens, the microscopic appearance is that of a syncytial mass. Mitotic figures appear in large numbers. In only a few areas do the cells take on an elongated or spindle form. Invasion of blood vessels is often seen.

There are two characteristics which positively identify the neuroblastoma. The first is the occasional arrangement of a score or more of cells into a *rosette* with peripheral distribution of the nuclei and central concentration of the cell cytoplasms. The second is the development of *neurofibrils* which can be seen with the phosphotungstic acid-hematoxylin stain. These delicate fibrils may appear anywhere through the tumor, but they are particularly apt to be found in the central portions of the rosettes, since they arise from the tail processes of cells in these formations.

While the histologic features already enumerated are typical of the common run of neuroblastomas, occasionally one finds a more malignant growth in which the cells are a little smaller and in which no rosettes or fibrils can be identified. This more embryonic type of neoplasm is classified as a "sympathogonioma." Conversely, a tumor with many of the features of a neuroblastoma may show some areas with differentiation into ganglion cells; to indicate a more favorable prognosis it can be designated as a "neuroblastoma-ganglioneuroma" or "neuroblastoma differentiating into ganglioneuroma."

Sites of Origin.—Neuroblastomas can originate in many parts of the body. Some arise in the adrenal gland, but others spring from sympathetic tissue anywhere along the retroperitoneal, retropleural, or even cervical spaces. In one of our specimens the primary lesion was near the bifurcation of the aorta, and presumably arose from the organ of Zuckerkandl. Others appeared to arise from the coeliac plexus. In the forty cases of neuroblastoma studied by Farber[5] there were the following distributions: retroperitoneal, nineteen; right adrenal, seven; left adrenal, six; retropleural, four; cervical region, four. It is evident from these statistics that the abdominal variety is not always located high in the renal fossa, but that it may occur at lower positions in either paravertebral gutter or even in front of the spine.

CLINICAL FINDINGS

Neuroblastoma is encountered in any part of childhood, but it is largely a tumor of the first few years of life. Our youngest patient was four days of age, and the oldest was nine years. Three fourths of them were less than four years of age.

Symptoms.—The most common initial complaint is related to an abdominal swelling which is generally painless. The appearance of *pain* is somewhat suggestive of neoplastic involvement of retroperitoneal nerves or invasion and obstruction of a kidney pelvis, ureter, or intestine. The history usually indicates that there has been *pallor,* increased *fatigue,* and possibly *weight loss* for several months. *Loss of appetite* is common. If metastases have occurred there may be pain over an enlarged liver, cough from pulmonary involvement, headache and vomiting from expanding nodules in the brain, protrusion of an eyeball from a retro-orbital growth, swelling of the head from a lesion of the calvarium, and possibly pain in an extremity from pathologic fracture or slipping of an epiphysis at a site of skeletal destruction.

Physical Findings.—In the great majority of cases, examination discloses *a firm, nodular mass* in one side of the abdomen which has a tendency to extend across the midline and which may even be connected with a smaller lump on the opposite side. This may be felt anywhere from the adrenal region down to the promontory of the sacrum, according to the site of origin. It is nontender, is obviously fixed to the posterior abdominal structures,

and does not move during inspiration. The *liver* may be enlarged or nodular if it contains metastases. In advanced cases evidence of *secondary lesions*
may be found elsewhere, such as protrusion of an eyeball, a soft raised mass
in the scalp, a MacEwen sign (in young individuals), palpable left cervical
lymph nodes (extension through thoracic duct), or tenderness over bones.
In a few cases there are changes dependent upon compression of the spinal
cord in the upper lumbar region.

The urinary sediment rarely has any abnormal elements; the finding
of red cells suggests that kidney or renal pelvis has been invaded. Some
degree of *anemia* is present in the vast majority of cases. This does not
necessarily mean that bone marrow has been involved or replaced by metastatic growth, nor does it necessarily imply that blood has been lost by way
of the urinary or intestinal tract. Indeed, it is hard to explain the cause for
anemia in many of these children.

ROENTGENOLOGIC EXAMINATION

Roentgenograms of the abdomen show a slightly opaque mass which,
however, has nothing characteristic whereby the type of tumor can be identified. It is practically impossible by *plain films* or *pyelograms* to differen-

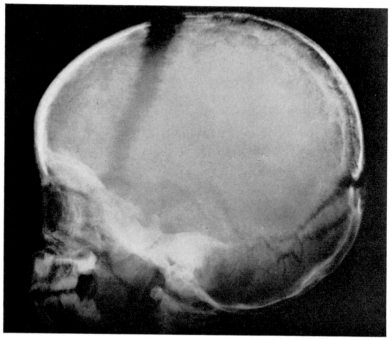

Fig. 264.—Roentgenogram from two-and-one-half-year-old boy (same as Fig. 262)
with metastases from retroperitoneal neuroblastoma. Mottled appearance of tables in
vertex of skull from bony metastases. Sutures separated because of metastases in brain.

tiate roentgenologically between neuroblastoma, embryoma of the kidney, and unattached retroperitoneal tumor. Small deposits of calcium are seen in some neuroblastomas, but these are also found in occasional embryomas of the kidney and in organizing hematomas of the adrenal glands. Pyelo-

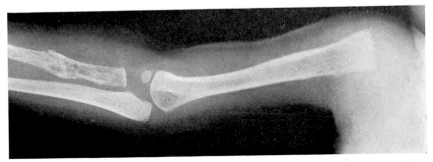

Fig. 265.—Skeletal metastases from a patient with neuroblastoma. Destructive lesions in radius; also in upper end of humerus with displacement of epiphysis.

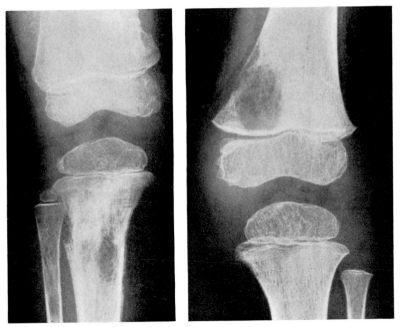

Fig. 266.—Roentgenograms from two children with skeletal metastases from abdominal neuroblastoma.

grams by intravenous or retrograde routes seldom give important additional information. They may visualize a kidney pelvis which is normal, displaced, or distorted.

While the roentgenographic changes of the primary abdominal lesion are not characteristic, the *metastases,* when present, will usually indicate the type of malignancy, particularly if they are found in association with an abdominal mass. The lungs or pleurae may be finely seeded. The cranial bones (when the patient is less than two years of age) may be separated and the sutures widened (Fig. 264). The skull, spine, ribs, pelvis, and the long bones of the extremities may be extensively peppered with small destructive lesions which have a moth-eaten appearance. The lesions are almost always symmetrically distributed on the two sides of the skeleton. The distal third of the arms and legs are rarely involved (in contradistinction to leukemic infiltrations). Proliferative bone lesions are sometimes found and in a few cases the sclerosing appearance in the spine and pelvis is somewhat similar to that seen in Paget's disease.[17]

DIFFERENTIAL DIAGNOSIS

A few of the conditions from which neuroblastoma must be differentiated might be enumerated:

Embryoma of the Kidney.—This occurs in children of about the same age distribution. There is a large mass which is almost always unilateral. By palpation it is usually well circumscribed, has a smooth contour, and is limited to one side of the abdomen. In contrast, the neuroblastoma has borders which are less well defined, a surface which is nodular or lobulated, and possibly an extension in front of or beyond the vertebral column. In the majority of cases this simple examination will rather clearly indicate which of the two conditions is present, but at times it is impossible to make the differential diagnosis by physical examination or indeed by any other means except with biopsy. x-Ray studies of the abdomen give little differential information. If chest or skeletal roentgenograms show metastases, the limitation of them to the lungs is more suggestive of embryoma, while the wider distribution to the lungs, brain, and particularly the skeleton are almost diagnostic of neuroblastoma.

Unattached Retroperitoneal Embryoma.—This term has been used to designate cystic or solid mixed growths which arise anywhere along the posterior abdominal or thoracic wall. They are believed to originate from remnants of the pronephros or mesonephros and hence may be found on either side of the vertebral column from the fourth cervical segment downward to the internal genitalia. They may reach an extremely large size. The description, "unattached," implies that they are not connected with the kidney, even though the histology is often similar to the renal embryomata. It is usually difficult to differentiate these retroperitoneal neoplasms from a neuroblastoma except by operation or autopsy. They are quite rare when compared to the relative frequency of neuroblastoma.

Other Tumors of the Adrenal Gland.—The adrenal gland may give rise to four different types of neoplasm, three from medullary and one from cortical tissue:

1. The *neuroblastoma,* which is a highly malignant, rapidly growing, widely disseminating neoplasm without any endocrinologic disturbances.

2. The *ganglioneuroma,* which is a benign, slowly growing, encapsulated neurologic tumor which does not metastasize and which does not produce any endocrinologic dysfunction.

3. The *chromaffinoma,* which is a benign (occasionally malignant) tumor[7] producing profound circulatory disturbances because of the formation of adrenalin and release of it in excessive amounts into the blood stream. These individuals have periods in which the blood pressure is elevated to as much as 200 mm. of mercury or more. The attacks appear at irregular intervals, and as often as several times a day. They are characterized by epigastric distress, excitability, sweating, headache, rapid pulse, and subse-

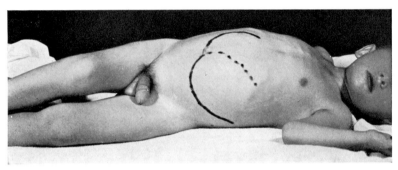

Fig. 267.—Three-year-old boy with a large carcinoma of adrenal cortex origin. Mass outlined by pencil marks. Note pubic hair and enlarged genitalia. (Such endocrine disturbances are never found with a neuroblastoma.)

quent exhaustion. The individual may die as a result of a hypertensive vascular accident or cardiac failure. The growths are usually circumscribed, can often but not always be felt in the adrenal region, and extirpation of them brings complete relief of symptoms.

4. *Adrenal cortical neoplasms,* which are malignant (occasionally benign) tumors[7] producing marked somatic and sexual changes by the formation and liberation of androgenic substances. They can be small and encapsulated (Fig. 268) but they are usually large, irregular, and fixed to adjacent structures. In most instances death results from local extension or pulmonary metastases. There are striking endocrinologic changes, characterized by a hypermasculinization and enlargement of the penis in the male (Fig. 267), masculinization with enlargement of the clitoris in the female (Fig. 268), a deepening of the voice in either sex, acne of the skin, enhancement of the somatic growth beyond the expected normal, mild to

moderate hypertension, advancement of the bony development (found by roentgenologic examination of wrists and epiphyses), and a greatly increased excretion of androgens in the urine. These obvious endocrinologic alterations serve to differentiate sharply the adrenal cortical tumors from the neuroblastomas.

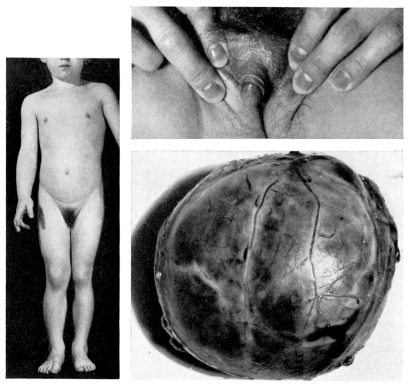

Fig. 268.—Three-year-old girl with masculinizing features produced by an adrenal cortex tumor. Note the square and muscular stature, the pubic hair, and the enlarged clitoris. Encapsulated, orange colored tumor removed from right adrenal. (Such endocrine disturbances are never produced by a neuroblastoma.)

TREATMENT

Excision of the Tumor.—If there is a presenting abdominal mass without clinical or roentgenologic evidence of metastases, abdominal *exploration* should be undertaken. It is best to do this through an anterior *transabdominal* approach, because only in this way can the operator estimate the full extent of the lesion and whether or not there are metastases in other abdominal viscera such as the liver. Removal of the primary tumor should not be begun until thorough inspection and palpation of the posterior and medial attachments have been made. All too frequently one undertakes dissection, only to find that the entire mass cannot be removed and that tumor tissue must be cut across which would start bleeding that is hard to control. Of course, every effort should be made to remove the lesion when possible, but in some instances a judicious withdrawal from the abdomen is a wiser choice. If the tumor is inoperable, a biopsy of it should be made to establish the correct diagnosis by microscopic study and to direct more intelligently subsequent x-ray therapy.

From one of our patients with the symptoms and signs primarily related to spinal cord compression, Dr. Franc D. Ingraham removed extradural tumor tissue which had locally extended from a neuroblastoma of the right extra-adrenal paravertebral region. At a second operation the abdominal portion of this was excised. Fortunately, the histology was one of a neuroblastoma differentiating into ganglioneuroma. A somewhat similar case has been reported by Cushing and Wolbach.[4]

Postoperative Roentgen Therapy.—*Local.*—Though we have no adequate statistics to support our beliefs, it is our contention that all neuroblastomas, even though apparently completely excised, should have postoperative local irradiation in order to kill any cells or bits of tissue which might be unwittingly left by the operator.

Limited Metastases.—A neuroblastoma with extensions or metastases limited to abdominal lymph nodes or the liver should not be regarded as a hopeless condition. Patients with such a condition should always have the benefit of x-ray irradiation. Justification for this statement rests upon observations from two children (Cases 6 and 7, in Table 39) whose livers at the time of operation were filled with metastases and yet who are alive and well, without evidence of tumor, three and one half and two years later, following x-ray irradiation.

Spray Irradiation of Widespread Metastases.—Whether or not metastatic lesions of the chest, skeleton, brain, and other parts of the body should be treated by x-ray irradiation has not yet been definitely settled. Certainly, if there is pain or other severe regional symptom which might be relieved by irradiation, this palliative therapy should be carried out. The neuroblastoma is a very radiosensitive tumor and small doses of x-ray are effective in destroying it. This has led to the belief that irradiation of the major part of the body and extremities of patients with metastases might kill off all existing tumor cells. Unfortunately, these spray treatments have depressing effects on the bone marrow so that severe anemia and leukopenia can result. Therefore, while widespread metastases can be effectively treated by x-rays, the secondary reaction on the tissues, particularly the bone marrow, may be of serious and even fatal consequence. It is not within the scope of the present work to set forth the details of x-ray treatment. The dosage and other factors employed in our cases are recorded in the publication of Wyatt and Farber.[17]

RESULTS OF TREATMENT

In the majority of children with untreated neuroblastoma, metastases develop and there is a rapid downhill course leading to death within a few months. There are insufficient data to set a definite time limit beyond which a surviving patient can be said to be cured. The extremely rapid proliferation of this neoplasm and the clinical data from our own and other series[2, 12] have made us feel that an individual who is well for a year after treatment (surgical, x-ray or a combination) can probably be regarded as a perma-

TABLE 39

DATA FROM SEVEN CASES WITH PROBABLE CURE OF ABDOMINAL NEUROBLASTOMA (FROM A SERIES OF THIRTY-TWO HISTOLOGICALLY VERIFIED CASES)

Case	Age and Sex	Site of Primary Neoplasm	Demonstrable Metastases	Treatment	Result
1	6 weeks, M.	Extra-adrenal, retroperitoneal	None	Tumor thought to be inoperable. Only biopsy performed ——— No x-ray	In excellent health. No demonstrable tumor or metastases 8½ years later
2	14 days, F.	Left adrenal	None	Complete surgical removal ——— No x-ray	Well. No evidence of recurrence 7½ years later
3	2 years, F.	Right. Extra-adrenal, retroperitoneal*	None	Complete removal ——— No x-ray	Excellent health. No evidence of tumor 6 years later
4	5 years, F.	Left adrenal	None	Complete surgical removal ——— No x-ray	Well. No evidence of recurrence 5½ years later
5	2 years, F.	Right. Extra-adrenal, retroperitoneal*	Extension into spinal canal	1. Excision from spinal cord 2. Excision from retroperitoneal tissues (incomplete) ——— x-Ray therapy	Excellent health. No evidence of tumor 4 years later
6	11 days, F.	Right adrenal	Extensive metastases in liver at operation	Removal of adrenal tumor. Biopsy of liver metastases ——— x-Ray therapy	Excellent health. No evidence of tumor 3½ years later
7	3 months, F.	Adrenal?	Massive metastases in liver at operation	Biopsy of liver metastases. Primary growth not removed ——— x-Ray therapy	Excellent health. No evidence of tumor 2 years later

* Histologic examination showed neuroblastoma differentiating into ganglioneuroma.

nent cure. It is admitted, however, that this is a working standard which is used for the present, and that it may have to be altered by future experience.

When evaluating the final results in a series of patients with neuroblastoma, one cannot conclusively attribute a success in any instance to surgery alone, to x-ray irradiation alone, or even to a combination of these therapeutic procedures. It is now known that a neuroblastoma can undergo *spontaneous hemorrhage and necrosis* and completely disappear without any treatment whatever. This was forcibly impressed upon us in a six-week-old boy who was explored and thought to have an inoperable growth; only a biopsy was performed. This child (Case 1, Table 39) has had no x-ray treatment, and yet he is completely well eight and one-half years later. In short, these highly cellular growths with an insufficient blood supply can become necrotic and die out, provided this process occurs before metastases have taken place.

In rare cases a neuroblastoma sympatheticum develops into a more slowly growing lesion—the *ganglioneuroma*. The rapidly growing neuroblastoma part may burn itself out or it may be destroyed by x-ray irradiation and leave the benign ganglioneuroma portion which can be subsequently excised. This happy sequence of events occurred in one of our cases and was also observed by Cushing and Wolbach.[4]

The optimum conditions for surgical treatment are found in the individual with an early lesion which is still *encapsulated* and which can be readily excised. Fig. 261 is a photograph of a hemorrhagic and encapsulated neuroblastoma removed from a fourteen-day-old girl who has had no x-ray therapy and who is alive and well seven and one-half years later.

In two of our patients, aged three months and eleven days, respectively, the livers were extensively replaced by histologically verified metastases. Both individuals have had subsequent x-ray irradiation and are in excellent health two years and three and one half years later. They now have no demonstrable metastases, in spite of the fact that they have been hospitalized and studied on several different occasions in the effort to detect recurrence.

Table 39 sums up some data from our seven cases which we regard as extremely hopeful, with the patients probably permanently cured.

BIBLIOGRAPHY

1. Bielschowsky, M.: Neuroblastic Tumors of Sympathetic Nervous System. In "Cytology and Cellular Pathology of the Nervous System," Wilder Penfield. New York: Hoeber, 1932, page 1085.
2. Blacklock, J. W. S.: Neurogenic Tumours of the Sympathetic System in Children. J. Path. and Bact., *39:* 27, 1934.
3. Chandler, F. A., and Norcross, J. R.: Sympathicoblastoma. J. A. M. A., *114:* 112, 1940.
4. Cushing, H., and Wolbach, S. B.: The Transformation of a Malignant Paravertebral Sympathicoblastoma into a Benign Ganglioneuroma. Am. J. Path., *3:* 203, 1927.
5. Farber, S.: Neuroblastoma. Abstract in Am. J. Dis. Child., *60:* 749, 1940.
6. Farber, S.: Incidence of Malignant Tumors in Infants and Children. (To be published.)
7. Gross, R. E.: Neoplasms Producing Endocrine Disturbances in Childhood. Am. J. Dis. Child., *59:* 579, 1940.
8. Hartung, A., and Rubert, S. R.: Roentgen Aspects of Sympathetic Neuroblastoma. Radiology, *24:* 607, 1935.
9. Hauser, H.: Radiosensitive Neuroblastoma. Am. J. Roentgenol., *31:* 234, 1934.
10. Holmes, G., and Dresser, R.: Roentgenologic Observations in Neuroblastoma. J. A. M. A., *91:* 1246, 1928.

11. Lehman, E. P.: Adrenal Neuroblastoma in Infancy—15-Year Survival. Ann. Surg., *95:* 473, 1932.
12. Redman, J. L., Agerty, H. A., Barthmaier, O. F., and Fisher, H. R.: Adrenal Neuroblastoma—Review of Literature. Am. J. Dis. Child., *56:* 1097, 1938.
13. Rypins, E. L.: Roentgen Diagnosis of Neuroblastoma in Children. Am. J. Roentgenol., *37:* 325, 1937.
14. Schrager, V. L.: Surgical Aspects of Neurogenic Tumors of the Abdomen. Surg., Gynec. and Obst., *68:* 1085, 1939.
15. Tileston, W., and Wolbach, S. B.: Primary Tumors of the Adrenal Gland in Children. Am. J. M. Sc., *135:* 871, 1908.
16. Wahl, H. R., and Craig, P. E.: Multiple Tumors of Sympathetic Nervous System; Report of Case Showing Distinct Ganglioneuroma, Neuroblastoma and Cystic Calcifying Ganglioneuroblastoma. Am. J. Path., *14:* 797, 1938.
17. Wyatt, G. M., and Farber, S.: Neuroblastoma Sympatheticum. A Note Concerning Radiological Appearances and Irradiation Treatment. Am. J. Roentgen. and Radium Therapy. (To be published.)

INDEX